Animal Welfare, Health and Management

Animal Welfare, Health and Management

Editor: Terry Caldwell

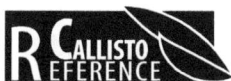

RCALLISTO
REFERENCE

www.callistoreference.com

Callisto Reference,
118-35 Queens Blvd., Suite 400,
Forest Hills, NY 11375, USA

Visit us on the World Wide Web at:
www.callistoreference.com

ISBN: 978-1-64116-140-4 (Hardback)

Cataloging-in-Publication Data

Animal welfare, health and management / edited by Terry Caldwell.
    p. cm.
Includes bibliographical references and index.
ISBN 978-1-64116-140-4
1. Animal welfare. 2. Animal health. I. Caldwell, Terry.
HV4708 .A55 2019
179.3--dc23

Table of Contents

Preface

The consideration of animal welfare is based on the philosophy that animals are sentient beings that are capable of pain, discomfort and emotional trauma. The standards of animal welfare vary in different contexts. Different parameters of longevity, disease, physiology, behavior, immunosuppression and reproduction are studied for determining the welfare of a particular animal or groups of animals. The study of animal health, welfare and management in zoos, laboratories, farms and in the wild is under the domain of animal welfare science. Some of the issues dealt within this field include animal testing, poaching, abandonment of pets, cruelty to animals, etc. This book provides significant information of this discipline to help develop a good understanding of animal welfare, health and management. It unravels the recent studies in these domains. It is meant for students and experts who are looking for an elaborate reference text on animal welfare studies.

This book is the end result of constructive efforts and intensive research done by experts in this field. The aim of this book is to enlighten the readers with recent information in this area of research. The information provided in this profound book would serve as a valuable reference to students and researchers in this field.

At the end, I would like to thank all the authors for devoting their precious time and providing their valuable contribution to this book. I would also like to express my gratitude to my fellow colleagues who encouraged me throughout the process.

Editor

Effects of the Truck Suspension System on Animal Welfare, Carcass and Meat Quality Traits in Pigs

Filipe Antônio Dalla Costa [1,2], Letícia S. Lopes [3] and Osmar Antônio Dalla Costa [2,3,*]

[1] Programa de Pós-Graduação em Zootecnia, Faculdade de Ciências Agrárias e Veterinárias, University of São Paulo State UNESP-FCAV, Jaboticabal 14884-900, Brazil; filipedallacosta@gmail.com

[2] Grupo de Estudos e Pesquisas em Etologia e Ecologia Animal-ETCO, UNESP/FCAV, Jaboticabal 14884-900, Brazil

[3] Embrapa Swine and Poultry, BR 153, Km 110, Concórdia 89700-991, Brazil; leticia.lopes@embrapa.br

* Correspondence: osmar.dallacosta@embrapa.br

Academic Editors: John J. McGlone and Anna K. Johnson

Simple Summary: Transportation is a complex stressor in which animals are exposed to a series negatively stimuli, such as vibration, new environmental conditions, variation in temperature and humidity, social mixing, noises among other poor factors, which can result in welfare problems and economic losses such as increased skin lesions, poorer pork quality traits. Transport stress may be reduced through a vehicle suspension system that provides a much smoother ride during transport, and consequently is less aversive to pigs. However, air suspension systems are more expensive and have bigger maintenance costs. This increase in transportation cost must be supported by the benefits from improvements in quality of freight transport; otherwise, the truckers will be paying unnecessarily for a similar or equivalent ride quality. Thus, finishing pigs were assessed after transport to slaughter by the same two double-decked trucks using two types of commercial vehicle suspension, leaf-spring and air suspension, to compare effects on blood cortisol and lactate at exsanguination, behaviour during lairage, and carcass (skin lesions) and pork quality traits. The use of leaf-spring suspension system negatively affects the welfare of pigs due to the increased carcass damage and resulted in poorer pork quality traits.

Abstract: The objective of this study was to assess the effects of two types of commercial suspension (leaf-spring (LS) vs. air suspension (AS)) installed on two similar double-decked trucks on blood cortisol and lactate concentration, lairage behavior, carcass skin lesions and pork quality traits of 120 crossbred pigs. The suspension type neither influenced pig behaviour in lairage nor blood cortisol and lactate concentrations ($p > 0.10$). However, when compared with the AS suspension system, the use of LS increased the number of skin lesions in the back and thigh ($p = 0.03$ and $p = 0.01$, respectively) and produced thigh with lower pH_u ($p < 0.001$) and yellower colour (higher b* value; $p = 0.03$), and paler back muscles (subjective colour; $p < 0.05$), with a tendency to lower pH ($p = 0.06$). Therefore, the use air suspension system can improve carcass and meat quality traits of pigs transported to slaughter.

Keywords: blood metabolites; transport; truck suspension; stress; lesions; meat quality

1. Introduction

The transport of pigs is an essential and inevitable process in the modern multi-site pig industry [1]. However, transportation is a stressful experience for pigs [2,3] that may result in economic losses due to mortality, carcass lesion and poor pork quality [2,4–6]. Within the effects of transport factors, the vibration of the truck plays an important role contributing to reduce the welfare of pigs during transport [7–11], travel sickness and stress [9,12], and increased skin lesions scores due to pigs' slips and falls while the vehicle is moving [7,11,12].

Nowadays, in the transport sector, where every cent has to be taken into account, higher purchase and maintenance costs must be supported by the benefits from improvements in animal welfare and pork; otherwise the truckers will be paying unnecessarily for a similar or equivalent ride quality. The vibrations of the truck caused by the truck design and condition, poor suspension system, floor, driving style and road conditions are some of the factors affecting the welfare of pigs during transport [7–10]. However, truck vibration may be reduced through the suspension system, leaf-spring or air type [9,10,13,14], whose objective is to enhance the contact of the vehicle with the road surface and indirectly reduce vehicle vibrations [8].

Excessive exposure to vibrations have been shown to result in travel sickness and stress [9,12], and increased skin damage scores due to pigs' slips and falls while the vehicle is moving [7,12]. However, when compared with the leaf-spring suspension, air suspensions proved to reduce vibrations of the truck up to five times more [13,15] and may thus provide livestock with more comfortable and smoother transport conditions [10,13]. According to Gebresenbet [13], a poor suspension system is one of the main factors causing vibration and loss of balance during livestock transport. Researches have mainly focused on effects of vibration on postural stability, behaviour during transport [9,12–14]; driving performance, truck speed, weight of shipment and road conditions on vibration level [9,13,15,16], and determination of vibration levels and frequencies of typical trucks during animal transport [10].

During transport, the level of truck vibration induces stress reactions such as increased heart rate, ectopic beats, cortisol and adrenocorticotropic hormone concentrations and postural behaviour changes that only occur under unusual environmental exposure [9,17,18]. The pork industry aims to obtain an optimal pork quality. However, the response to stressful situations increases the rate of glycolysis [19,20], which produces lactic acid early post mortem by an anaerobic metabolism [21]. Stressed pigs prior to slaughter show a rapid glycolysis of muscle glycogen with increased lactic acid production before the slaughter. Consequently, a lower pH is reached earlier while the carcass temperature still high and the pork quality traits are impaired due to the increase in protein denaturation [22–24]. Conversely, longer-term stress during hours until the slaughter moment reduces muscle glycogen stores and leads to a lower production of lactic acid post mortem. Hence, even after 24 h, the ultimate pH is still high, which reduces the pork quality traits [24,25]. Based on this, the physical activity due to difficulties in keeping balance and slips and falls during transport may affect the rate of glycolysis, resulting in an impaired meat quality. However, little is known about the effects of the suspension system on physiologic parameters of stress, behaviour and meat quality of pigs transported to abattoir. The aim of this study was to evaluate the effects of two types of commercial suspension systems, leaf-spring and air suspension, on the blood indicators of pigs' welfare, behaviour during lairage, number of skin lesions in the back and thigh, and meat quality traits under commercial conditions.

2. Materials and Methods

All experimental procedures performed in this study were approved by the institutional animal care committee on the basis of the current guidelines of the São Paulo State University's Animal Research Ethics Board (protocol number 6119-08).

2.1. Description of Study Site

The study was conducted in a commercial abattoir located in Southern Brazil (Rio Grande do Sul state) under federal inspection service. It is located 27°21′06″W (latitude) and 53°23′46″S (longitude) and at 531 m above sea level. The climate of the area is mild with an average rainfall of 20 mm for the studied period. However, there was no rain during the period from loading, transport, unloading until the slaughter. Transport trials were run during the winter of 2008 (June) at a relatively mild air temperature (to avoid thermal stress) with an average ambient temperature during the transport of 14 °C (range from 13 to 19 °C) and a thermo-humidity index of 57.3 (range from 55.7 to 66.1).

All farms were located within a radius of 56 km (54.4 ± 1.9 km) from the abattoir and consisted of only one growing-finishing facility with similar design, and capacity to finish over 450 pigs (±25) per cycle (170 days). Pigs were kept in pens (10.4 ± 0.4 pigs/pen) on concrete floor at an average density of 1.15 m²/pig. The topography of the area of transport from farms to abattoir was generally flat with a few steep slopes.

2.2. Animals, Loading Facilities and Handling of Pigs on the Farm

The number of skin lesions was visually counted on the left side of the body of each pig (120 pigs) used along all measurements, written down through a paper and pencil spreadsheet, and the proportion of pigs showing lesions at the farm on the day before transport, at unloading and slaughter was calculated. A total of 120 from 960 crossbred pigs (BW of 113 ± 1.1 kg) originating from five commercial swine growing-finishing farms were fasted for 12 h before loading and loaded in groups of 5–6 pigs by a trained loading crew using paddles and rattles always from 23 h to 24 h. At each farm, pigs had to climb an adjustable loading ramp (11.6 ± 0.5 m long), which could be set up to reach the bottom and the fixed upper deck (15° and 21° slope, respectively) of the truck. The loading order of the two trucks was switched in each farm (i.e., starting by the leaf-spring suspension truck in the first farm and by the air suspension truck in the next one consecutively). Two pigs per compartment for each treatment were used in this study (2 pigs/6 compartments/2 trucks/5 farms = 120 pigs). At each farm, the loading procedure took on average 20 min (±2 min).

2.3. Transport Conditions and Vehicle Features

Pigs were transported to a commercial slaughter plant using two similar double-decked trucks (Triel-HT, Erechim, Brazil) on each continuous journey (5 journeys) of 114 min (±22.7) on average and at a mean speed of 30 km/h on the same route. In each truck, pigs were distributed into 6 compartments (3 per deck) holding 16 pigs each at a density of 230 kg/m². The average transport distance was 54.4 km (±1.9), consisting of 12.8 km (±3.9) on earth road and 41.6 km (±3.2) on paved road. The driver for each truck tested was the same throughout of the study and switched treatments each journey to reduce driver variations on the response of the pigs to transport as previously suggested in other studies [3,9,26,27].

The trucks had neither drinking nipples nor showers. Both trucks (Volkswagen 24.250 2008, Volkswagen Caminhões e Ônibus, Resende, Brazil) were fixed upper metallic deck trailer models equipped with six compartments (2.92 m length × 2.4 m width × 1 m height), loading surface of 42 m² (6 compartments × 2.92 m × 2.4 m), drum braking system, natural ventilation, metallic open sides, and a grid cross slating floor (aluminum). Of the two trucks, one was equipped with a leaf-spring suspension system (LS; Volkswagen Caminhões e Ônibus, Resende, Brazil) and the other with an air suspension system (AS; Scania Latin America Ltda., São Bernardo do Campo, Brazil). The LS uses a semi-elliptic leaf spring system attached to the vehicle axle and consisting of several layers of flexible steel strips that are joined to cushion from impacts, whereas, the AS consists of valves, air pipes and woven and rubber-like material air-spring bags. The air originates from the truck air compressor and reservoir and pressurizes the air-spring bags that, similar to a spring, cushion from impacts during travel while increasing the contact of tires with the road surface.

2.4. Handling of Pigs at the Slaughter Plant

Pigs were immediately unloaded on arrival at the slaughter plant through an adjustable in slope metal ramp (5 m length, slope ≤ 15°) with anti-skid floor using paddles. Pigs were kept in separate pens (no social mixing; 5 m length × 4 m width × 1.5 m wall height) according to the treatment (LS vs. AS) for 3 h at a density of 0.6 m²/100 kg. All pens had a concreted floor and walls with solid metallic gate to conduct the pigs in/out a proportion of one nipple drinking to fifteen pigs with a flow of 2 L/min was respect. The ambient temperature at the abattoir ranged from 13–18 °C during the period of data collection, which was controlled with a sprinkling and forced ventilation system. At the end of lairage, pigs were driven to slaughter using paddles, boards and rattles and electrically stunned (head-only electrical stunning; 700 V, 1.3 A, 5 s; Valhalla, Stork RMS b.v., Lichtenvoorde, Holland) before exsanguination in the horizontal position within 30 s. This abattoir slaughters up to 2000 pigs/day and operated at 280 pigs/h during the data collection of this study.

2.5. Behavioral Observations during Lairage

The behavior of pigs in lairage was assessed in each pen by one trained observer using the scan sampling method consisting of direct observations at 15 min intervals along the 3 h period and analyzed by the hour. The recorded behaviors are listed in Table 1. The proportion of pigs expressing each behaviour was calculated per period of 60 min.

Table 1. Ethogram of pigs' behavior during lairage.

Behaviour	Description
Standing	Pig on all fours limbs extended and stopped.
Walking	Pig on all four limbs and moving around.
Seated	Pig seated on the caudal region of body with forelimbs extended.
Lying down	Pig with lateral or ventral body surface in contact with the floor and without support of the fore and hindquarters.
Fighting	Two or more pigs performing a sequence of aggressive physical contacts for more than 3 s, such as biting, head knocking, pushing and shoving each other, with no grater intervals than 10 s.

2.6. Blood Parameters

A sub-sample of 120 pigs (2/compartment/truck or treatment, totalizing 12 pigs/truck or treatment/replicate or journey) was used for the analysis of blood stress indicators in the bleeding blood. Blood samples (10 mL) were collected in a tube (Vacuplast, Cral Artigos para Laboratório Ltd., São Paulo, Brazil) for cortisol analysis. Another 2 mL of blood was collected in a tube containing 3.0 mg of sodium fluoride and 6.0 mg of Na2EDTA solution to extract plasma for lactate concentration analysis. Samples were immediately centrifuged at 4 °C for 12 min at 1400 g. Plasma was transferred into 1.5 mL Eppendorf tubes and stored at −80 °C until lactate concentration analysis. Serum samples were kept at room temperature (~23 °C) for 1 h before refrigeration at 4 °C. The following day, serum samples were centrifuged at 4 °C for 12 min at 1400 g, the supernatant was transferred into 1.5 mL Eppendorf tubes and stored at −80 °C until analysis. Plasma lactate levels were measured using a commercially available kit (Lactat PAP Enzyme Farbtest, Rolf Greiner Biochemica, Flacht, Germany) and their plasma concentration determined with a microplate reader. The quantitative determination of cortisol was made using a commercial kit (Coat-A-Count Cortisol Kit, Diagnostic Products Corporation, Los Angeles, CA, USA) with a microplate reader and expressed in ng/mL. The intra-assay CV was 26.08% and 22.43% for lactate and cortisol concentration, respectively.

2.7. Carcass Handling and Skin Lesion Assessment

After slaughter, carcasses were eviscerated, split and chilled (1–4 °C for 24 h) according to standard commercial practices. In the cooler, lesions were assessed on each left carcass side and classified as fighting-type lesions (1 = less than 10 lesions; 2 = 11 to 20 lesions; and 3 = greater than 20 lesions) or mounting-type lesions (score 1 = less than 5 lesions; 2 = 6 to 10 lesions; and 3 = greater than 10 lesions) by visual assessment of shape and size according to the photographic standards of the Institut Technique du Porc (ITP) [28] as described by Faucitano [29]. According to the ITP scale, lesions due to biting during fighting are 5 to 10 cm in length, comma shaped, and concentrated in high number in the anterior (head and shoulders) and posterior (thigh) regions of the carcass. Long (10 to 15 cm), thin (0.5- to 1-cm-wide), comma shaped lesions densely concentrated on the back of pigs caused by the fore claws were classified as mounting type lesions. And large dark brown rectangular marks usually found on the middle, back and hind regions were classified as handling lesions.

2.8. Meat Quality

Meat quality was evaluated in the *Longissimus dorsi* (back) and *Semimembranosus* (thigh) muscle of the same pigs previously evaluated. Muscle pH was assessed at 45 min (pH_i) and 24 h (pH_u) post mortem using a pHmeter (HI 8314 model, Hanna Instruments, São Paulo, Brazil) fitted with a spear tip electrode (HI 1217D, Hanna Instruments, São Paulo, Brazil) and an automatic temperature compensation probe (Tec 530, Hanna Instruments, São Paulo, Brazil) by insertion into the *Longissimus dorsi* (LD; between the 13th and 14th rib) and *Semimembranosus* (SM) muscles. At 24 h of slaughter, objective and subjective colour, and drip loss measurements were taken in the LD and SM muscles. Instrumental colour (L*, a* and b* values) was measured using a Minolta Chromameter (CR-400; Minolta Camera Ltd., Osaka, Japan) equipped with a 25 mm aperture, 0° viewing angle, and D65 illuminant. Visual colour was evaluated through the Japanese Pork Color Standards (JPCS; ranging from 1 = pale to 6 = dark color) [30]. Percentage of drip loss was measured using a modified EZ-driploss method [31]. Following this method, at 24 h post mortem, two muscle cores samples of 25 mm diameter were taken from the center of 2.5 cm thick LD (at the level of the 13th/14th last rib) and SM muscle chops using a specific drip loss knife, weighed and placed into funnel-shape plastic drip loss containers (KABE Labortechnik, Umbrecht-Elsenroth, Germany) and stored for 48 h at 4 °C. Muscle core samples were carefully collected from their containers using a tweezers after the 48 h storage period, surface moisture of cores were carefully dabbed prior being reweighed, and then drip loss percentage was determined by dividing the difference between initial and final core weights by the initial core weight. The back and thigh muscles were classified according to pH_u, drip loss and light reflectance (L*) variation (Table 2). To assess cooking losses, four LD muscle chops (150 g each) were individually vacuum-packed in heat resistant sealed plastic bags (nylon polyethylene bag 16 × 30 × 0.1 cm) 10 micron thick with a vacuum of 0.8 bar with a double seal using a DZ-4000 vacuum packer machine (Cetro Solutions in packing, Taiwan, China), and cooked in water bath at 80 °C for 1 h. After cooking, chops were then placed on absorbent paper to remove surface moisture and weighed when the internal temperature reached 20–25 °C. The weight loss was calculated by difference between initial and final weight [32]. The same LD muscle chops were then cooled at 2–4 °C for 12 h and used for the determination of Warner-Bratzler shear force. Five rectangular cores (1 × 1 × 2 cm), parallel to the longitudinal orientation of the muscle fibers, were taken in each chop and analyzed using a Warner-Bratzler device attached to a TAXT2i Texture Analyzer (Stable Micro Systems, Survey, UK).

Table 2. Meat quality classification [3,33].

Classes [1]	pH_u	Driploss	L*
PSE	<6.0	>6.0	>50
RSE	<6.0	>6.0	45–50
PFN	<6.0	<6.0	>50
RFN	5.5–6.1	<6.0	<50
DFD	≥6.1	<3.0	<44

[1] PSE: pale, soft, exudative; RSE: red, soft, exudative; PFN: pale, firm, non-exudative; RFN: red, firm, non-exudative; DFD: dark, firm, dry.

2.9. Statistical Analysis

Data was analysed as randomized complete block design to check effects of treatments by analysis of variance in ANOVA. Values of blood cortisol and lactate concentration were log-transformed (Ln) for data normalization before analysis. Frequencies of lesions were transformed and expressed as the square root of (x + 1). The model included effects of block (two decks: upper and lower × three position of compartments: front, middle, rear), day of transport (1, 2, 3, 4 and 5), farm, treatments, interaction between farm and block, and error (correspondent to randomized variation on the observations in the day of farm and vehicle suspension system), supposedly homoscedastic, independent and normally distributed. Variance analysis using GLM SAS (2003) was applied to study the effects of truck suspension using the group as experimental unit for the analysis of behaviour data, and the individual as the experimental unit for the analysis physiological and meat quality data, and transport was the adopted repetition. For the analysis of pig behaviour data during the lairage period, the experiment was conducted according to a randomized block design (farm) with two treatments (trucks) in the plot and 3 repeated measures over times (1st, 2nd, and 3rd hour of lairage). The likelihood ratio and chi-square tests were used to compare the skin lesion-type categories. The tests were performed using the FREQ procedure of SAS (2003) with Student's t test protected by the significance of the F test for mean comparison. A probability level of $p < 0.05$ was chosen as the limit for statistical significance in all tests and probability levels of $p \leq 0.10$ were considered as a tendency. There was no significant effect and interaction of farm, block and farm, or block in any of the studied variables ($p > 0.10$).

3. Results and Discussion

3.1. Behaviour during Lairage

Overall, in this study lairage time had an effect on pig behaviors ($p < 0.05$), with the proportion of standing, walking and sitting pigs decreasing with time after the first hour of lairage and that of pigs lying down increasing to almost all pigs at the end of lairage. However, no effect of the truck suspension system, deck and compartment position was observed on these behaviours in this study ($p > 0.10$; Table 3).

Table 3. Effects of truck suspension system on behavior [1] of pigs during lairage.

Behaviour (%)	Period (h)	Truck Suspension System [2]		Mean
		AS	LS	
Standing	1	47.08 ± 10.32 [A]	49.58 ± 6.23 [A]	48.33 ± 5.70 [A]
	2	12.08 ± 4.08 [B]	12.08 ± 7.05 [B]	12.08 ± 3.84 [B]
	3	5.83 ± 3.39 [B]	1.25 ± 0.83 [B]	3.54 ± 1.81 [B]
	Mean	21.67 ± 6.03	20.97 ± 6.25	
Lying down	1	40.42 ± 14.53 [A]	41.67 ± 8.36 [A]	41.04 ± 7.91 [A]
	2	83.75 ± 4.99 [B]	82.50 ± 10.43 [B]	83.13 ± 5.45 [B]
	3	91.67 ± 4.80 [B]	97.92 ± 1.61 [B]	94.79 ± 2.60 [B]
	Mean	71.94 ± 7.81	74.03 ± 7.58	
Seated	1	5.42 ± 1.56 [A]	5.83 ± 1.67 [A]	5.63 ± 1.08 [A]
	2	2.92 ± 1.06 [B]	2.92 ± 1.06 [B]	2.92 ± 0.71 [B]
	3	1.67 ± 0.78 [B]	0.83 ± 0.83 [B]	1.25 ± 0.56 [B]
	Mean	3.33 ± 0.7	3.19 ± 0.86	
Walking	1	5.42 ± 2.60	2.92 ± 1.56	4.17 ± 1.49 [A]
	2	1.25 ± 1.25	0.83 ± 0.83	1.04 ± 0.71 [B]
	3	0.00 ± 0.00	0.00 ± 0.00	0.00 ± 0.00 [B]
	Mean	2.22 ± 1.08	1.25 ± 0.64	
Fighting	1	1.67 ± 1.67	0.00 ± 0.00	0.83 ± 0.83
	2	0.00 ± 0.00	1.67 ± 1.67	0.83 ± 0.83
	3	0.83 ± 0.83	0.00 ± 0.00	0.42 ± 0.42
	Mean	0.83 ± 0.60	0.56 ± 0.56	

[1] See Material and methods (Table 1) for more details; [2] LS Truck = Leaf-spring suspension system; AS Truck = Air suspension system; [A,B] Different letters indicate statistically significant differences ($p \leq 0.05$) by Student's t test protected by the significance of the F test in the column.

After the first hour of lairage, there was a significant reduction in the expression of standing, walking, and sitting; and consequently an increase in the frequency of the pigs lying down. After one hour of lairage, more than 80% of pigs were lying, and practically all pigs were lying within 3 h. The level of vibration is affected by the vehicle suspension system [9], which may hamper pigs to keep their posture and prevent them lying down during transport. Swaying behaviour and loss of balance can also increase with transport time [9]. In this condition, due to the physical exhaustion and stress [13,26,34], pigs would prefer settling and lying down to rest instead of doing other activities (i.e., standing, walking and fighting) during the lairage, as found in other studies [35]. However, other transport conditions (i.e., road conditions, proper density, and relatively mild air temperature-driven behaviour) used in this study may have compensated the vibration level and reduced any effects on the pigs' behaviour during lairage [9,10,26,35]. Indeed, both drivers had already applied for training of animal welfare and defensive driving, which may have reduced potential differences of truck vibration on pigs' behaviour during lairage [9,26].

3.2. Physiological Response

In this study, the type of suspension system had no effects on blood cortisol (9.16 ± 0.49 vs. 7.95 ± 0.54 µg/dL for LS and AS, respectively; $p > 0.10$) and lactate levels (14.33 ± 0.71 and 14.26 ± 0.86 mmol·L^{-1} for LS and AS, respectively; $p > 0.10$) at exsanguination. Vibration values are greater in the upper deck in vertical and lateral position, while the lower deck presents greater vibration on driving direction [9]. Even with these differences, no effects of deck and compartment position were found ($p > 0.10$). Differently from a previous study, increased blood cortisol levels were observed in piglets subjected to vibrations [7]. After the beginning of vibration simulation, Perremans et al. [18] found a quick increase in blood cortisol levels, which returned to baseline levels within one hour after the end of stimulus. As blood lactate concentration returns to basal levels within 2 h after physical exercise [36,37], the lack of effect of truck suspension system on blood lactate may indicate that all pigs, regardless of the transport conditions, recovered from handling and transport stress thanks to the adequate lairage conditions (i.e., sufficient space allowance to lie down and ambience). Nonetheless, in both groups, the blood lactate levels at exsanguination were greater than the resting level of blood lactate for market-weight pigs (>4 mM; [38]), reflecting a general state of fatigue in all pigs transported. The CV values found are high, which may reflect an individual effect on these variables, and contributed to the lack of significant differences between treatments.

3.3. Skin and Carcass Lesion

The transport conditions of pigs can impact directly on carcass lesions. In agreement with previous studies [3,5,39], in this study, the overall proportion of pigs presenting skin lesions increased from farm to slaughter (29% to 62%) as a result of the additive effects of loading, transportation, unloading and lairage.

There was a significant effect of truck suspension system on the number of carcass lesions located in the back and thigh ($p \leq 0.05$; Table 4). Pigs transported in LS truck showed a greater number of carcass lesions caused by animal mounting than in LS ($p \leq 0.05$; Table 4). A tendency to more carcass lesions caused by handling was observed ($p \leq 0.10$; Table 4). Aradom et al. [9] found different vibration values according to the deck position (upper vs. lower). However, in this study, different from Barton-Gade et al. [13] and Dalla Costa et al. [5], who found higher number of bruises in pigs transported in the rear transport compartment, no effect of the deck (upper vs. lower) or compartment position (front, middle, rear) on number of skin lesions in the back and thigh was found ($p > 0.10$ for both).

Table 4. Number [1] of carcass lesions (mean ± SE) in pigs transported by trucks with different suspension systems.

Site of Carcass	Truck Suspension System [2]		p-Value
	LS Truck	AS Truck	
Back	5.32 ± 0.62	3.73 ± 0.41	0.03 *
Thigh	2.26 ± 0.28	1.47 ± 0.15	0.01 *
Shoulder	3.22 ± 0.66	3.35 ± 0.88	0.90
Lesion Type			
Handling	2.78 ± 0.28	2.18 ± 0.23	0.08 †
Fight	5.80 ± 1.13	4.35 ± 1.09	0.32
Mounting	2.06 ± 0.22	1.38 ± 0.18	0.02 *

[1] Number of lesions expressed in root of (x + 1); [2] LS Truck = Leaf-spring suspension system; AS Truck = Air suspension system; † $p < 0.10$, * $p < 0.05$ indicate significant statistical difference.

During transport, pigs may have difficulties in keeping posture and, consequently, lose balance and fall. Because pigs tend to stand up during the uncomfortable conditions of transport, especially during short journeys [40,41], increased carcass lesions are observed due the loss of balance and slips and falls [42]. Rough driving styles and poor suspension system are the main factors causing vibration and loss of balance during animal transport [16]. The truck equipped with AS may have provided smoother transport conditions for the pigs [8–10], and consequently, reduced the number of pigs slipping and falling, stepping on each other and striking themselves against the walls of the truck compartments [18]. Based on this, pigs facing better transport conditions can have a lower incidence of lesions as a result of exposure to a lower frequency of loss of balance. The cumulative effect of slips and falls during transport is likely to explain the increased number of lesions observed in the back and thigh. When a pig slips and falls down and has some difficulties in standing up again due to the vibration level and loss of balance, there is a considerable chance of other pen mates tramp this pig which may contribute to increasing the number and severity of skin lesions classified as mounting. Indeed, the fall of one pig can results in slips and falls of other pen mates from the same compartment. The stocking density adopted was within the regulation of EU for both trucks (230 kg/m^2) [43]. However, the greater number of carcass lesions classified as mounting observed in LS truck is suggestive of more pigs stepping on each other in order to keep balance during the transport than in the AS truck. Indeed, the fall of one pig can cause the loss of balance or fall of other pen mates' pigs. Overall, a loss of balance and fall means welfare problems in the form of bruises, injuries and physical fatigue.

A confounding effect of handling during loading/unloading, mixing unfamiliar pigs, social conflicts and driving should be considered with regard to carcass lesions. However, in order to avoid this problem, the experimental design of the study was done to make both groups receive the same treatments during all steps of preslaughter handling, and so, they have the same random influences. All procedures of loading and unloading were done by a trained crew, which was previously advised to have the same behaviour in all loading and unloading in order to avoid any interference on pigs' behaviour and welfare between treatments. Indeed, all procedures were watched by a technical team, aiming to identify any critical point during these phases and clear difference on the handling between treatments, but no differences were noticed. In order to reduce the response to transport driving behaviour, the loading order and driver used were switched in each treatment, and both drivers used here had previously took training of animal welfare and defensive driving [9,26,27]. Thus, based on this, even with the effect of mixing that was not possible to be avoided under commercial conditions and influence both groups equally, the differences found were mainly due to the effects of treatments.

3.4. Meat Quality

There was no significant effect of suspension, deck and compartment position system on meat quality classification ($p > 0.10$; Table 5). However, pigs transported by LS truck had lower JPCS scores in *Longissimus dorsi*, and lower pH_u mean and higher value of color b* in *Semimembranosus* muscles than pigs transported by AS truck (Table 6). The pH_u mean in *Longissimus dorsi* and JPCS score in *Semimembranosus* tended to be lower in pigs transported by LS truck. In agreement with this study, Warriss et al. [44] reported potential effects of vibration on muscle pH, and glycogen reserves in broiler chickens. When stimulated for 3 h of vibration, the pH in both white (*Pectoralis superficialis*) and red (*Biceps femoris*) muscles decreased.

Table 5. Meat quality classification [1] according to effect of truck suspension system (LS or leaf-spring suspension vs. AS or air suspension system) as assessed in the *Longissimus dorsi* and *Semimembranosus* muscles [2].

Muscle	Classes [3]	Truck Suspension System	
		LS	AS
Longissimus dorsi (Back)	PSE	6 (10.00%)	5 (8.33%)
	RSE	20 (33.33%)	17 (28.33)
	PFN	4 (6.67%)	4 (6.67)
	RFN	30 (50.00%)	34 (56.67)
	DFD	-	-
Semimembranosus (Thigh)	PSE	2 (3.33%)	2 (3.33%)
	RSE	22 (36.67%)	16 (26.67%)
	PFN	3 (5.00%)	5 (8.33%)
	RFN	33 (55.00%)	37 (61.67%)
	DFD	-	-

[1] See Material and methods (Table 2) for more details; [2] Number and percentage of back and thigh muscles classified in each treatment; [3] PSE: pale, soft and exudative; RSE: red, soft and exudative; PFN: Pale, Firm, non-exudative; RFN: red, firm and non-exudative; DFD: dark, firm and dry.

The variation in pork pH_u and JPCS score may be explained by the greater occurrence of mounting behaviour found in LS truck, as observed in carcass lesions (Table 4). Pigs transported in LS truck had a pH_u value lower than 5.5 in *Loguissimus dorsi*, which may indicate a mild pork quality defect. Conversely, even in red muscles such as the *Semimembranosus*, values of pH_u did not exceed the threshold of 6.3, which when exceeded is indicative of dark, firm and dry (DFD) pork [13]. Except for the visual colour score, the Minolta L* value, which is an indicator of colour lightness, was not affected by truck suspension system in this study. This lack of difference in Minolta L* value may be caused by the confounding effect of the light reflectance of marbling fat, which does not influence visual colour score. Because of fat colour reflectance, higher marbling scores may have resulted in higher L* values, while visual colour sores are not influenced by marbling scores [44,45]. The distribution shown in Table 5 is similar to other studies [3,46] that evaluated the meat quality in pig abattoirs in Brazil under very similar conditions of this study. The most desirable meat quality classification for the pork chain is red, firm and non-exudative (RFN), which had the highest incidence in agreement to the literature [3,46]. The variation in meat quality classification depends on the level of pre-slaughter stress, which can affect the muscle glycogen level. Stressful conditions at the moment of slaughter increase the muscle metabolism continually after death, and hence, a lower pH_i ($pH_i < 6.0$) is found in a drop rate increased by two to four times due to the increased production of protons and lactate in the early post mortem period [47,48]. Conversely, stress during different stages of pre-slaughter period may lead to low glycogen content at the time of slaughter, which reduces the amount of protons and lactic acid produced, and then, restricts the pH fall [49]. According to Henckel et al. [48], the pH_u values only increase due to muscle glycogen content lower than 53 μmol/g at slaughter. Usually, these phenomenon results in increased PSE and DFD meat, respectively. However, the incidence of PSE defect in pork was low, and the no incidence of DFD defect was found in this study.

Table 6. Values (mean $\pm$ SE) of pork quality parameters of pigs transported by trucks with different suspension system.

Muscle	Variable [1]	Suspension System [2]		*p*-Value
		LS Truck	AS Truck	
Longissimus dorsi (Back)	pH_1	6.41 ± 0.03	6.36 ± 0.03	0.1910
	pH_u	5.45 ± 0.07	5.56 ± 0.04	0.0641 [†]
	T_1	28.50 ± 0.19	28.62 ± 0.14	0.5138
	L*	47.57 ± 0.31	47.30 ± 0.29	0.4959
	a*	7.35 ± 0.17	7.47 ± 0.18	0.5129
	b*	-0.43 ± 0.20	-1.96 ± 0.96	0.1040
	JPCS	2.68 ± 0.07	2.97 ± 0.09	0.0065 *
	DL, %	4.86 ± 0.31	5.13 ± 0.27	0.5424
	WLC, %	39.50 ± 0.19	39.99 ± 0.37	0.1773
	SS, Kgf	4.32 ± 0.19	4.53 ± 0.13	0.4015
Semimembranosus (Thigh)	pH_1	6.52 ± 0.02	6.52 ± 0.03	1.0000
	pH_u	5.53 ± 0.03	5.61 ± 0.04	0.0003 *
	T_1	28.76 ± 0.19	28.82 ± 0.13	0.7698
	L*	46.75 ± 0.26	46.43 ± 0.34	0.3587
	a*	6.83 ± 0.23	6.96 ± 0.17	0.5957
	b*	-1.29 ± 0.24	-1.73 ± 0.17	0.0318 *
	JPCS	3.01 ± 0.07	3.17 ± 0.08	0.0916 [†]
	DL, %	2.55 ± 0.23	2.70 ± 0.23	0.6489

[1] pH_1 = pH 45 min post mortem; pH_u = pH 24 h post mortem (pH_u); T_1 = muscle temperature at 45 min post mortem; L = luminosity; a = red color; b = yellow color; JPCS = Japanese Pork Color Standards; DL = Drip loss; WLC = water loss by cooking; SS = shearing strength; [2] LS Truck = Leaf-spring suspension system; AS Truck = Air suspension system; [†] $p < 0.10$, * $p < 0.05$ indicate significant statistical difference in the same line by Student's *t* test, protected by the significance of the F test.

4. Conclusions

The current study indicates that the truck suspension system can affect the welfare of pigs in the form of injuries, which results in reduced pork quality traits and losses to the pork chain. Thus, based on these results, the welfare and meat quality traits of pigs were better in AS truck than LS. The authors hope these results will stimulate further researches and lead to development, identification and use of technologies to improve welfare of animals during transport and, consequently, make the pig industry more sustainable.

Acknowledgments: The authors appreciate the assistance of Luiz Carlos Ajala, Édio Luís Klein and Dirceu da Silva, for data collection at the slaughter plant and laboratory analysis. Sincere thanks go to the CNPQ (National Council of Technological and Scientific Development) for granting a PhD scholarship to Filipe Dalla Costa to conduct his studies and EMBRAPA Swine and Poultry for financial support, manpower, and facilities usage. Many thanks also go to Neville George Gregory and Luigi Faucitano for the critical review of the manuscript.

Author Contributions: Filipe Antônio Dalla Costa designed the experiment and wrote the paper. Letícia S. Lopes designed the experiment, analyzed the data and had creative input into the writing. Osmar Antônio Dalla Costa conceived and designed the experiments, collected the field data, analyzed the data, contributed reagents/materials/analysis tools, and had creative input into the writing.

Conflicts of Interest: The authors declare no conflict of interest.

References

1. Kephart, R.; Johnson, A.; Sapkota, A.; Stalder, K.; McGlone, J. Establishing bedding requirements on trailers transporting market weight pigs in warm weather. *Animals* **2014**, *4*, 476–493. [CrossRef] [PubMed]

2. Pereira, T.L.; Corassa, A.; Komiyama, C.M.; Araújo, C.V.; Kataoka, A. The effect of transport density and gender on stress indicators and carcass and meat quality in pigs. *Span. J. Agric. Res.* **2015**, *13*, 1–11. [CrossRef]

3. Dalla Costa, F.A.; Paranhos da Costa, M.J.R.; Faucitano, L.; Dalla Costa, O.A.; Lopes, L.S.; Renuncio, E. Ease of handling, physiological response, skin lesions and meat quality in pigs transported in two truck types. *Arch. Med. Vet.* **2016**, *48*, 299–304. [CrossRef]

4. Guàrdia, M.D.; Estany, J.; Balasch, S.; Oliver, M.A.; Gispert, M.; Diestre, A. Risk assessment of DFD meat due to pre-slaughter conditions in pigs. *Meat Sci.* **2005**, *70*, 709–716. [CrossRef] [PubMed]

5. Dalla Costa, O.A.; Faucitano, L.; Coldebella, A.; Ludke, J.V.; Peloso, J.V.; Dalla Roza, D.; Paranhos da Costa, M.J.R. Effects of the season of the year, truck type and location on truck on skin lesions and meat quality in pigs. *Livest. Prod. Sci.* **2007**, *107*, 29–36. [CrossRef]

6. Čobanović, N.; Bošković1, M.; Vasilev, D.; Dimitrijević, M.; Parunović, N.; Djordjević, J.; Karabasil, N. Effects of various pre-slaughter conditions on pig carcasses and meat quality in a low-input slaughter facility. *S. Afr. J. Anim. Sci.* **2016**, *46*, 380–390. [CrossRef]

7. Pierce, C.; Singh, S.P.; Burgess, G. Comparison of leaf spring to air cushion trailer suspensions in the transportation environment. *Packag. Technol. Sci.* **1992**, *5*, 11–15. [CrossRef]

8. Warriss, P.D. The welfare of slaughter pigs during transport. *Anim. Welf.* **1998**, *7*, 365–381.

9. Aradom, S.; Gebresenbet, G. Vibration on animal transport vehicles and related animal behaviours with special focus on pigs. *J. Agric. Sci. Technol.* **2013**, *3*, 231–245.

10. Gebresenbet, G.; Aradom, S.; Bulitta, F.S.; Hjerpe, E. Vibration levels and frequencies on vehicle and animals during transport. *Biosyst. Eng.* **2011**, *110*, 10–19. [CrossRef]

11. Šímová, V.; Večerek, V.; Passantino, A.; Voslářová, E. Pre-transport factors affecting the welfare of cattle during road transport for slaughter—A review. *Acta Vet. Brno* **2016**, *85*, 303–318. [CrossRef]

12. Randall, J.M. Human subjective response to lorry vibration: Implications for farm animal transport. *J. Agric. Eng. Res.* **1992**, *52*, 295–307. [CrossRef]

13. Barton-Gade, P.; Christensen, L.; Brown, S.N.; Warris, P.D. Effect of tier and ventilation during transport on blood parameters and meat quality in slaughter pigs. In *EU-Seminar: New Information on Welfare and Meat Quality of Pigs as Related to Handling, Transport and Lairage Conditions*; Landbauforschung Völkenrode: Mariensee, Kulmbach, Germany, 1996; Volume 166, pp. 101–116.

14. Randall, J.M.; Stiles, M.A.; Geers, R.; Schütte, A.; Christensen, L.; Bradshaw, R.H. Vibration on pig transporters: Implications for reducing stress. In *EU-Seminar: New Information on Welfare and Meat Quality of Pigs as Related to Handling, Transport and Lairage Conditions*; Landbauforschung Völkenrode: Mariensee, Kulmbach, Germany, 1996; pp. 143–159.

15. Singh, S.P. Vibration levels in commercial truck shipments. *Am. Soc. Agric. Eng.* **1991**, *91*, 1–12.

16. Perremans, S.; Randall, J.M.; Rombouts, G.; Decuypere, E.; Geers, R. Effect of whole-body vibration in the vertical axis on cortisol and adrenocorticotropic hormone levels in piglets. *J. Anim. Sci.* **2001**, *79*, 975–981. [CrossRef] [PubMed]

17. Perremans, S.; Randall, J.M.; Allegaert, L.; Stiles, M.A.; Rombouts, G.; Geers, R. Influence of vertical vibration on heart rate of pigs. *J. Anim. Sci.* **1998**, *76*, 416–420. [CrossRef] [PubMed]

18. Jama, N.; Maphosa, V.; Hoffman, L.C.; Muchenje, V. Effect of sex and time to slaughter (transportation and lairage duration) on the levels of cortisol, creatine kinase and subsequent relationship with pork quality. *Meat Sci.* **2016**, *116*, 43–49. [CrossRef] [PubMed]

19. Ritter, M.J.; Ellis, M.; Bertelsen, C.R.; Bowman, R.; Brinkmann, J.; DeDecker, J.M.; Keffaber, K.K.; Murphy, C.M.; Petterson, B.A.; Schlipf, J.M.; et al. Effects of distance moved during loading and floor space on the trailer during transport on losses of market weight pigs on arrival at the packing plant. *J. Anim. Sci.* **2007**, *85*, 3454–3461. [CrossRef] [PubMed]

20. Hoffman, L.C.; Laubscher, L.L. A comparison between the effects of day versus night cropping on the quality parameters of red hartebeest (*Alcelaphus buselaphus*) meat. *S. Afr. J. Wildl. Res.* **2011**, *41*, 50–60. [CrossRef]

21. Choi, Y.M.; Jung, K.C.; Choe, J.H.; Kim, B.C. Effects of muscle cortisol concentration on muscle fiber characteristics, pork quality, and sensory quality of cooked pork. *Meat Sci.* **2012**, *91*, 490–498. [CrossRef] [PubMed]

22. Geverink, N.A.; Bradshaw, R.H.; Lambooij, E.; Wiegant, V.M.; Broom, D.M. Effects of simulated lairage conditions on the physiology and behaviour of pigs. *Vet. Rec.* **1998**, *143*, 241–244. [CrossRef] [PubMed]

23. Terlouw, C. Stress reactions at slaughter and meat quality in pigs: Genetic background and prior experience: A brief review of recent findings. *Livest. Prod. Sci.* **2005**, *94*, 125–135. [CrossRef]

24. Gajana, C.S.; Nkukwana, T.T.; Marume, U.; Muchenje, V. Effects of transportation time, distance, stocking density, temperature and lairage time on incidences of pale soft exudative (PSE) and the physico-chemical characteristics of pork. *Meat Sci.* **2013**, *95*, 520–525. [CrossRef] [PubMed]

25. Peeters, E.; Deprez, K.; Beckers, F.; de Baerdemaeker, J.; Aubert, A.E.; Geers, R. Effect of driver and driving style on the stress responses of pigs during a short journey by trailer. *Anim. Welf.* **2008**, *17*, 189–196.

26. Schwartzkopf-Genswein, K.S.G.; Faucitano, L.; Dadgar, S.; Shand, P.; González, L.A.; Crowe, T.G. Road transport of cattle, swine and poultry in North America and its impact on animal welfare, carcass and meat quality: A review. *Meat Sci.* **2012**, *92*, 227–243. [CrossRef] [PubMed]

27. Institut Technique Du Porc. *Notation des Hématomes sur Couenne—Porcs Vivant ou Carcasses*; ITP: Le Rheu, France, 1996.

28. Faucitano, L. Causes of skin damage to pig carcasses. *Can. J. Anim. Sci.* **2001**, *81*, 39–45. [CrossRef]

29. Nakai, H.; Saito, F.; Ikeda, T.; Ando, S.; Komatsu, A. Standards models of pork color. *Bull. Natl. Inst. Anim. Ind.* **1975**, *30*, 69–74.

30. Correa, J.A.; Méthot, S.; Faucitano, L. A modified meat juice container (EZ-DripLoss) procedure for a more reliable assessment of drip loss and related quality changes in pork meat. *J. Muscle Foods* **2007**, *18*, 67–77. [CrossRef]

31. Honikel, K.O. Reference methods for the assessment of physical characteristics of meat. *Meat Sci.* **1998**, *49*, 447–457. [CrossRef]

32. Faucitano, L.; Ielo, M.C.; Ster, C.; Fiego, D.L.; Methot, S.; Saucier, L. Shelf life of pork from five different quality classes. *Meat Sci.* **2010**, *84*, 466–469. [CrossRef] [PubMed]

33. Tarrant, P.V.; Kenny, F.J.; Harrington, D.; Murphy, M. Long distance transportation of steers to slaughter: Effect of stocking density on physiology, behaviour and carcass quality. *Livest. Prod. Sci.* **1992**, *30*, 223–238. [CrossRef]

34. Bradshaw, R.H.; Parrott, R.F.; Forsling, M.L.; Goode, J.A.; Lloyd, D.M.; Rodway, R.G.; Broom, D.M. Stress and travel sickness in pigs: Effects of road transport on plasma concentrations of cortisol, beta-endorphin and lysine vasopressin. *Anim. Sci.* **1996**, *63*, 507–516. [CrossRef]

35. Correa, J.A.; Gonyou, H.W.; Torrey, S.; Widowski, T.M.; Crowe, T.G.; La Forest, J.P.; Faucitano, L. Welfare and carcass and meat quality of pigs being transported for 2 hours using two vehicle types during two seasons of the year. *Can. J. Anim. Sci.* **2013**, *93*, 43–55. [CrossRef]

36. Edwards, L.N.; Grandin, T.; Engle, T.E.; Porter, S.P.; Ritter, M.J.; Sosnicki, A.A.; Anderson, D.B. Relationship of blood lactate and meat quality in market hogs. In Proceedings of the Reciprocal Meat Conference, Lubbock, TX, USA, 20–23 June 2010; Available online: https://www.researchgate.net/publication/260983276_Relationship_of_blood_lactate_and_meat_quality_in_market_hogs (accessed on 21 August 2016).

37. Edwards, L.N.; Engle, T.E.; Grandin, T.; Ritter, M.J.; Sosnicki, A.; Carlson, B.A.; Anderson, D.B. The effects of distance traveled during loading, lairage time prior to slaughter, and distance traveled to the stunning area on blood lactate concentration of pigs in a commercial packing plant. *Prof. Anim. Sci.* **2011**, *27*, 485–491.

38. Dalla Costa, O.A.; Ludke, J.V.; Paranhos da Costa, M.J.R.P.; Peloso, J.V.; Coldebella, A.; Triques, N. Effect of fasting time at farm and transport conditions of slaughter pigs on lairage resting behaviour and skin injuries. *Ciênc. Anim. Bras.* **2009**, *10*, 48–58.

39. Mormède, P. Assessment of pig welfare. In *The Welfare of Pigs: From Birth to Slaughter*; Faucitano, L., Schaefer, A., Eds.; Wageningen Academic Publishing: Wageningen, The Netherlands, 2008; pp. 33–64.

40. Warriss, P.D.; Brown, S.N.; Edwards, J.E.; Knowles, T.G. Effect of lairage time on levels of stress and meat quality in pigs. *Anim. Sci.* **1998**, *66*, 255–261. [CrossRef]

41. Goumon, S.; Faucitano, L.; Bergeron, R. Effect of ramp configuration on easiness of handling, heart rate and behavior of near-market pigs at unloading. *J. Anim. Sci.* **2013**, *91*, 3889–3898. [CrossRef] [PubMed]

42. Gebresenbet, G. Status of research in animal transport: Evaluation and recommendation. *Swed. Gov. Off. Rep.* **2003**, *6*, 267–305.

43. The Council of the European Union. *Council Regulation (EC) No. 1/2005. No 1/2005 of 22 December 2004 on the Protection of Animals during Transport and Related Operations and Amending Directives 64/432/EEC and 93/119/EC and Regulation (EC) No 1255/97*; The Council of the European Union: Brussels, Belgium, 2005. Available online: https://www.agriculture.gov.ie/media/migration/animalhealthwelfare/transportofliveanimals/Council%20Regulation%201%20of%202005.pdf (accessed on 25 November 2016).

44. Warriss, P.D.; Brown, S.N.; Knowles, T.G.; Edwards, J.E.; Duggan, J.A. Potential effect of vibration during transport on glycogen reserves in broiler chickens. *Vet. J.* **1997**, *153*, 215–219. [CrossRef]

45. Jones, S.D.M.; Tong, A.K.W.; Campbell, C.; Dyck, R. The effects of fat thickness and degree of marbling on pork colour and structure. *Can. J. Anim. Sci.* **1994**, *74*, 155–157. [CrossRef]

46. Van der Wal, P.G.; Olsman, W.J.; Garssen, G.J.; Engel, B. Marbling, intramuscular fat and meat colour of Dutch pork. *Meat Sci.* **1992**, *32*, 351–355. [CrossRef]

47. Araújo, A.P. Pre-Slaughter Management and Welfare of Pigs in Brazilian Abattoirs. Ph.D. Thesis, Faculdade de Medicina Veterinária e Zootecnia, University of São Paulo State, Botucatu, Brazil, 2009.

48. Henckel, P.; Karlsson, A.H.; Oksbjerg, N.; Søholm, P.J. Control of post mortem pH decrease in pig muscle: Experimental design and testing of animal models. *Meat Sci.* **2000**, *55*, 131–138. [CrossRef]

49. Henckel, P.; Karlsson, A.; Jensen, M.T.; Oksbjerg, N.; Petersen, J.S. Metabolic conditions in porcine longissimus muscle immediately pre-slaughter and its influence on peri-and *post-mortem* energy metabolism. *Meat Sci.* **2002**, *62*, 145–155. [CrossRef]

Factors Which Influence Owners When Deciding to Use Chemotherapy in Terminally Ill Pets

Jane Williams [1,*], Catherine Phillips [2] and Hollie Marie Byrd [2]

[1] Animal Health Research Group, Hartpury University Centre, Gloucester GL19 3BE, UK
[2] Veterinary Nursing Research Group, Hartpury University Centre, Gloucester GL19 3BE, UK;
   Catherine.phillips@hartpury.ac.uk (C.P.); hollie1111@aol.com (H.M.B.)
* Correspondence: jane.williams@hartpury.ac.uk

Academic Editor: Clive J. C. Phillips

Simple Summary: Cancer is as common amongst pets as it in humans. Chemotherapy can be integrated into treatment regimes for terminally ill pets to attempt to shrink tumours to extend life expectancy, but it does not cure cancer and it can have negative side effects including vomiting, depression and behavioral changes. To date, little research has been undertaken to explore owners' decisions whether or not to treat their animals with chemotherapy. Seventy-eight dog and cat owners completed an online questionnaire to determine if they would opt for chemotherapy if their pet was diagnosed with cancer, and asked how they thought their pet's quality of life would be affected. Fifty-eight percent of respondents would not use chemotherapy largely due to their previous experience of it. Seventy-two percent over estimated pet survival time post chemotherapy, with most people believing it would lead to remission or a cure. Owners expected their pets to be less active, sleep more and play less, reducing their quality of life. Common side effects associated with chemotherapy were not rated as acceptable. The results suggest pet owners would benefit from an increased understanding of the positive and negative impacts of chemotherapy when initially discussing treatment options with the veterinary team.

Abstract: Chemotherapy is a commonly integrated treatment option within human and animal oncology regimes. Limited research has investigated pet owners' treatment decision-making in animals diagnosed with malignant neoplasia. Dog and cat owners were asked to complete an online questionnaire to elucidate factors which are key to the decision making process. Seventy-eight respondents completed the questionnaire in full. Fifty-eight percent of pet owners would not elect to treat pets with chemotherapy due to the negative impact of the associated side effects. Seventy-two percent of respondents over estimated pet survival time post chemotherapy, indicating a general perception that it would lead to remission or a cure. Vomiting was considered an acceptable side effect but inappetence, weight loss and depression were considered unacceptable. Owners did expect animals' to be less active, sleep more and play less, but common side effects were not rated as acceptable despite the potential benefits of chemotherapy. Based on the results, veterinary teams involved with oncology consultations should establish if clients have prior experience of cancer treatments and their expectations of survival time. Quality of life assessments should also be implemented during initial oncology consultations and conducted regularly during chemotherapy courses to inform client decision making and to safe guard animal welfare.

Keywords: veterinary medicine; oncology; client decision-making; cancer; pets

1. Introduction

Chemotherapy is a commonly integrated treatment option within human and animal oncology regimes [1–3] which aims to reduce the growth of tumours and spread of malignant neoplastic cells. It is defined as the ingestion or injection of cytotoxic drugs to destroy neoplastic or cancer cells [4]. In animals five cancer treatment approaches are taken: palliative care, surgery, chemotherapy (±surgery), radiotherapy or euthanasia [5]. Within veterinary practice, the treatment approach for animals diagnosed with malignant and terminal neoplasia will be informed by discussion with the veterinary team including an overview of therapeutic options, their side effects and benefits, prognosis and survival time, and impact on the pet's quality of life. Despite this, research suggests chemotherapy is often elected for by pet owners due to their prior experience or knowledge of its positive (perceived effective) application in human cancer treatment [6,7].

Neoplasia affects approximately 0.02% dogs and 0.01% cats in the UK per annum [8,9]. The prognosis for animals suffering from malignant neoplasia varies upon the clinical approach taken but generally is poor. For example, the average survival time post-diagnosis for dogs with lymphoma without treatment is 4 to 6 weeks [10]. Research has shown this can be extended with treatment, for example Wang et al. [11] reported survival times of between 5 and 7.5 months with treatment [11]. It should however be noted that survival times will vary between individuals, the type of malignancy present and the oncology regime undertaken.

The decision making process during oncology treatment can lead to ethical dilemmas for owners and the veterinary team. The status of animals in society is inconsistent, ranging from owners who treat their pets as family members [12] and will spare no expense upon them, to others who will abandon animals when they become an inconvenience [13]. The Royal College of Veterinary Surgeon's Code of Professional Conduct requires veterinary surgeons to provide owners of animals undergoing chemotherapy with an outline of all potential treatment options, associated fees and side effects, and the subsequent prognosis for their pet [14]. The priority for the veterinary team is to safeguard the welfare of their animal patient but they also need to support the owner/s through an emotive decision. However, the owner ultimately has the responsibility to make a decision which safeguards the welfare of their pet [15] and as such needs to understand the full implications of their choice. Within human medicine, terminally ill patients and their care givers often feel doctors have 'given up' on them if chemotherapy is not offered as treatment option or is withdrawn during the latter stages of palliative care [16]. A similar scenario may exist within veterinary medicine but this has not been investigated to date. Interestingly, Giuffrida and Kerrigan [17] report that the owners of terminally ill pets value the quality of life of their pet over extended survival times. This suggests that an open and transparent approach from the veterinary team when discussing with the owner the risks, benefits, impact of the treatment involved and the outcome with consideration of quality of life, is essential to support informed consent for subsequent treatment protocols or if they decide to opt for euthanasia [18–20].

Chemotherapy Treatment

The use of chemotherapy within therapeutic oncology programmes in the veterinary sector is becoming more commonplace [21]. Despite this no large scale studies to date have investigated the prevalence, incidence or severity of potential side-effects associated with the treatment in animals, or if clinical symptoms reported as side effects may be due to alternative aetiologies. Therefore owners may refer to human medicine and their own experiences to judge the impact of chemotherapy protocols within their pets. A full review of the impact of chemotherapy on survival times in animals is beyond the scope of this review due to the range of different protocols, multitude of cancer types and confounding factors which can affect prognosis. Illustrations of survival times are provided however readers unfamiliar with oncology are advised that these provide specific examples and do not represent the entirety of the field. Chemotherapy has been shown to extend the lifespan of terminally ill dogs diagnosed with malignant neoplasia on average by 185 days (histiocytic sarcoma) [22], 301 days (appendicular osteosarcoma) [23] and 216 to 342 days (lymphoma) [24]. Similar results have been found in cats that have undergone chemotherapy for extranodal lymphoma recording survival times ranging from 70 days to 749 days [25]. Surgical removal of malignant neoplastic masses without an accompanying chemotherapy course can also exert a beneficial impact on survival, however survival time is often reduced compared to animals with the same diagnosis who undergo surgery and chemotherapy (mammary carcinoma) [26]. Therefore, chemotherapy is considered to extend survival time for the terminally ill pet compared to surgical reduction alone and has a clear benefit as part of an oncology treatment regime [27]. Weeks et al. [28] surveyed the expectations of terminally ill patients with lung and colorectal cancer, finding 69% and 81% of patients respectively felt that chemotherapy would cure their cancer. Prior experience of chemotherapy may influence pet owners' decision making and although surveys suggest quality of life is of key importance [17], when faced with losing their pet, extended survival times, which chemotherapy offers, alongside the incorrect perception that chemotherapy could facilitate a cure, may influence owner choices.

Chemotherapy can cause detrimental side effects in animals [29] and humans [28]. The treatment is non-discriminatory and can have a toxic effect on diseased and healthy tissue [30], resulting in myelosuppression, gastrointestinal toxicosis and nausea in human patients [31–33]. Within dogs, analogous side effects have been reported post chemotherapy treatment including gastrointestinal disease, myelosuppression, cardiotoxicity, dyspnoea and neutropenia resulting in immunological challenges predisposing patients to secondary infections [34,35]. Cognitive changes are also often reported by human patients post chemotherapy treatment, termed "chemobrain"; symptoms include difficulty comprehending normal tasks, lack of concentration, memory issues and lack of awareness of what they are doing [36]. Canine patients will often vomit after treatment and are thought to experience nausea leading to anorexia during chemotherapy [37,38]. As a result of regular emesis, patients can experience weakness, fatigue, anaemia and fever-type symptoms which can result in weight loss. Behavioural changes, reported within quality of life assessments in neoplasia cases [29], with pets becoming progressively more lethargic and depressed (unresponsive, inactive and withdrawn with altered eating and sleeping patterns) resulting in reduced interaction with their owners and the environment which can be upsetting for owners. However it should be remembered that the remit of chemotherapy is to shrink or prevent spread of tumours, and many of the perceived negative side effects should be considered alongside the beneficial effect this treatment can have on prognosis and survival time in canine and feline cancer patients.

Quality of life assessments are often employed to make judgments on an animal's welfare status [29,39,40]. Yeates and Main [41] advocate that a quality of life assessment should be included by the veterinary team when considering therapeutic options for animals suffering from malignant neoplasia. Integrating Quality of Life (QOL) assessments can inform owner decision making, to ensure an ethical balance between *quality* and *quantity* of life is achieved, and the welfare of the animal affected is fully considered [40,41]. The quality of life process can also provide a baseline measure for subsequent assessments. Quality of life assessments, conducted via owner questionnaires, have been conducted in cats [39,42] and dogs undertaking chemotherapy [43,44]. Generally, owners across species were very perceptive to clinical changes in their pets but did not appear to demonstrate equal acuity when identifying QOL changes. This may reflect the tool used, as many quality of life assessments rarely progress beyond evaluation of clinical parameters and fail to integrate other qualities such as cognition, normal functionality, and con-specific interaction within them [44].

To date, research evaluating chemotherapy use in pets has centred on retrospective reviews of veterinary records to evaluate clinical symptoms, therapeutic approaches and subsequent survival times in neoplastic animals. For examples refer to Finlay et al. [45] and Wright et al. [19]. Whilst this information is critical to enable informed dialogue from the veterinary team to the client, assessment of the factors which influence the decision making process pet owners undertake when deciding whether to consent to a course of chemotherapy has been neglected. Therefore, this study aimed to explore factors which may influence owners' decision to elect to undertake chemotherapy in animals, to help inform the approaches taken by the veterinary profession.

2. Method

A mixed methods approach was used to survey current and previous owners of dogs or cats in the UK, to ascertain what factors would influence the decision making process to elect to undertake chemotherapy treatment in a terminally ill pet. Ethical approval was obtained from the University of the West of England (Hartpury) Ethics Committee (Project Identification Code: ETHICS2016-04).

2.1. Participants

Participants were recruited via social media: Facebook and Twitter, between November 2015 and February 2016 due to the capacity for social media to acquire a large number of participants [46]. Subjects were required to be over 18 years of age and to currently own or have previously owned a cat or dog, to be eligible for participation. No previous experience with neoplasm in terminally ill animals or humans was essential. Only fully completed questionnaires progressed to data analysis.

2.2. Survey Design

A questionnaire was designed in Google Forms™. The questionnaire included open and closed questions (Supplementary Materials). Likert scales were also integrated within the questionnaire to allow participants to rank the importance of key themes surveyed. These were complemented by the use of open questions to encourage participants to answer with unprompted responses to facilitate a truer expression of the emotions and feelings they had on the use of chemotherapy in animals [47]. Three key themes were adapted from previous research [39,40,43] and were embedded within the questionnaire: owner perception of the benefits and side effects of chemotherapy (Table 1), rating of quality of life (scale 1: low to 10: high) pre, peri and post chemotherapy, and views on survival times and life expectancy with and without chemotherapy treatment.

Table 1. Quality of life assessment questions.

Participants Were Asked to Rate if They Found the Potential Impact of Chemotherapy in Animals, for the Questions Listed, as Acceptable or Unacceptable.
My pet does not play during chemotherapy
My pet's activity is the same during chemotherapy
My pet sleeps more than usual during chemotherapy
My pet eats normally during chemotherapy
My pets seem depressed during chemotherapy
My pet has more good days then bad during chemotherapy
My pet trembles and shakes occasionally during chemotherapy
My pet grooms normally during chemotherapy
My pet experiences vomiting during chemotherapy
My pet drinks normal amounts during chemotherapy
My pet has diarrhoea during chemotherapy
My pet is aware and happy when I'm present during chemotherapy
My pet is less active during chemotherapy

2.3. Data Analysis

Data from completed questionnaires were transferred to Microsoft™ Excel version 2013 (Microsoft Corporation, Redmond, WA, USA). Frequency analysis of categorical data was performed across the cohort, then data were organised by gender and age within gender to highlight any emergent trends within the subgroups. Grounded theory analysis was applied to the narrative obtained from open questions to enable emergent themes from the data to be recognised [48].

3. Results

A total of 78 questionnaires were completed in their entirety and went forward to analysis. The majority of respondents were female ($n = 68$); these represented a variety of age ranges: 18–24 years:

23%, 25–35 years: 26%, 36–49 years: 27% and over 50 years: 22%. Male participants (n = 10) demonstrated an older age demographic: 18–24 years: 10%, 25–35 years: 40% and over 50 years: 50%. The majority of respondents had some prior experience of chemotherapy (female respondents: 53%; male respondents: 60%), this was within a friend or family member for 39% of female respondents and 40% of male respondents, and in a pet for 14% of female respondents and 20% of male respondents (Figure 1). Fifty-five percent of respondents (female respondents: 57%; male respondents: 30%) stated they were familiar with the side effects that accompanied chemotherapy in animals, with slightly more, 57%, aware of the side effects associated with chemotherapy in human patients (female respondents: 61%; male respondents: 40%).

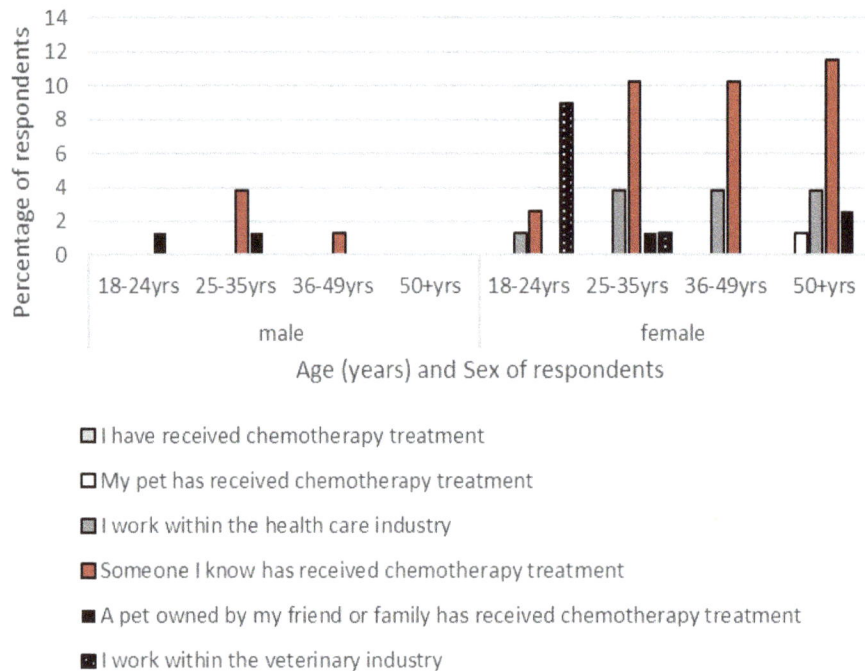

□ I have received chemotherapy treatment

□ My pet has received chemotherapy treatment

▨ I work within the health care industry

■ Someone I know has received chemotherapy treatment

■ A pet owned by my friend or family has received chemotherapy treatment

▨ I work within the veterinary industry

Figure 1. Participants' previous experiences with chemotherapy treatment (CT).

The majority of participants (58%) believed that the benefits of chemotherapy did not counterbalance the impact of the potentially negative side effects which animals may experience during treatment. However, when respondents were asked to rate the acceptability of defined side effects and benefits of chemotherapy, mixed opinions were recorded (Figures 2 and 3, respectively). Interestingly, respondents thought that pets' QOL would be enhanced after chemotherapy (median rating: 7; interquartile range (IQR): 2) compared to prior to (median rating: 5; IQR: 3) and during treatment (median rating: 5; IQR: 3). All respondents indicated that they believed chemotherapy would extend an animal's life expectancy and 72% felt that chemotherapy would extend survival time over one year (Figure 4).

Respondents expectations on the quality of life dogs and cats experience during chemotherapy regimens varied (Figure 5). The results indicate the majority of owners wanted their animal to retain a *normal* quality of life with regards to eating, drinking, behaviour and activity levels, and low expression of known side effects associated with chemotherapy: vomiting, diarrhoea and depression.

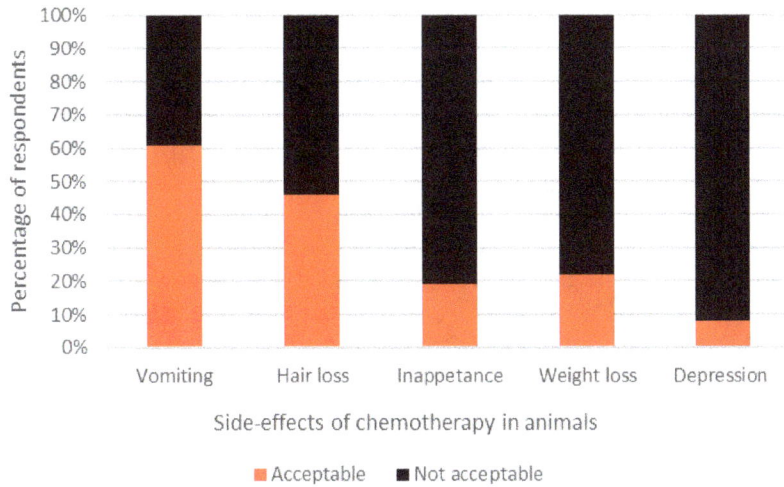

Figure 2. Acceptability of side effects associated with chemotherapy treatment in dogs and cats.

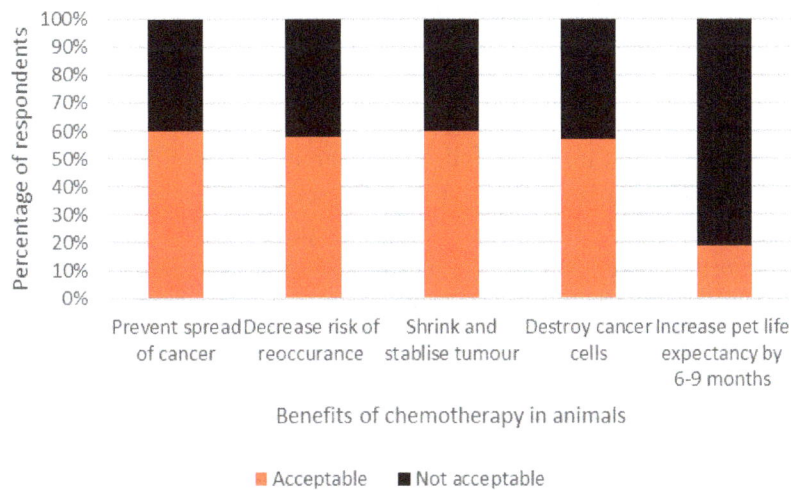

Figure 3. Acceptability of beneficial effects associated with chemotherapy treatment in dogs and cats.

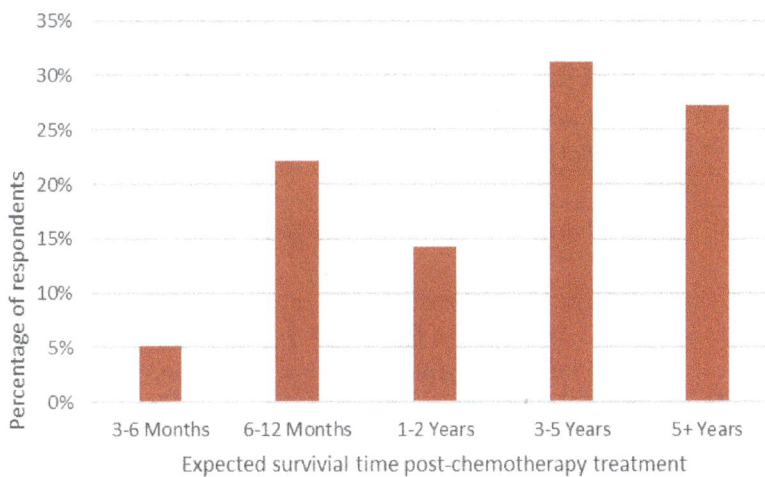

Figure 4. Perceived survival time post-chemotherapy treatment in dogs and cats.

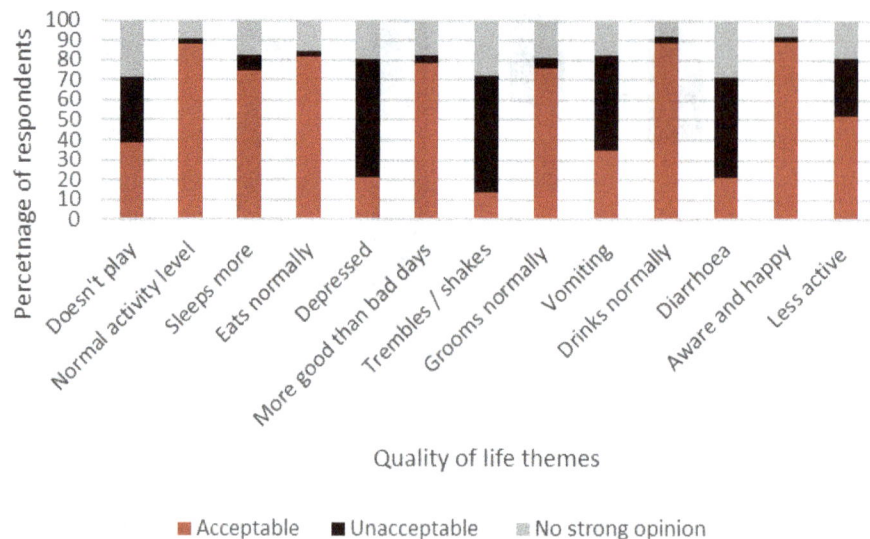

Figure 5. Dog and cat owners' expectations of pets' quality of life during and after chemotherapy.

When asked if survival time would influence the decision to undertake chemotherapy in their pet, a total of 52 out of 78 respondents (67%) disagreed, or strongly disagreed to the statement "I would opt for chemotherapy treatment if my pet will live for an extra 3 months with the chemotherapy". Generating mixed comments such as *"cancer if the lesser evil"* and *"months is enough time as long as it is enjoyable"*. Whilst 40 respondents (52%) agreed, or strongly agreed to the statement *"I would opt for chemotherapy treatment if my pet will live for an extra 12 months with chemotherapy"*, although others felt: *"one year is not enough"*. Forty-two percent of participants (45% female; 30% male) would elect for chemotherapy if their pet was diagnosed with a malignant tumour knowing the potential benefits of the treatment. This reduced to 35% (35% female; 40% male) when considering the side effects of chemotherapy treatment. These participants generally believed the *"benefits (of chemotherapy) outweigh the side effects" "it (chemotherapy) will give the animal vital time"* and *"the side effects don't appear to be drastic"*, *"any cancer treatment should be available to animals"*, *"chemotherapy is a wonderful idea even with limited knowledge"*, with one commenting *"anything is better than putting the animal to sleep"*. In contrast, respondents who would not elect for chemotherapy in their pet felt *"that after seeing what it does to a person, I am unsure as to how ethical it is to do this to an animal that doesn't understand"* and, *"having seen a relative undergo chemo, I would be less inclined to agree to chemo for my dogs"*. When making a decision to treat animals with CT, the use of prior knowledge obtained by the participants exerted an influential impact on some respondents' decision making: *"after seeing what it does to humans, I don't think it is ethical"*, *"I would find it hard as my sister and niece have been through it"*, *"cancer is the lesser evil"* and *"surgery is a quicker resolution"*.

4. Discussion

Most of the participants had some experience of chemotherapy in humans and/or animals, which appears to inform decision making when considering if they would elect to place a terminally ill pet upon a course of chemotherapy. Previous experience has been identified to contribute to the decision making process in human medicine [49–51]. The results here suggest that owners' beliefs and prior experience of chemotherapy, especially their perception of side effects over potential benefits of the treatment, will influence their decision to use chemotherapy in their pets. It would be worthwhile for veterinary teams to allocate time to fully understand owners' historic experiences of chemotherapy as these will influence the treatment regime selected.

Similar traits to those observed in human oncology patients and their carers appear to also occur within animal owners. The majority of respondents believed their pet's quality of life would improve post-chemotherapy but many (72%) overestimated average survival time post-treatment. Fewer owners would have elected for chemotherapy if the result was a shorter 3-month extended survival compared to a 12-month survival period for their pet, which suggests quality of life is a key consideration in decision-making. However it should be noted that "agree" and "strongly agree" responses were summed to obtain these figures, therefore the results may over represent the strength of feeling of those who took part. Respondents also quantified the benefits of chemotherapy in terms of the treatment being a cure rather a palliative intervention. These opinions mimic those found in human cancer patients and their caregivers [28]. Human cancer patients have indicated a preference to be fully informed before undertaking treatment to provide time to adapt to their diagnosis and make a fully informed decision [52–54]. A similar approach would be advocated in pet owners as proxy representatives of the animal, as our results suggest that owners consider what treatment approach to adopt from their perspective rather than their pets. It is therefore also important to eliminate any potential disconnect that exists between owners' perception of the severity of side effects and the reality of what to expect within chemotherapy regimens. Veterinary teams should ensure their approach in terminal cases includes knowledge transfer of the fundamental characteristics and effects of chemotherapy, with a clear focus on how an animal's quality of life will be affected and the likely incidence and expression of side effects, to enable owners to possess sufficient knowledge and understanding to make a fully informed decision. Paradoxically in human chemotherapy, patients who feel they have a good relationship with open communication with their clinician are at higher risk of having unrealistic expectations of the long term benefits of chemotherapy [28]. Therefore, it would be beneficial to integrate a period of reflection into the decision making process and perhaps a multi-person approach is warranted to ensure clients engage with information transfer. Without these opportunities, owners may select chemotherapy to facilitate more time with their pet, despite a poor understanding of the impact of chemotherapy on the animal which could lead to increased distress during treatment protocols and after the animal's death akin to feelings observed in human care givers post-bereavement [16].

The majority of respondents expected aspects of an animal's quality of life to reduce during and after a course of chemotherapy treatment, with pets sleeping more, being less playful and showing reduced activity levels. Interestingly, despite 55% of respondents stating they were aware of the side effects associated with chemotherapy in animals, most owners did not feel these side effects were acceptable when judging a pet's quality of life. Respondents also did not feel the common side effects of chemotherapy (vomiting, diarrhoea and behavioural changes) would be acceptable, as well as wanting affected animals to experience more good than bad days. Previous work [46] found that although owners of animals undergoing chemotherapy were very perceptive of clinical changes they did not recognise signs which represented a reduced quality of life, despite the same people prioritising quality of life over extended life expectancies [17]. The results suggest a disconnect exists between owners' expectations of what their pet's quality of life should be during chemotherapy and what it is likely to be. Similarly, most owners here equated the therapy with an extended survival time beyond average life expectancies post diagnosis or that it represented a cure, commenting: "(chemotherapy) *saves them, extends life, is a cure, chemotherapy increases their quality of life, the benefits outweigh the side effects, and having side effects for a short time and to live a lot longer* and *healthier is better*". A similar paradox occurs within human oncology [16,28] with misconceptions of the clinical impact of chemotherapy (quality of life and life expectancy) common amongst patients receiving palliative care and their care-givers. It is imperative to note that chemotherapy can lengthen survival times and offer a better quality of life for neoplastic animals, a concept that should not be lost in client-veterinary communication. Therefore it is important that the veterinary team supporting decision making in owners and understand that such paradoxes exist as they could potentially misinform a client's judgement of a pet's quality of life and welfare, and the subsequent decision to not elect for chemotherapy or to agree to the treatment.

Quality of life assessments are key tools that can be used to benefit patients, clinicians, caregivers or owners, and can inform the medical/veterinary therapeutic decision making process [55]. The majority of assessments are disease specific and tend to focus on clinical parameters [39]. Examples in human medicine include the EuroQol [56], Sickness Impact Assessment (SIP) [57] and the SF-36 [58]. Readers are recommended to refer to Vols et al. [29] and Belshaw et al. [40] for reviews of quality of life tools used within veterinary medicine. Specific oncology quality of life assessment tools are also available (for example: De Haes et al. [59]). There is general agreement that an effective quality of life assessment should contain six fundamental dimensions [59]:

1. Physical functioning (physiological, biomechanical and neural parameters, and the ability to perform routine tasks—quantitative assessment),
2. Psychological functioning (cognitive abilities, mental health status, mood and personality—quantitative and qualitative assessment). It should be noted these facets are difficult to assess within animals and general behavioral changes may need to be considered to provide a measure of psychological function,
3. Social functioning (environmental interaction and relationships—qualitative assessment),
4. Role activities (motivation, communication, play and exercise—quantitative and qualitative assessment),
5. Overall life satisfaction (enjoyment and fulfilment—qualitative assessment), and,
6. Perception of health status (overall rating—quantitative and qualitative assessment).

The key goal of quality of life assessment as a tool to inform owners' decision making prior to electing for an animal to start chemotherapy treatment or during chemotherapy regimens, is the ability of the assessment to quantify clinically meaningful changes. Clinically meaningful changes can be defined as those which influence a patient's management or that result in a reduction or improvement in functionality, or an increase or decrease in clinical symptoms [55]. Interpretation of change can in itself be challenging as it is difficult to quantify if a change in score of ±0.1 or ±1.0 equates to a clinically meaningful change. In veterinary oncology, quality of life assessments are predominately questionnaire based and rarely go beyond clinical parameters [47]. More work needs to be done to define reliable and valid tools and parameters which capture the full repertoire of changes that occur in an animal's quality of life, specifically here with reference to the terminally ill oncology patient [17]. The development of effective quality of life assessments would provide a baseline measure to facilitate comparison between individuals in the clinical environment. Additionally, quality of life assessments should be used as a precursory tool to facilitate client-veterinary discussions over the prognosis and treatment options available, and enable clients to make truly informed decisions whether selecting palliative care or euthanasia [17]. Therefore, we would recommend that veterinary teams integrate a quality of life assessment into the initial consultation process for the oncology patient and implement regular quality of life assessments for the duration of their treatment to optimise animal welfare.

The study does have limitations as questionnaires cannot fully explore the complexity that underpins the perception and feelings of the respondents surveyed. The results presented here represent the views of this sample and their perception of chemotherapy as a treatment, and these may not be an accurate representation of broader pet owners' feelings and opinions. Further work incorporating larger numbers would be warranted. Future research using focus groups, interviews and case studies drawn from individuals who were or had experienced chemotherapy directly with their pet is essential to gain a broader insight into the owner decision making process, owner views of chemotherapy and its impact on pets, and the influences of the veterinary team upon this.

5. Conclusions

The veterinary team has a duty of care to their clients and their pets to ensure the full complexities of oncology and chemotherapy are communicated during consultations. Prior experience of chemotherapy appears to directly influence owner decision making when considering whether to undertake a course of chemotherapy in a pet. Owners generally overestimated the impact of chemotherapy on pet survival times post treatment potentially establishing false expectations which could result in enhanced distress post bereavement. Owners rate pets' quality of life as key when choosing whether to engage with chemotherapy, however this assessment appears focused on clinical parameters and not functional tasks, personality expression or changes in behaviour. Based on the results, veterinary teams involved with oncology consultations should establish if clients have prior experience of cancer treatments and their expectations of survival time. Quality of life assessments which evaluate patient health status via clinical parameters, physical, psychological and social function, interaction and life satisfaction should also be implemented during initial oncology consultations and conducted regularly during chemotherapy courses to inform client decision making and to safe guard animal welfare.

Acknowledgments: We would like to thank the participants for engaging with our project.

Author Contributions: Project design, planning and data collection was undertaken by Jane Williams and Hollie Marie Byrd. Data analysis, manuscript writing up and editing was performed by Jane Williams, Catherine Phillips and Hollie Marie Byrd.

Conflicts of Interest: The authors declare no conflict of interest.

References

1. Adelstein, D.J.; Saxton, J.P.; Rybicki, L.A.; Esclamado, R.M.; Wood, B.G.; Strome, M.; Lavertu, P.; Lorenz, R.R.; Carroll, M.A. Multiagent concurrent chemoradiotherapy for locoreginally advances squamous cell head and neck cancer: Mature result from a single institution. *J. Clin. Oncol.* **2006**, *24*, 1064–1071. [CrossRef] [PubMed]

2. Wilkowski, R.; Thoma, M.; Weingandt, H.; Duhmke, E.; Heinemann, V. Chemoradiation for ductal pancreatic carcinoma: Principles of combining chemotherapy with radiations, definition of target volume and radiation dose. *J. Pancreas* **2005**, *6*, 216–230.

3. Rakovitch, E.; Tsao, M.; Ung, Y.; Pignol, J.P.; Cheung, P.; Chow, E. Comparison of the efficacy and acute toxicity of weekly versus daily chemoradiotherapy for non-small-cell lung cancer: A meta-analysis. *Int. J. Radiat. Oncol. Biol. Phys.* **2004**, *58*, 196–203. [CrossRef]

4. Macmillian Cancer Support. What Is Chemotherapy? Available online: Https://www.macmillan.org.uk/information-and-support/treating/chemotherapy/chemotherapy-explained/what-is-chemotherapy.html (accessed on 27 January 2016).

5. Wolfesberger, B.; Tonar, Z.; Fuchs-Baumgartinger, A.; Walter, I.; Skalicky, M.; Witter, K.; Thalhammer, J.G.; Pagitz, M.; Kleiter, M. Angiogenic markers in canine lymphoma tissues do not predict survival times in chemotherapy treated dogs. *Res. Vet. Sci.* **2012**, *92*, 444–450. [CrossRef] [PubMed]

6. Withrow, S.J. Why worry about cancer in pets? In *Withrow and MacEwen's Small Animal Clinical Oncology*, 4th ed.; Withrow, S.J., Vail, D.M., Eds.; Saunders Elsevier: Philadelphia, PA, USA, 2007; pp. xv–xvii.

7. Dobson, J.M. Introduction: Cancer in cats and dogs. In *BSAVA Manual of Canine and Feline Oncology*, 3rd ed.; Dobson, J.M., Duncan, B., Lascelles, X., Eds.; British Small Animal Veterinary Association: Guarantee, UK, 2011; pp. 1–5.

8. Animal Heath Trust Cancer Research. Available online: http://www.aht.org.uk/cms-display/science_oncology.html (accessed on 20 January 2016).

9. International Cat Care. Cancer in Cats. Available online: http://icatcare.org/advice/cat-health/cancer-cats (accessed on 20 January 2016).

10. Animal Cancer Trust. Types of Cancer. Available online: http://www.animalcancertrust.co.uk/types-of-cancer (accessed on 2 March 2016).

11. Wang, S.L.; Lee, I.J.; Liao, A.T. Comparison of efficacy and toxicity of doxorubicin and mitoxantrone in combination of chemotherapy for canine lymphoma. *Can. Vet. J.* **2016**, *57*, 271–276. [PubMed]

12. Pirrone, F.; Pierantoni, L.; Mazzola, S.M.; Vigo, D.; Albertini, M. Owner and animal factors predict the incidence of, and wner reaction towards, problematic behaviours in companion dogs. *J. Vet. Behav. Clin. Appl. Res.* **2015**, *10*, 295–301. [CrossRef]

13. Arkow, P. Application of ethics to animal welfare. *Appl. Anim. Behav. Sci.* **1998**, *59*, 193–200.

14. Royal College of Veterinary Surgeons. Communication and Consent. Available online: http://www.rcvs.org.uk/advice-and-guidance/code-of-professional-conduct-for-veterinary-surgeons/supporting-guidance/communication-and-consent (accessed on 27 January 2016).

15. Jacobs, H.H. Ethics in pediatric end-of-life care: A nursing perspective. *J. Pediatr. Nurs.* **2005**, *20*, 360–369. [CrossRef] [PubMed]

16. Wright, A.L.; Zhang, B.; Keating, N.L.; Weeks, J.C.; Prigerson, H.G. Associations between palliative chemotherapy and adult cancer patients' end of life care and place of death: Prospective cohort study. *Br. Med. J.* **2014**. [CrossRef] [PubMed]

17. Giuffrida, M.A.; Kerrigan, S.M. Quality of life measurement in prospective studies of cancer treatments in dogs and cats. *J. Vet. Intern. Med.* **2014**, *28*, 1824–1829. [CrossRef] [PubMed]

18. Macdonald, J.; Gray, C. "Informed consent"—How do we get it right? *Vet. Nurs. J.* **2014**, *29*, 101–103. [CrossRef]

19. Wright, I.M. Complications and consent. *Equine Vet. Educ.* **2014**, *26*, 292–293. [CrossRef]

20. Panting, G. Informed consent. *Orthop. Trauma* **2010**, *24*, 441–446. [CrossRef]

21. Hamilton, A. Chemotherapy: What progress in the last 5 years? *J. Clin. Oncol.* **2005**, *23*, 1760–1775. [CrossRef] [PubMed]

22. Cannon, C.; Borgatti, A.; Henson, M.; Husbands, B. Evaluation of a combination chemotherapy protocol including lomustine and doxorubicin in canine histiocytic sarcoma. *J. Small Anim. Pract.* **2015**, *56*, 425–429. [CrossRef] [PubMed]

23. Shapiro, W.; Fossum, T.W.; Kitchell, B.E.; Couto, C.G.; Theilen, G.H. Use of cisplatin for treatment of appendicular osteosarcoma in dogs. *J. Am. Vet. Med. Assoc.* **1988**, *192*, 507–511. [PubMed]

24. Elliott, J.W.; Cripps, P.; Marrington, A.M.; Grant, I.A.; Blackwood, L. Epirubicin as part of a multi-agent chemotherapy protocol for canine lymphoma. *Vet. Comp. Oncol.* **2013**, *11*, 185–198. [CrossRef] [PubMed]

25. Taylor, S.S.; Goodfellow, M.R.; Browne, W.J.; Walding, B.; Murphy, S.; Tzannes, S.; Gerou-Ferriani, M.; Schwartz, A.; Dobson, J.M. Feline extranodal lymphoma: Response to chemotherapy and survival in 110 cats. *J. Small Anim. Pract.* **2009**, *50*, 584–592. [CrossRef] [PubMed]

26. McNeil, C.J.; Sorenmo, K.U.; Shofer, F.S.; Gibeon, L.; Durham, A.C.; Barber, L.G.; Baez, J.L.; Overley, B. Evaluation of adjuvant doxorubicin-based chemotherapy for the treatment of feline mammary carcinoma. *J. Vet. Intern. Med.* **2009**, *23*, 123–129. [CrossRef] [PubMed]

27. Wendelburg, K.M.; Price, L.L.; Burgess, K.E.; Lyons, J.A.; Lew, F.H.; Berg, J. Survival time of dogs with splenic hemangiosarcoma treated by splenectomy with or without adjuvant chemotherapy: 208 cases (2001–2012). *J. Am. Vet. Med. Assoc.* **2015**, *247*, 393–403. [CrossRef] [PubMed]

28. Weeks, J.C.; Catalano, P.J.; Cronin, A.; Finkelman, M.D.; Mack, J.W.; Keating, N.L.; Schrag, D. Patients' expectations about effects of chemotherapy for advanced cancer. *N. Engl. J. Med.* **2012**, *367*, 1616–1625. [CrossRef] [PubMed]

29. Vols, K.K.; Heden, M.A.; Kristensen, A.T.; Sandoe, P. Quality of life assessment in dogs and cats receiving chemotherapy—A review of current methods. *Vet. Comp. Oncol.* **2016**. [CrossRef]

30. Boden, E.; Andrews, A. *Black's Veterinary Dictionary (Online)*; Bloomsbury: London, UK, 2015.

31. Shehadeh, N.J.; Ensley, J.F.; Kucuk, O.; Black, C.; Yoo, G.H.; Jacobs, J.; Lin, H.S.; Heilbrun, L.K.; Smith, D.; Kim, H. Benefit of postoperative chemoradiotherapy for patients with unknown primary squamous cell carcinoma of the head and neck. *Head Neck* **2006**, *28*, 1090–1098. [CrossRef] [PubMed]

32. Hume, K.R.; Johnson, J.L.; Williams, L.E. Adverse effects of concurrent carboplatin chemotherapy and radiation therapy in dogs. *J. Vet. Intern. Med.* **2009**, *23*, 24–30. [CrossRef] [PubMed]

33. Morrow, G.R.; Roscoe, J.A.; Hickok, J.T.; Andrews, P.L.; Matteson, S. Nausea and emesis: Evidence for a biobehavioural perspective. *Support. Care Cancer* **2002**, *10*, 96–105. [CrossRef] [PubMed]

34. Axiak-Bechtal, S.; Fowler, B.; Yu, D.H.; Amorim, J.; Tsuruta, K.; DeClue, A. Chemotherapy and remission status do not alter pre-existing innate immune dysfunction in dogs with lymphoma. *Res. Vet. Sci.* **2014**, *97*, 230–237. [CrossRef] [PubMed]

35. Lane, A.E.; Black, M.L.; Wyatt, K.M. Toxicity and efficacy of a novel doxorubicin and carboplatin chemotherapy protocol for the treatment of canine appendicular osteosarcoma following limb amputation. *Aust. Vet. J.* **2012**, *90*, 69–74. [CrossRef] [PubMed]

36. Myers, J.S. Cancer and chemotherapy related cognitive changes: The patient experience. *Semin. Oncol. Nurs.* **2013**, *29*, 300–307. [CrossRef] [PubMed]

37. Navari, R.M. 5-HT3 receptors as important mediators of nausea and vomiting due to chemotherapy. *Biochim. Biophys. Acta* **2015**, *1848*, 2738–2746. [CrossRef] [PubMed]
38. Xenoulis, P.G. Nausea: Is it a big "little problem" in animals? *Vet. J.* **2015**, *203*, 267. [CrossRef] [PubMed]
39. Tzannes, S.; Hammond, M.F.; Murphy, S.; Sparks, A.; Blackwood, L. Owners perception of their cats quality of life during COP chemotherapy for lymphoma. *J. Feline Med. Surg.* **2008**, *10*, 73–81. [CrossRef] [PubMed]
40. Belshaw, Z.; Asher, L.; Harvey, N.D.; Dean, R.S. Quality of life assessment in domestic dogs: An evidence-based rapid review. *Vet. J.* **2015**, *206*, 203–212. [CrossRef] [PubMed]
41. Yeates, M.; Main, D. Assessment of companion animal quality of life in veterinary practice and research. *J. Small Anim. Pract.* **2009**, *50*, 274–281. [CrossRef] [PubMed]
42. Lynch, S.; Savary-Bataille, K.; Leeuw, B.; Argyle, D.J. Development of a questionnaire assessing health-related quality-of-life in dogs and cats with cancer. *Vet. Comp. Oncol.* **2010**, *9*, 172–182. [CrossRef] [PubMed]
43. Reynolds, C.A.; Oyama, M.A.; Rush, J.E.; Rozanski, E.A.; Singletary, G.E.; Brown, D.C.; Cunningham, S.M.; Fox, P.R.; Bond, B.; Adin, D.B.; et al. Perceptions of quality of life and priorities of owners of cats with heart disease. *J. Vet. Intern. Med.* **2010**, *24*, 1421–1426. [CrossRef] [PubMed]
44. Hamilton, M.J.; Sarcornrattana, O.; Illiopoulou, M.; Xie, Y.; Kitchell, B. Questionnaire-based assessment of owner concerns and doctor responsiveness: 107 canine chemotherapy patients. *J. Small Anim. Pract.* **2012**, *53*, 627–633. [CrossRef] [PubMed]
45. Finlay, J.; Wyatt, K.; Black, M. Evaluation of the risks of chemotherapy in dogs with thrombocytopenia. *Vet. Comp. Oncol.* **2017**, *15*, 151–162. [CrossRef] [PubMed]
46. Salmons, J. *Doing Qualitative Research Online*; Sage Publications: London, UK, 2016.
47. Bruce, I. *Questionnaire Design How to Plan, Structure and Write Survey Material for Effective Market Research*, 3rd ed.; Kogan Page Limited: New Delhi, India, 2013.
48. Charmaz, C. *Constructing Grounded Theory: A Practical Guide through Qualitative Analysis*; Sage Publications: London, UK, 2006.
49. Li, S.Y.W.; Rakow, T.; Newell, B.R. Personal experience in doctor and patient decision making: From psychology to medicine. *J. Eval. Clin. Pract.* **2009**, *15*, 993–995. [CrossRef] [PubMed]
50. Karimian, Z.; Kojuri, J.; Sagheb, M.M.; Mahboudi, A.; Saber, M.; Amini, M.; Dehghani, M.R. Comparison of residents' approaches to clinical decisions before and after the implementation of evidence based medicine course. *J. Adv. Med. Educ. Prof.* **2013**, *2*, 170–175.
51. Roykenes, K. "My math and me": Nursing students' previous experiences in learning mathematics. *Nurse Educ. Pract.* **2016**, *16*, 1–7. [CrossRef] [PubMed]
52. Wisk, T.M. Informed consent. *Plast. Surg. Nurse* **2006**, *26*, 203. [CrossRef]
53. Sinding, C.; Hudak, P.; Wiernikowski, J.; Aronson, J.; Miller, P.; Gould, J.; Fitzpatrick-Lewis, D. "I like to be an informed person but..." negotiating responsibility for treatment decisions in cancer care. *Soc. Sci. Med.* **2010**, *71*, 1094–1101. [CrossRef] [PubMed]
54. Oostendorp, L.J.M.; Ottevanger, P.B.; Van De Wouw, A.J.; Honkoop, A.H.; Los, M.; Van Der Graaf, W.T.A.; Stalmeier, P.F.M. Patients' preferences for information about the benefits and risks of second-line palliative chemotherapy and their oncologist's awareness of these preferences. *J. Cancer Educ.* **2016**, *31*, 443–448. [CrossRef] [PubMed]
55. Crosby, R.D.; Kalotkin, R.L.; Williams, R. Defining clinically meaningful change in health related quality of life. *J. Clin. Epidemiol.* **2003**, *56*, 395–407. [CrossRef]
56. Brooks, R. EuroQoL the current state of play. *Health Policy* **1996**, *37*, 53–72. [CrossRef]
57. Bergner, M.; Bobbit, R.A.; Carter, C.A. The sickness impact profile: Development and final revision of a health status measure. *Med. Care* **1981**, *19*, 787–803. [CrossRef] [PubMed]
58. Ware, J.E.; Sherbourne, C.D. The MOS short form health survey (SF-36). *Med. Care* **1992**, *30*, 473–483. [CrossRef] [PubMed]
59. De Haes, J.L.J.M.; Olscheski, M.; Fayers, P.M. *Measuring Quality of Life of Cancer Patients with the Rotterdam Symptom Checklist (RSCL): A Manual*; Groningen Northern Centre for Health Care Research: Groningen, The Netherlands, 1996.

3

Conscientious Objection to Animal Experimentation in Italian Universities

Ilaria Baldelli [1,2], Alma Massaro [3], Susanna Penco [4], Anna Maria Bassi [4], Sara Patuzzo [5,*] and Rosagemma Ciliberti [6]

[1]   Dipartimento di Scienze Chirurgiche e Diagnostiche Integrate (DISC), Università di Genova, 16132 Genova, Italy; ilaria.baldelli@unige.it

[2]   Unità Operativa di Chirurgia Plastica e Ricostruttiva, IRCCS Azienda Ospedaliera Universitaria San Martino -IST Genova, 16132 Genoa, Italy

[3]   Dipartimento di Antichità, Filosofia, Storia, Geografia (DAFIST), Università di Genova, 16126 Genova, Italy; almamassaro@gmail.com

[4]   Dipartimento di Medicina Sperimentale (DIMES), Università di Genova, 16132 Genova, Italy; Susanna.Penco@unige.it (S.P.); ambassi@medicina.unige.it (A.M.B.)

[5]   School of Medicine and Surgery, University of Verona, P.le L. A. Scuro 10, 37134 Verona, Italy

[6]   Dipartimento di Scienze della Salute (DISSAL), Università di Genova, 16132 Genova, Italy; rosellaciliberti@yahoo.it

*   Correspondence: sara.patuzzo@univr.it

Academic Editor: Clive J. C. Phillips

Simple Summary: This paper examines the trend of Italian academic faculties in complying with the obligation to inform university students of their right to exercise their conscientious objection to scientific or educational activities involving animals, hereafter written as "animal CO", as established by Law 413/1993, "Norme sull'obiezione di coscienza alla sperimentazione animale" ("Rules on conscientious objection to animal experimentation"), thereafter "Law 413/1993". Despite an increasing interest in the principles of animal ethics by the international community, this law is still largely disregarded more than 20 years after its enactment. The Ethics Committees, Animal Welfare Committees, as well as the Italian Ministry of Education, University and Research should preside over and monitor the Universities' compliance with the duty to disclose animal CO.

Abstract: In Italy, Law 413/1993 states that public and private Italian Institutions, including academic faculties, are obliged to fully inform workers and students about their right to conscientious objection to scientific or educational activities involving animals, hereafter written as "animal CO". However, little monitoring on the faculties' compliance with this law has been performed either by the government or other institutional bodies. Based on this premise, the authors have critically reviewed the existing data and compared them with those emerging from their own investigation to discuss limitations and inconsistencies. The results of this investigation revealed that less than half of Italian academic faculties comply with their duty to inform on animal CO. Non-compliance may substantially affect the right of students to make ethical choices in the field of animal ethics and undermines the fundamental right to express their own freedom of thought. The Italian Ministry of Education, Universities and Research, ethics committees and animal welfare bodies should cooperate to make faculties respect this law. Further research is needed to better understand the reasons for the current trend, as well as to promote the enforcement of Law 413/1993 with particular regard to information on animal CO.

Keywords: animal ethics; 3Rs; conscientious objection; veterinary education; science education; non-animal methods

1. Introduction

An increased awareness of the ethical issues relating to research involving animals can be found in the Italian Law 413/1993 [1], originally referred to as Law 116/1992, "Attuazione della direttiva CEE n. 609/86 in materia di protezione degli animali utilizzati a fini sperimentali o ad altri fini scientifici" ("Implementation of the Directive CEE n. 609/86 on the protection of animals for experimental or scientific purposes"), now replaced by Law 26/2014, "Attuazione della direttiva 2010/63/UE sulla protezione degli animali utilizzati a fini scientifici" ("Implementation of the Directive 2010/63/UE on the protection of animals for scientific purposes"), thereafter "Law 26/2014". Law 413/1993 introduced the opportunity for physicians, researchers, students and healthcare providers to not take part in experimental research that involved animals by exercising conscientious objection to scientific or educational activities involving animals, hereafter written as "animal CO". Furthermore, their decision not to take part in such activities would not expose them to possible adverse consequences arising from their refusal to participate in otherwise legally enforceable acts. Workers had the right to perform alternative activities which did not include animals, while retaining the same qualifications and remuneration. Similarly, students who opted for animal CO had the right to receive educational and teaching activities without animals.

It is important to note that the Italian law uses the expression "animal experimentation" with a general meaning that covers all scientific practices, including educational activities involving animals. Therefore, the Italian law is inadequate as it has chosen poor wording, which is not sufficiently descriptive. In the same way, when the Italian law states the right to opt for animal CO, it applies the same inaccurate reference to the general field of "animal experimentation", implicitly including the specific sector of educational animal use.

Law 413/1993 aims to safeguard personal freedom to express ethical choices, according to fundamental ethical principles and human rights recognized at an international level [2], as stated in the Universal Declaration of Human Rights; the European Convention for the Protection of Human Rights and Fundamental Freedoms; and in the International Covenant on Civil and Political Rights adopted by the United Nations General Assembly.

In this light, in addition to Law 413/1993 on animal CO, Italian legislation provides two other laws that safeguard the right of healthcare professionals to exercise their conscientious objection: Law 194/1978, "Norme per la tutela sociale della maternità e sull'interruzione volontaria della gravidanza" ("Rules for social protection of maternity and on voluntary interruption of pregnancy") [3]; and Law 40/2004, "Norme in materia di procreazione medicalmente assistita" ("Rules on medically assisted procreation") [4].

According to Law 413/1993, all public and private entities who are authorized to perform scientific or educational activities must inform all workers and students of their right to exercise animal CO and provide a specific declaration form that can be repealed at any time. However, with specific attention to academic faculties, Law 413/1993 does not provide details about how this information should be communicated, for instance by posting the full text of the law on the faculties' websites or during lectures with an explanation by professors. Consequently, monitoring of the faculties' compliance with their information duty appears to be difficult. Currently, a starting control has been conducted by the following bodies and associations.

In 2009, the Italian National Bioethics Committee (NBC), a government agency whose aim is to provide for opinions on bioethical issues, published a specific investigation [5]. Later, two non-governmental agencies, the Hans Ruesch Foundation (HRF), and the Associazione Radicale Antispecista Parte in Causa (ARA), carried out further research [6,7].

In this paper, the authors critically reviewed data from the NBC, HRF and ARA reports and compared them with those emerging from their own investigation. The purpose of the analysis was to verify the legal compliance by academic faculties to inform students on their right to choose conscientious objection in situations where medical education involved the use of animals. In addition, the authors discuss the ethical implications that this sensitive issue enshrines.

2. Previous and New Investigations

2.1. The NBC Investigation

In 2009, the NBC published the report "Metodologie alternative, Comitati etici e obiezione di coscienza alla sperimentazione animale" ("Alternative Methods, Ethics Committees and Conscientious Objection to Animal Experimentation") [5]. The report was based on replies to a questionnaire sent to 128 different scientific faculties at Italian universities and contained the following three questions:

Q1.   Have your students been informed of their right to conscientious objection as stated in Article 3, Paragraph 5 of Law 413/93, which states: "All public and private establishments that legally carry out animal experimentation are obliged to inform all workers and students of their right to exercise conscientious objection with regards to animal experimentation. The establishments themselves are also obliged to set up a form for the declaration of conscientious objection to animal experimentation by the current Law"?

Q2.   Have there been any cases of students making such a request?

Q3.   Have you employed teaching methods that do not involve activities or interventions of animal experimentation to pass exams, as required by Article 4, Paragraph 3 of Law 413/93, which states: "University authorities shall make optional all laboratory activities where animal experimentation is foreseen. Within the start of the academic year that follows the coming into force of this Law, courses shall be offered that do not require activities related to animal experimentation as part of their final exam requirements. Universities' student administration offices shall give maximum dissemination of students' right of conscientious objection to animal experimentation"?

As the NBC report stated, the duty to inform students of their right to animal CO has been partially ignored: 87 faculties out of 128 have informed their students, whereas 41 did not. Of the 41, 28 faculties justified the lack of dissemination of the law due to the absence of animal experimentation in their educational courses.

2.2. The Hans Ruesch Foundation (HRF) Investigation

After the NBC investigation, the HRF—an independent association that promotes the development of information on scientific activities involving animals—decided to promote and control the effective fulfillment of the faculties previously interviewed by the NBC.

First, the HRF asked the 41 faculties—that had previously declared to the NBC not to have informed their students—to comply with the information provisions set out by the Law 413/1993 via registered mail. Out of these 41 faculties, 14 responded that they subsequently would, whilst 27 faculties did not reply at all [6].

An additional audit of the faculties' websites was carried out for all 87 "yes" responses to Q1 of the questionnaire sent out by the NBC. Furthermore, the HRF considered the presence of the text of Law 413/93 and the application form in the faculties' website as a sign of compliance.

The results showed that only 10 of the cited 87 faculties published the text of Law 413/1993 on their websites.

Therefore, the HRF sent the 77 faculties that had not posted the information on their websites a formal request to comply with Law 413/93. Of these 77 faculties, 14 fulfilled the formal request and 62 did not. No further information about the remaining faculty is provided in the report.

The final results of the HRF report stated that only 41 out of 128 faculties were compliant (32%).

2.3. The "Nothing to Object?" ARA Campaign

The aim of the ARA, with its campaign titled "Nothing to object?" was to continue the HRF investigation [7]. Like the HRF, the ARA posited that the requirement for compliance with Law 413/1993 was the presence of information concerning the law and the declaration form on animal CO on the faculties' websites.

Out of a sample size of 90 websites monitored, 81 did not provide any information. Therefore, the ARA sent these 81 faculties a formal request to comply with Law 413/1993. Of these 81 faculties, 39 subsequently complied with the regulations. In conclusion, out of the 90 faculties examined by the ARA, 48 (53%) were found to be compliant.

2.4. Our Own Investigation

In order to clarify the situation, we decided to carry out our own investigation into this matter. Along the lines of the HRF and ARA reports, we considered the presence of the text of Law 413/1993 and the declaration form on animal CO on the faculties' websites as a criterion of "maximum dissemination". With the expression "maximum dissemination", we intended that complete information on animal CO would be clearly available and accessible, as well as easily consultable. Therefore, in 2016 we analyzed the websites of the 128 faculties previously examined by the NCB (through a questionnaire) and by HRF (through a check of the websites) using a double standardized methodology. First, accessibility to information was evaluated by consulting relevant sections, such as "Research", "Courses", "Services", "Student Section", and "Animal Legislation". Next, expressions, such as "animal experimentation", "conscientious objection", "alternative methods" and "Law 413/1993" were used to fill in the search box of the websites. This consultation was not simple as the faculties were absorbed into research departments as a consequence of the reforms of the Italian university system governed by Law 240/2010, "Norme in materia di organizzazione delle università, di personale accademico e reclutamento, nonché delega al Governo per incentivare la qualità e l'efficienza del sistema universitario" ("rules on organization of Universities, academic staff and enrolment, as well as the government mandate to promote the quality and efficacy of the academic system"). For this reason, the majority of the faculties' websites were replaced. In these cases, the department websites and "Course" sections were checked.

To sum up, 37 (28.9%) out of 128 faculties were found to be compliant. In 18 faculties (14.1%), the information was not sufficiently accessible to students, especially if they were not aware of its existence. More than half of the faculties (69) did not provide any information. In four cases, the websites were not functioning properly. The results of our investigation are summarized in Table 1.

Table 1. Results of our investigation about the information on the Law 413/1993 on Faculties' websites.

Law Fulfillment	Information on Law	No. of Websites	%
Adequate	Easy *website consultation* [1] and effective *search box* [2]	32	29%
	Easy *website consultation* only	5	
Inadequate	Poor *website consultation* and effective *search box*	3	14%
	Poor *website consultation* only	4	
	Effective *search box* only	11	
None	Absence of any information	69	54%
Not evaluable	Run time error of the website	4	3%
		128	100%

[1] Accessibility to the information by consulting the website; [2] Accessibility to the information by using the search box.

3. Discussion

3.1. The NBC Investigation

The review of the NBC report highlighted an overlooked inaccuracy. In the report, only 10 faculties appeared to have responded positively to question Q2 "Have there been any cases of students making a request of conscientious objection?"; however, our analysis showed that Milano-Science and Lecce-Science had provided the answers "very rarely" and "rarely" rather than "no", resulting in a total of 12 affirmative responses. Another problem derived from the NBC investigation regarded the use of the expression "animal experimentation". As we have specified before, the NBC, according to

Italian regulation, used this expression with a general meaning which included educational activities involving animals. This broader definition may have led some faculties to believe that Q1 referred solely to experimental practices involving animals, thus justifying the absence of information on their websites. The use of this generic and ambiguous term in the Italian system may have affected the awareness and response of those wishing to exercise their right to animal CO. Indeed, their choices may differ according to the different ways in which animals are used. It is worth noting that the first time the NBC questionnaire was submitted, teaching practices involving animals were allowed in universities. According to several universities and countries (including Germany, Czech Republic, Norway and Holland) [8], practices involving animals were banned by Law 26/2014 "in educational activities carried out in primary and secondary schools, as well as in university courses" (art. 5, point 2) [9]. The overall prohibition did not state which educational activities animal use was banned, rather, it included two exceptions: one for degree courses in veterinary medicine, and the other for postgraduate courses in medicine and in veterinary medicine.

3.2. The HRF Investigation

The results of the HRF investigation also revealed some inaccuracies. First, among the 62 faculties that had responded inappropriately "yes" to Q1 (as no information was present on their websites), two faculties (the Faculty of Pharmacy in Camerino and Faculty of Veterinary Science in Cagliari) were mistakenly counted as the Faculty of Pharmacy in Camerino had provided a response other than "yes" to Q1 and the Faculty of Veterinary Science in Cagliari was not included in the tables provided in the original HRF report. Furthermore, the wording "Pisa-Science" was probably used to indicate both the Faculty of Science in Pisa and the Faculty of Science of the "Scuola Normale Superiore" in Pisa. Finally, the HRF failed to provide any indication to responses to Q1 from three faculties: The Faculty of Medicine in Milan; the Faculty of Science in Varese; and the Faculty of Medicine in Catania.

3.3. Our Own Investigation and Overall Analysis

With regard to our investigation, a limiting factor was the criterion used to ensure maximum dissemination adopted by the HRF and ARA reports: the presence of the text of Law 413/1993 and the declaration form on animal CO on the faculties' websites. The faculties' websites could not be considered as the sole information source used by those faculties to inform students of their right to exercise animal CO. Indeed, faculties may use different delivery modes such as internal journals, information provided to students during enrolment, lectures, seminars, meetings and workshops. However, currently, faculty websites can be reasonably considered as the principal vehicle that university students consult. Students, in fact, regularly visit their faculty's website to access information regarding their timetables, exam enrolments, teaching staff contact details, and other information necessary for their studies and their active participation in faculty life in general.

From a general comparative analysis of all the above cited reports, the results of the NBC, HRF and ARA show that in both 2009 and 2012, the level of compliance with Law 413/1993 remained at less than 50% of the faculties examined and non-compliance continued despite explicit requests. Our most recent report (2016) revealed serious inadequacies as information on Law 413/1993, where present, was often difficult to retrieve for those students not purposefully searching for it. Furthermore, information on animal CO was often positioned in sections that are not always visited by students. This situation of inadequacy may also be a consequence of the reforms introduced by Law 240/2010, which saw the migration of faculty websites to those of the new departments, resulting in a loss of information. In addition, Law 26/2014, which established a non-specific ban on animal experimentation for teaching purposes, may actually have contributed to reduce the awareness level of compliance with Law 413/1993. From this point of view, such an explanation provided by many faculties for their non-compliance with the duty of information would appear to justify the current situation. In addition, another reason for the continuing non-compliance by some faculties could derive from the misinterpretation of the poor wording of Law 413/1993.

3.4. Educational Animal Use and the Right to Animal Conscientious Objection

The authorized use of animals in educational activities brings up very controversial issues, especially considering it often involves the invasive use of animals. This is particularly questionable within the veterinary educational programs where in these cases, the ethical justification of the authorization is to promote medical knowledge useful to the betterment of all animals in society. However, this argument, which is grounded on the concept of the "right sacrifice of few for all", raises several discussions. In general, the practical reason of using animals in education is to ensure that students are gain adequate skills that could not be achieved by alternative means, nevertheless, some studies also criticize this approach [10]. Furthermore, stressing the choice to invest in alternative methods constitutes a real path for the reduction of animal use. At an educational level, the reduction or the replacement of animal use can be carried out by using videos, computer simulations, inanimate models such as mechanical and plasticized specimens, and "ethically-sourced cadavers" from animals euthanized for medical reasons [11].

It is fundamental to remember that the right to animal CO should be granted to all students in the above-mentioned cases where animals are involved in teaching activities. Furthermore, it is worth noting that in addition to the cases where a ban is provided, students may be guided by teachers to use animals in the elaboration of their theses. As already clarified, an effective way to protect students' right to opt for animal CO is to provide them with the specific information set out by the Italian legislation.

Finally, we believe that students have the right to choose animal CO regardless of whether they actually take part in activities involving animals. In fact, students may opt for animal CO simply to declare their individual ethical position regarding the possible use of animals in a particular setting (in this case, universities). Furthermore, as well as providing information regarding the possibility of exercising animal CO, universities could also inform students that, according to Law 14/2014, not all academic practices that involve animals and cause moral conflicts are subject to the right of conscientious objection. In particular, this right is not foreseen in animal slaughter methods and practices (not included in the animal experimentation practices set forth by Italian regulation) studied in veterinary science degrees [12]. Indeed, the role of a veterinary doctor is regarded as fundamental in guaranteeing food safety and animal welfare at the time of slaughter [13].

4. Conclusions

In spite of these limits, we believe that all investigations have made a valuable contribution to an issue that has been neglected for far too long. In fact, whilst opportunities to express conscientious objection to human issues such as voluntary termination of pregnancy and to medically-assisted procreation have benefited from extensive information campaigns, the same cannot be said of animal CO.

Such scarce attention reveals a lack of sensibility to animal ethics issues that contrasts with the principles of animal ethics in the so-called 3Rs (Reduction, Refinement, Replacement), which underpin European law dedicated to protecting animals used in scientific activities [14,15]. Respect of these principles plays an important role in raising personal awareness amongst students on ethical issues [11–17]. As seen in the literature [18], students who are encouraged to contemplate ethical issues can actively contribute to the development of rules that respect different ethical points of view.

Appropriate strategies should be developed so that the issue of animal ethics and the right to exercise animal CO receives adequate attention.

Careful monitoring of compliance by faculties regarding their duty of information could be carried out by bioethical committees such as the cited NBC; or by animal welfare bodies established by Law 26/2014 under Directive 2010/1963/EU with the specific purpose to safeguard animal welfare, as well as by the Italian Ministry of Education, University and Research. Additionally, the Ministry should officially reprimand non-compliant faculties that do not uphold their obligations of information and reward compliant faculties with special funds. These benefits could be released with the purpose to balance any additional costs that universities would incur in order to ensure adequate alternative scientific activities and programs.

With regard to the scientific literature, we hope for greater attention on animal issues and the development of further investigations such as a direct survey on students' knowledge in this field to better understand the reasons for Italian non-compliance with national law provisions.

Author Contributions: Rosagemma Ciliberti, Anna Maria Bassi and Alma Massaro conceived and designed the study; Ilaria Baldelli and Susanna Penco performed the review of the existing data and analyzed the new data; Rosagemma Ciliberti, Alma Massaro, Ilaria Baldelli and Sara Patuzzo wrote the paper. Rosagemma Ciliberti and Sara Patuzzo equally coordinated the study.

Conflicts of Interest: The authors declare no conflict of interest.

References

1.   Italian Government. Legislative Decree 413/1993. Available online: http://www.dimes.unipg.it/LEGGE% 20413.pdf (accessed on 4 October 2016).
2.   Patuzzo, S.; Pulice, E. Towards a European Code of medical ethics. Ethical and legal issues. *J. Med. Ethics* **2016**, *43*, 41–46. [CrossRef] [PubMed]
3.   Italian Government. Law 194/1978. Available online: http://www.salute.gov.it/imgs/c_17_normativa_ 845_allegato.pdf (accessed on 4 October 2016).
4.   Italian Government. Law 40/2004. Available online: http://www.iss.it/rpma/index.php?id=75&tipo=12& lang=1 (accessed on 4 October 2016).
5.   Metodologie Alternative, Comitati Etici e Obiezione di Coscienza Alla Sperimentazione Animale. Available online: http://presidenza.governo.it/bioetica/pareri_abstract/met_alltenative_sper_animale_18122009.pdf (accessed on 4 October 2016).
6.   Rapporto Sull'ostruzionismo Dell'università Italiana alla Legge Sull'obiezione di Coscienza alla Vivisezione. Available online: http://www.hansruesch.net/articoli/ObiezioneCoscienza.pdf (accessed on 4 October 2016).
7.   Parte in Causa. Available online: https://associazioneparteincausa.wordpress.com/2015/01/26/primo-rapporto-sulla-campagna-nulla-da-obiettare-per-il-rispetto-della-legge-sullobiezione-di-coscienza-alla-sperimentazione-animale/ (accessed on 4 October 2016).
8.   Bekoff, M.; Meaney, C.A. *Encyclopedia of Animal Rights and Animal Welfare*; Greenwood Press: New York, NY, USA, 2013.
9.   Martini, M.; Penco, S.; Baldelli, I.; Biolatti, B.; Ciliberti, R. An ethics for the living world: Operation methods of Animal Ethics Committees in Italy. *Ann. Ist. Super. Sanità* **2015**, *51*, 244–247. [PubMed]
10. Knight, A. The effectiveness of humane teaching methods in veterinary education. *Altex* **2007**, *24*, 91–109. [PubMed]
11. Knight, A. Conscientious objection to harmful animal use within veterinary and other biomedical education. *Animals* **2014**, *4*, 16–34. [CrossRef] [PubMed]
12. Gandini, G.; Acocella, F.; Bontempo, V.; Fonda, D.; Fossati, P.; Modina, S.; Pirrone, F.; Zetti, M.; Costa, P.; Tallacchini, M. Lo Studente e Gli Animali: Riflessioni Bioetiche e Indicazioni d'Uso. 2014. Available online: http://www.veterinaria.unimi.it/files/_ITA_/Organizzazione/ceta_studente_e_animali_riflessioni_ bioetiche.pdf (accessed on 4 October 2016).
13. Ciliberti, R.; Molinelli, A. Towards an GMO discipline: Ethical remarks. *Vet. Res. Commun.* **2005**, *29*, 27–30. [CrossRef] [PubMed]
14. Balcombe, J. A global overview of law and policy concerning animal use in education. In *Progress in the Reduction, Refinement and Replacement of Animal Experimentation*; Balls, M., van Zeller, A.M., Halder, M.E., Eds.; Elsevier Science: Amsterdam, The Netherlands, 2000; pp. 1343–1350.
15. Ciliberti, R.; Martini, M.; Bonsignore, A.; Penco, S. Break with tradition: Donating cadavers for scientific purposes and reducing the use of sentient beings. *Ann. Ist. Super. Sanità* **2016**, *52*, 261–268. [PubMed]
16. Whittaker, A.; Anderson, G. A policy at the University of Adelaide for student objections to the use of animals in teaching. *J. Vet. Med. Educ.* **2013**, *40*, 52–57. [CrossRef] [PubMed]

17. Kramer, M.G. Humane education, dissection, and the law. *Anim. Law* **2009**, *13*, 281–298.

18. Sachana, M.; Theodoris, A.; Cortinovis, C.; Pizzo, F.; Kehagias, E.; Albonico, M.; Caloni, F. Student perspectives on the use of alternative methods for teaching in veterinary faculties. *Altern. Lab. Anim.* **2014**, *42*, 223–233. [PubMed]

4

Does a 4–6 Week Shoeing Interval Promote Optimal Foot Balance in the Working Equine?

Kirsty Leśniak [1,*], Jane Williams [1], Kerry Kuznik [1] and Peter Douglas [2]

[1] Centre for Performance in Equestrian Sport, Hartpury College, Gloucester GL19 3BE, UK; jane.williams@hartpury.ac.uk (J.W.); kerrykuznik@hotmail.co.uk (K.K.)
[2] PE Douglas DWP, Ivybridge, Devon PL21 0NP, UK; peter.douglas@hotmail.com
* Correspondence: Kirsty.lesniak@hartpury.ac.uk

Academic Editor: Clive J. C. Phillips

Simple Summary: Hoof shape is linked to an increased risk of lameness in the horse and has been shown to adapt to different loading patterns associated with the workload and shoeing interval length. This study investigated how different measurements of the hoof wall and the hoof pastern axis angle changed with work in riding school horses, across a four to six week shoeing/trimming interval. The dorsal hoof wall, and weight bearing and coronary band lengths reduced in size post-shoeing/trimming. This, combined with the increase to the inner and outside hoof wall heights on the digital images despite trimming, suggests that shoeing/trimming increased the vertical orientation of the hoof during the shoeing interval investigated. At the same time, increases in the dorsal hoof wall angle, heel angle, and heel height occurred, promoting a more correct dorsopalmar balance. The changes observed are consistent with the workload of the horses studied. The results suggest that a regular farriery interval of no more than six weeks could prevent excess loading of the structures within the hoof, reducing long term injury risks through cumulative, excessive loading in riding school horses.

Abstract: Variation in equine hoof conformation between farriery interventions lacks research, despite associations with distal limb injuries. This study aimed to determine linear and angular hoof variations pre- and post-farriery within a four to six week shoeing/trimming interval. Seventeen hoof and distal limb measurements were drawn from lateral and anterior digital photographs from 26 horses pre- and post-farriery. Most lateral view variables changed significantly. Reductions of the dorsal wall, and weight bearing and coronary band lengths resulted in an increased vertical orientation of the hoof. The increased dorsal hoof wall angle, heel angle, and heel height illustrated this further, improving dorsopalmar alignment. Mediolateral measurements of coronary band and weight bearing lengths reduced, whilst medial and lateral wall lengths from the 2D images increased, indicating an increased vertical hoof alignment. Additionally, dorsopalmar balance improved. However, the results demonstrated that a four to six week interval is sufficient for a palmer shift in the centre of pressure, increasing the loading on acutely inclined heels, altering DIP angulation, and increasing the load on susceptible structures (e.g., DDFT). Mediolateral variable asymmetries suit the lateral hoof landing and unrollment pattern of the foot during landing. The results support regular (four to six week) farriery intervals for the optimal prevention of excess loading of palmar limb structures, reducing long-term injury risks through cumulative, excessive loading.

Keywords: equine; hoof; shoeing; hoof angle; conformation; morphometric measurements

1. Introduction

Equine distal limb lameness is commonly associated with poor foot conformation and hoof imbalance [1–4], with hoof-related lameness being a key cause of poor performance and early retirement in the sport [5,6] and as a pleasure horse [6–8].

Research has identified that the biomechanical function of the distal limb can alter as a result of changes in the hoof shape. Consequently, this influences the forces acting on the hoof's structural components [9,10], as well as the distal interphalangeal joint (DIPJ) and proximal interphalangeal joint (PIPJ) moments [6], the leverage on the toe at breakover, and the forces acting on the navicular bone [2]. An example of such biomechanical influences are those which facilitate the breakover of the stride, achieved through the shortening of the toe. The alternation in hoof orientation achieved through the shortening of the toe is suggested to result in improved angulation between the proximal and middle phalanx, thus elevating the position of the navicular bone and consequentially reducing the loading of the deep digital flexor tendon (DDFT) [11,12]. The principles behind this biomechanical influence have been utilised by veterinarians and farriers in the application of heel wedges or rocker shoes for the treatment of conditions such as DDFT tendinopathies and navicular syndrome [13]. Hoof conformation refers more to the geometric morphology of the static foot [14,15]. The term balance is recognised as not only a consideration of the geometric shape of the hoof, but also the way in which this interacts with the rest of the limb and the ground with which it is in contact [15]; this includes dorsopalmar balance, which refers to hoof pastern axis alignment. Consequently, the impact of trimming and shoeing the feet can affect the health, performance, and longevity of the equine athlete [8]. Therefore, the principal role of the farrier is to balance the feet of the horse to facilitate optimal movement, prevent injury, and to improve performance [8,16]. Farriery should always include trimming the feet and can include applying horse shoes. The majority of modern horses are shod to cope with the demands of their workload, to enhance performance, and to extend career longevity [8]. Despite advances in research, farriery largely remains a profession based on traditional empirical craftsmanship, rather than scientific evidence [4,17]. Regular farrier treatments are recommended to maintain or improve the athletic performance capacity of the horse [6,18]. However an 'optimal' shoeing/trimming interval has not been defined. Moleman et al. [6] suggested that the shoeing/trimming interval length should be determined for individual horses by their farrier, to meet their specific needs. The interval length may also be influenced by the knowledge, understanding, and potentially financial constraints of horse owners and keepers.

Anecdotally, within the equine industry, shoeing/trimming interval lengths are commonly between four to eight weeks. However, intervals can vary beyond eight weeks, especially within the leisure horse population. Within research, the length of recommended shoeing/trimming intervals vary between four to six weeks, or six to eight weeks [4,6,7,18,19]. The majority of studies to date have evaluated changes in the hoof associated with eight week intervals [4,8]. An eight week interval has been connected with increases in the dorsal hoof wall length (DHWL) and a reduction in the dorsal hoof wall angle (DWHA), which places the DIPJ under increased strain [6]. If the aim of farriery is to restore the balance of the hoof, correct conformational defects, and optimise distal limb biomechanics, then the ideal shoeing/trimming interval should facilitate consistency in the loading of the foot, and by default, the associated structures of the distal limb. Therefore, shorter intervals between four to six weeks may benefit the horse if they can be shown to limit changes within the foot, and by association, the distal limb. Currently, there is a paucity of evidence-based knowledge concerning the linear and angular changes that occur within the hoof associated with shoeing/trimming intervals, in order to confirm the potential benefits of this practice (four to six week interval) [6,20]. Therefore, the aim of this study was to determine how linear and angular hoof morphometric measurements varied pre- and post-farriery with a four to six week shoeing/trimming interval, in horses which were free from lameness and regularly shod/trimmed. We hypothesised that the foot of the horse would be more symmetric and balanced, and that the hoof pastern axis (HPA) would present in correct alignment post-farrier treatment compared to pre-farrier treatment, but that the differences observed would not be significant pre- and post-farriery.

2. Method

Twenty-six horses of mixed breed, gender, age (12 ± 9.9 years), and height (157 cm ± 2.3 cm), which did not display any stereotypic behaviours and were resident at Hartpury College, Gloucestershire, UK, were selected for inclusion in the study. All subjects were on loan for use within the College's riding school and were subjected to the same exercise and management regime: two 45-minute flat, jump, or lunge lessons per day (ProWax, Andrew Bowen, Singleton, Lancashire, UK), with one day off per week, and stabled (rubber matting and shavings) with restricted grass turnout. The horses included in the study were deemed in good health and functionally fit for work by experienced equestrian professionals who had daily access to an equine veterinary surgeon, to examine horses presenting with lameness. The horses declared unfit for work by the veterinary surgeon were removed from the study. Each individual received regular farrier treatment (hot shod; full set or front shoes) by one main farriery team (WCF (Worshipful Company of Farriers) qualified), at shoeing intervals between four and six weeks. Farriery was performed by one of four farriers under the direction and supervision of a lead farrier, to promote a consistent approach. All horses had been previously exposed to farrier treatment and were not undergoing any corrective farriery. Ethical approval for the study was granted by the University of the West of England (Hartpury) Ethics Committee (Project Identification Code: ETHICS2016-03).

Data were collected between September and December, when horses presented for their next farrier treatment. Digital images were taken of each horse's left forelimb and hoof, to enable a comparison of morphometric measurements of key anatomical features and angles (Table 1) pre- and post-farriery treatment, with old and new or refitted shoes, respectively [6,21,22].

Table 1. Location of anatomical markers.

1.	Midpoint of dorsal hoof wall, proximal margin	
2.	Midpoint of dorsal hoof wall, distal margin	
3.	Dorsal aspect of the radiocarpal joint	
4.	Dorsal aspect of the carpometacarpal joint	
5.	Dorsal aspect of the metacarpal phalangeal joint	
6.	Lateral aspect of the radiocarpal joint	
7.	Lateral aspect of the carpometacarpal joint	
8.	Lateral aspect of the metacarpal phalangeal joint	

2.1. Protocol

Prior to data collection, horses had their rugs removed and limbs cleaned. Key anatomical landmarks were used to orientate the placement of circular markers on the left forelimb and hoof, to ensure that the same anatomical regions were measured within all of the horses (Table 1) and to facilitate subsequent measurements from the digital images. Horses were stood square, with equal weight bearing on all four limbs, on a concrete surface and within a calibrated and marked out grid, to enable repetition and accuracy of positioning. Scale markers were used to mark out the area, to allow for image calibration and accurate digital measurement [2]. Horses also stood in front of a black board in the marked out area, to provide a contrast with the foot and forelimb [21]. Lateral and anterior digital photographic images of the left forelimb were obtained by using three digital cameras (Panasonic DMC-FZ45; 14.1 MP, Panasonic, Bracknell, UK and Ireland), as shown in Figure 1. For the acquisition of the lateral view of the limb, camera A was attached to a tripod (Velbon DV-7000, Velbon, Maidenhead, UK) (height 170 cm, base wide 82 cm), which was positioned centrally to the marked out area and four metres (m) back from the wall. Lateral images of the hoof were obtained by camera (B) at a 0.3 zoom, positioned just above ground level and one metre back from the horizontal scale marker, midway in line with the marked out grid on the floor laterally in line with the hoof. Camera (C) was positioned one metre back from the vertical scale marker at a 0.3 zoom and held just above ground level, in order to take images of the dorsal hoof aspect from an anterior view of the horse [6]. Images from camera A confirmed that horses were standing square; the images from cameras B and C were used to facilitate measurements.

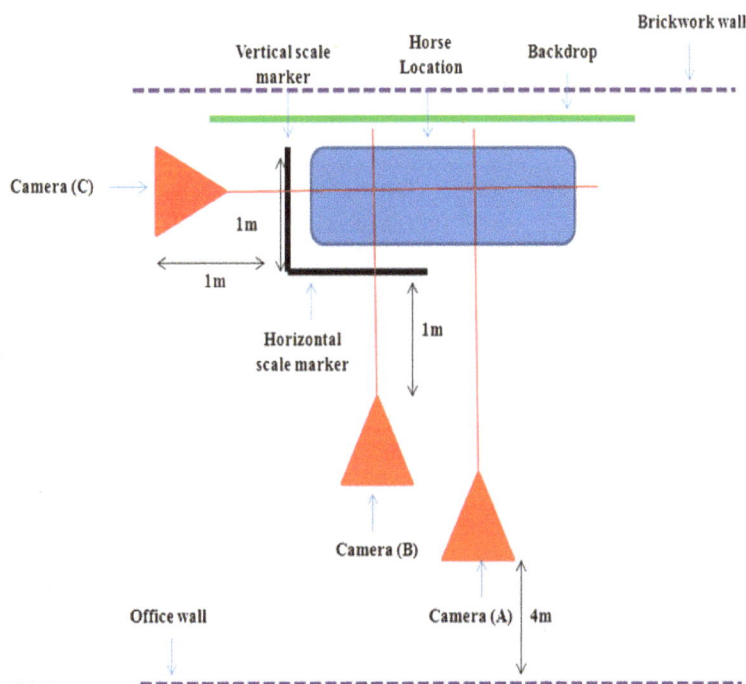

Figure 1. Layout of cameras, scale markers, backdrop, and positioning of the horse for digital image collection.

2.2. Data Processing and Analysis

The photographic images were imported into Dartfish™ software version 7 (Dartfish, Fribourg, Switzerland), to facilitate the angular and linear measurements outlined in Tables 2–4. Hoof angle displacement, the fetlock joint angle, and vertical displacement were determined by plumb line measurements. All measurements were repeated three times for each photographic image and their mean was calculated. Mean data were exported to Microsoft Excel, Version 15 (Microsoft, Washington, DC, USA), for categorical organisation, and to allow the mean and standard deviation to be determined for each variable, across the cohort. Van Heel et al. [4] utilised force plate determination of Centre of Pressure (CoP) to propose an equation which successfully predicts the shift of CoP relative to the toe, from the hoof measurements.

Van Heel et al.'s [4] predictive equation for CoP is as follows:

$$\Delta d = a_{old}.\cos\alpha_{old} - a_{new}.\cos\alpha_{new}$$

where, in the current study, a_{new} is the length of the dorsal hoof wall post-farriery, α_{new} is the hoof angle post-farriery, a_{old} is the length of the dorsal hoof wall pre-farriery (after four to six weeks), and α_{old} is the hoof angle pre-farriery. d is the predicted location of CoP at midstance, relative to the point of rotation at the toe.

Using the Van Heel et al. [4] equation, the shift in distance that occurred for the CoP after farrier treatment was calculated pre- and post-farriery treatment for each individual horse and to provide mean measurements for pre- and post-farriery CoP for the cohort. A series of paired t-tests analysed whether differences existed between the variables examined from the pre- to the post-farrier treatment periods using Statistics Package for the Social Sciences (SPSS) Version 20 (IBM Corp., Armonk, NY, USA). Paired t-tests were also used to identify whether differences were present between the medial and lateral hoof angles and lengths in the foot, both prior to shoeing, and after the horses had been shod. A series of Pearson's product correlations examined whether any linear relationships occurred between the variables measured both pre- and post-farriery treatment. Significance was set at $p \leq 0.05$.

Table 2. Angular and linear morphometric variables measured from the 2D lateral view images of the hoof [22,23].

Lateral Hoof Measurements		
Variable	**Abbreviation**	**Description**
Dorsal hoof wall length	DHWL	Length of dorsal hoof wall from hair line at the coronary band to ground level
Weight bearing length lateral	WBL-L	Length from the dorsal to the palmar point of the hoof wall in contact with the ground surface
Coronary band length	CBL	Length from the dorsal to the palmar point of the coronary band
Dorsal hoof wall angle	DHWA	Angle between the dorsal hoof wall and the ground plane
Heel angle	HLA	Angle between the palmer aspect of the hoof wall and the ground surface
Dorsal coronary band height	DCBH	Vertical height between the dorsal region of the coronary band and the solar plane
Palmer coronary band height	PCBH	Vertical height between the palmer region of the coronary band and the solar plane

Table 3. Angular and linear morphometric variables measured from the 2D dorsal view images of the hoof.

Dorsal Hoof Measurements		
Variable	**Abbreviation**	**Description**
Weight bearing length dorsal	WBL-D	Coronary band width between the lateral and medial hoof walls at the distal region of the hoof
Coronary band width	CBW	Support length between the lateral and medial hoof walls at the proximal region of the hoof
Medial dorsal hoof wall length	MDHWL	Length of the medial hoof wall from hairline to ground
Midline dorsal hoof wall length	CDHWL	Length of the hoof wall at the midpoint of the hoof from hairline to ground
Lateral dorsal hoof wall length	LDHWL	Length of the lateral hoof wall from hairline to ground
Medial hoof angle	MHA	Angle between the medial hoof wall and solar plane
Lateral hoof angle	LHA	Angle between the lateral hoof wall and solar plane

Table 4. Angular and linear morphometric variables measured from the 2D lateral view of the limb.

Lateral Limb Measurements			
	Variable	**Abbreviation**	**Description**
1.	Vertical displacement (Yellow)	VD	
2.	Fetlock joint angle (Pink)	FJA	
3.	Hoof angle displacement (Red)	HAD	

3. Results

3.1. Hoof Measurements

Significant differences were reported after shoeing for the majority of the lateral view, anterior view, and HPA measurements (Table 5).

Table 5. Differences between hoof measurements pre- and post-farriery. Bold probability values denote statistical significance. (Length, width and height in cm; angles in degrees).

	Variable	Mean ± Standard Deviation		p Value	Increase/Decrease
		Pre-Farriery	**Post-Farriery**		
	DHWA	52.1° ± 3.47°	54.36° ± 3.99°	**$p = 0.0001$**	Increased
	HLA	45.49° ± 7.59°	49.96° ± 5.55°	**$p = 0.0001$**	Increased
	DHWL	7.81 ± 1.35 cm	7.56 ± 0.91 cm	$p > 0.05$	Decreased
Lateral View	WBL-L	11.58 ± 1.16 cm	11.04 ± 1.4 cm	**$p = 0.0001$**	Decreased
	CBL	10.88 ± 0.96 cm	10.15 ± 1.09 cm	**$p = 0.0001$**	Decreased
	DCBH	7.22 ± 1.21 cm	7.43 ± 0.78 cm	$p > 0.05$	Increased
	PCBH	2.70 ± 0.63 cm	3.24 ± 0.56 cm	**$p = 0.0001$**	Increased
	CBW	5.39 ± 1.00 cm	5.09 ± 1.09 cm	**$p = 0.05$**	Decreased
	WBL-D	6.84 ± 1.44 cm	6.14 ± 1.29 cm	**$p = 0.001$**	Decreased
	CDHWL	3.87 ± 0.61 cm	4.14 ± 0.94 cm	$p > 0.05$	Increased
Anterior View	MDHWL	3.57 ± 0.69 cm	3.84 ± 0.74 cm	**$p = 0.03$**	Increased
	LDHWL	3.72 ± 0.68 cm	4.09 ± 0.80 cm	**$p = 0.009$**	Increased
	MHA	78.96° ± 5.81°	80.17° ± 5.41°	$p > 0.05$	Increased
	LHA	73.17° ± 4.20°	72.79° ± 4.07°	$p > 0.05$	Decreased
	HAD	189.49° ± 4.89°	183.28° ± 2.89°	**$p = 0.0001$**	Decreased
Lateral limb	FJA	212.71° ± 8.03°	212.81° ± 8.48°	$p > 0.05$	Increased
	VD	184.04° ± 2.72°	183.39° ± 2.11°	$p > 0.05$	Decreased

3.2. Medio-Lateral Variation

Significant medio-lateral variation was reported between the linear and angular measurements in the hoof (Figure 2). The mean LDHWL (3.72 ± 0.68 cm) was found to be 4% longer ($p = 0.01$) than the mean MDHWL (3.57 ± 0.69 cm), prior to farriery. Medio-lateral variation in DHWL demonstrated an increased significant difference after shoeing ($p = 0.0001$), with the mean LDHWL (4.09 cm ± 0.80 cm) being 7% longer than the mean MDHWL (3.84 ± 0.74 cm). Similar results occurred for the hoof angle; significant differences were found between the mean MHA and mean LHA prior to farriery

(p = 0.0001), with the MHA (78.96° ± 5.81°) being 7% greater than the LHA (73.17° ± 4.20°). Again, a more significant difference was recorded after shoeing (p = 0.0001), with the direction of difference remaining consistent, with MHA (80.80° ± 5.41°) being 10% greater than LHA (72.79° ± 4.07°).

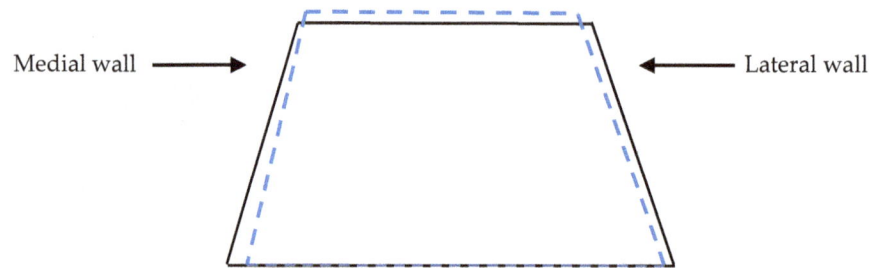

Figure 2. Pre-trimming (solid black line) and post trimming (blue dotted line); note the more upright angle of the medial wall, acutely angled lateral wall, and increased wall lengths.

3.3. Centre of Pressure

The calculated shift in the CoP distance found that the predicted CoP was located, on average, 0.5 cm back from the point of rotation of the toe across the cohort after shoeing.

3.4. Measurement Correlations

Significant correlations were found between twenty-eight pairs of variables measured prior to farriery treatment, and these ranged in strength and direction (Table 6). After shoeing, the number of correlations within the morphometric measurements of the hoof reduced, with only twenty-three pairs shown to be significantly associated (Table 6).

Table 6. Significantly correlated variables pre- and post-farriery. Bold regression co-efficient values denote strong (>0.75) relationships.

Variables		Pre-Farriery		Post-Farriery	
		r co-eff	*p* Value	*r co-eff*	*p* Value
DHWA	WBL-L	−0.39	0.050	−0.45	0.022
LHA	PCBH	0.42	0.031	-	-
DHWL	CBL	0.57	0.002	-	-
DHWL	DCBH	**0.93**	0.0001	0.40	0.043
DHWL	PCBH	**0.75**	0.0001	0.65	0.0001
DHWL	LDHWL	-	-	0.50	0.009
WBL-L	CBL	0.68	0.0001	**0.86**	0.000
WBL-L	PCBH	0.46	0.019	-	-
WBL-L	CBW	0.66	0.0001	0.46	0.018
WBL-L	WBL-D	0.67	0.0001	-	-
WBL-L	LDHWL	-	-	0.38	0.053
CBL	DCBH	0.59	0.001	-	-
CBL	PCBH	0.61	0.001	-	-
CBL	CBW	0.59	0.002	0.52	0.007
CBL	WBL-D	0.65	0.0001	-	-
CBL	CDHWL	-	-	0.41	0.040
CBL	MDHWL	-	-	0.41	0.036
CBL	LDHWL	-	-	0.50	0.010
DCBH	PCBH	**0.84**	0.0001	-	-
PCBH	HAD	−0.41	0.039	-	-
CBW	WBL-D	**0.95**	0.0001	**0.87**	0.0001
CBW	CDHWL	0.54	0.005	**0.78**	0.0001

Table 6. *Cont.*

Variables		Pre-Farriery		Post-Farriery	
		r co-eff	*p* Value	*r co-eff*	*p* Value
CBW	MDHWL	0.67	0.0001	**0.76**	0.0001
CBW	LDHWL	0.58	0.002	**0.82**	0.0001
WBL-D	CDHWL	0.53	0.005	**0.79**	0.0001
WBL-D	MDHWL	0.64	0.0001	**0.76**	0.0001
WBL-D	LDHWL	0.53	0.006	**0.79**	0.0001
CDHWL	MDHWL	**0.91**	0.0001	**0.93**	0.0001
CDHWL	LDHWL	**0.86**	0.0001	**0.92**	0.0001
CDHWL	LHA	0.44	0.026	-	-
MDHWL	LDHWL	**0.91**	0.0001	**0.92**	0.0001
MDHWL	MHA	−0.41	0.040	-	-
FJA	VD	−0.70	0.0001	-	-
MHA	FJA	-	-	−0.44	0.025
VD	MHA	-	-	0.51	0.008
HLA	VD	-	-	0.41	0.035

4. Discussion

Correct (balanced) hoof conformation is essential to prevent lameness [24]. For example, Wright [25] recorded that 45.2% of horses demonstrating lameness were mediolaterally imbalanced. Balance is related to the shape and size of the hoof and is influenced by the relationship between the skeletal structures of the limb and the hoof [1,14]. Therefore, to achieve appropriate hoof balance, an understanding of the interaction between hoof conformation, movement, and the athletic activity of the horse is required [19].

DHWL was reduced by less than expected in the horses studied. Kummer et al. [8] reported that the DHWL shortened, on average, by 1 cm ($n = 40$) during an eight to ten week shoeing interval. Extrapolation from these results would suggest that the four to six week interval applied here would have been expected to reduce DHWL by 0.5 to 0.75 mm, which is much greater than was found (0.25 ± 0.97 cm). The discrepancies between these results are likely reflective of the differing study durations (Kummer et al. [8] collected repeated data over 12 months), the addition of a biotin supplement to Kummer et al.'s [8] study population, and the differing load and variation of work requirement (dressage and show jumpers in to Kummer et al.'s [8] study, compared to riding school horses here).

DHWA is defined as the angle formed at the junction of the DHW and the weight bearing surface of the foot [8,26] and a correct angle is essential to achieve an optimal hoof pastern axis. Despite still being documented in practitioner aimed literature until recently, the historic ideal DHWA of 45° for the front feet has been contradicted in science and practice [26,27]. Variability in DHWA is reported [28]; however, it is widely recognised that the ideal angle for the front feet should range between 50° to 55°. This is within the same range as that suggested for the hind feet [27,29], although wide variation (45° to 60°) in forelimb DHWA exists within the literature [2,8,10,22,30]. The DHWA mean values pre- and post-farriery fall within 'normal' DHWA ranges: 48.6° to 58.4°. The range reported here is comparable with previous research: Thomason et al. [31] ($n = 10$) reported a DHWA ranging from 48° to 57° and a mean angle of 51.8°; and Dyson et al. [22] ($n = 19$) reported a mean DHWA of 52.4°, ranging 43.4°–64.7°.

The decrease in DHWA associated with a four to six week interval (2.26° decrease, approximately 0.94° per two weeks) is analogous to the 3.3° decrease reported by Moleman et al. [6] across an eight week shoeing interval, but is greater than the 2.5° decrease (approximately 0.57° per two weeks) reported across an 8–10 week shoeing interval by Kummer et al. [8]. Force distribution in the hoof is related to DHWA, with more acute angles increasing loading in the heels. For example, a 39° DHWA angle results in 75% of loading weight within the heels, compared to 57% loading when the angle is increased to the 'normal' 55° [32]. Therefore, longer shoeing/trimmer intervals which result in decreased DHWAs will increase palmar loading, resulting in the weakening and collapse of the heels, and will amplify loading of the suspensory apparatus, leading to an increased susceptibility to injury [33,34].

Changes reported in the lateral view suggest that angular modifications of the distal limb are occurring at the level of both the MCP and DIP joints. The reduced DHWL, increased DHW and heel angle, the decrease in the weight bearing length, and increase in the palmar coronary band height, suggest that although the toe shortened, the length of the heel was not altered during the shoeing/trimming procedure. Following trimming, the weight bearing length decreased in the anterior view, whilst the medial and lateral wall lengths, as measured from the digital images, increased. The changes which occurred in the MCP and DIP joint angulations across the lateral view could also explain the increase in medial and lateral wall lengths from the anterior view images. We believe that the decrease in the coronary band lengths observed from both the lateral and anterior view 2D images occurred as a result of the change in positioning of the hoof capsule post-shoeing/trimming. The dorsal wall shortens by a relatively greater amount than the heels, which results in the hoof assuming a more vertical orientation. This is supported by the differences found between the lateral and medial hoof wall length; 73% of participants had a longer lateral wall pre-shoeing, and this increased to 88% of the population post-shoeing. Furthermore, the mean difference between the two sides increased following routine shoeing, from 7% to 10%. Guidance in achieving mediolateral balance of the equine foot refers to the trimming of the medial and lateral walls, to ensure that the live sole of the foot is level with the ground [35] and the hoof is in balance with the limb column [27], as opposed to the postulation that balance is attained through the attainment of symmetrical wall lengths [29]. More recent studies have found that subtle asymmetries manifested as a more upright medial wall and a more angled lateral wall are common within the domestic horse population [8,36–39] and reflect the lateral landing and unrollment pattern of the foot observed in sound horses [17,40]. Our results support the practice of trimming according to the live sole, with a more inclined conformation, without altering the mediolateral balance of the foot, to promote soundness and not change the wall lengths. Use of the live sole as guidance ensures that following lateral landing and unrollment, loading of the foot produces equal pressure across the circumference of the foot to the ground, through the anatomical structures in the distal limb [10]. The differences reported in the medial and lateral wall lengths can also reflect the difference in the angles between the walls and the weight bearing surface of the foot (Figure 3).

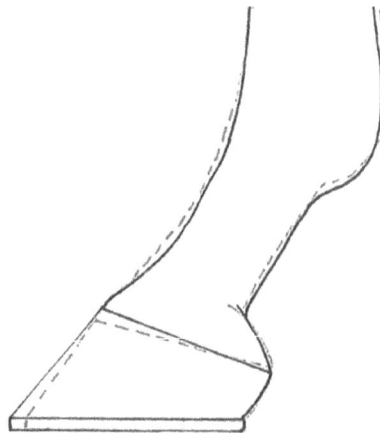

Figure 3. Pre-trimming (solid black line) and post trimming (blue dotted line); the solid line also represents the increased vertical orientation observed post-shoeing/trimming. Note the more upright angle of both the heel angle and DHW angle, and the shortening of the toe.

Pre-shoeing, only 31% of horses presented with a greater LHA, though this decreased to 12% post-shoeing. The more slanted lateral wall presented a more acute angle with the sole compared to the angle on the more upright medial wall, which was more obtuse, by between 1° and 7°. Approximately 25% of participants presented with a longer medial than lateral wall pre-shoeing, suggesting that the loading pattern that they exhibited differed from normal lateral landing and unrollment. These differences potentially infer a more medial landing posture, indicating that some degree of low level lameness was inherent in the study population; a potential inherent career risk of riding school horses [41]. Further to the influence of the loading pattern, mediolateral balance can also be influenced by the individual farrier, with significant differences previously observed between individuals [42]. The current study did not evaluate the influence of individual farriers and therefore this could account for some of the differences found.

Interestingly, although MHAs and LHAs changed post-shoeing, these changes were not significant. A similar number of horses presented with an increase and decrease in LHA; however, a greater proportion of the sample (58%) demonstrated an increase in MHA post-shoeing. The lack of significant results is attributed to the large individual variations seen between the horses examined.

The hoof pastern axis (HPA) is defined by plotting a line down from the middle of the metacarpophalangeal joint, through the centre of the proximal and distal interphalangeal joints, and through the axis of the phalanges [10,26]. A straight alignment is accepted as ideal and considered optimal for physiological function [11,42]. The shortening of DHWL through trimming of the toe within the current population, accompanied by an increase in both the heel angle and the coronet band at the heels, placed the hoof capsule in a more vertically orientated position. At the same time, there is a consequential increase in the heel angle and a corresponding reduction in HPA displacement, combined with a concurrent increase in the fetlock joint angle and decrease (not significant) in vertical limb displacement. These changes in joint angulations suggest that a four to six week shoeing interval contributes toward promoting consistency in HPA through addressing the fetlock joint angle [6] and vertical displacement. However, for these horses, the four to six week interval did not stop the foot from becoming broken backwards (where DHWA is more acute than the angle of the dorsal pastern.), and so the changes observed may just be mechanical and a static response to trimming of the toe. If the foot moves towards a more broken back angulation throughout the duration of even a four to six week shoeing interval, where a more traditional six to eight week interval is used, the broken back angulation might reach a level whereby loading of the navicular region and the suspensory apparatus, specifically the DDFT, may be detrimental and enhance the risk of injury.

The forelimb CoP is known to deviate in a palmar direction across an eight week shoeing interval, whilst breakover remains relatively consistent [4,17]. The centre of pressure (CoP) within the current study was predicted to be, on average, 0.5 cm in a palmar direction to the point of rotation of the toe across the cohort, which is less than half of that of the 1.3 cm observed over an eight-week interval by Van Heel et al. [4]. The shoe of a shod horse prevents the wear of the toe, but not of the heel, and therefore, as the toe lengthens, the angle of both the toe and the heel decrease, resulting in the palmar movement of the CoP, and an increased loading in the DIP joint and the DDFT.

Moleman et al. [6] identified similar growth patterns at the toe across an eight week shoeing interval, but found none at the heel and no significant change in PIP joint moment. Consequentially, the change of motion is thought to be located in the DIPJ, increasing loading on the DDFT and navicular bone, which act to stabilise the DIPJ in order to maintain a dynamic equilibrium during locomotion [6,11,43]. The shortening of the DHWL achieved during trimming reverses these mechanics through the correction of deviation of the CoP away from the central foot axis [44], to a more dorsal location, and thereby reduces the load on the suspensory apparatus. The reduced palmar shift in the CoP observed within the shorter four to six week interval examined here, suggests that this time frame would exert a protective effect on DIPJ and DDFT loading, compared to longer shoeing intervals.

Limitations

The current study applied a pragmatic and observational research approach to investigate the impact of shoeing practices on hoof morphology in riding school horses. Whilst the study has strong external validity, it should be noted that the real-world design possesses a number of limitations, and therefore, the results should be interpreted with caution. Many factors can influence hoof growth. These include, but are not limited to, horse breed, height, diet, disease, time of year, the environmental effects of pasture quality, and lameness. The horses integrated here were subject to consistent management practices and were considered fit for riding school work by experienced equestrian professionals and the supporting veterinary team. The presence of low grade lameness has been previously identified in riding school horses to affect loading patterns and, subsequently, hoof growth, which could explain some of the variation observed within our results [41]. Subjects did vary in breed and height, which could have influenced the results obtained. Similarly, although every effort was made to ensure that horses were standing square prior to digital photography through the use of handlers and the positioning grid [2] in order to prevent positional rotation of the distal limb and foot, there is a possibility that the measurements taken integrate some degree of rotation. Force plate analysis is recommended for future studies, to accurately assess that horses are standing square and that equal loading is exhibited in each of the four limbs. Measurements of both the right and left hooves are also advocated in future research, to facilitate comparative analysis. Previous research [42] has associated morphometric differences in hoof measurements post trimming with individual farrier techniques and personal interpretations of the HPA. A team of farriers was utilised here. Furthermore, all farriers worked under the direction of one lead farrier and trimmed and shod horses according to their instructions, promoting a more consistent approach, which should limit the impact of individual technique. However, to ensure that the changes observed here are not related to individual farriery techniques, we would advise future research to use a consistent farrier or to assess the impact of individual farriers within data analysis.

5. Conclusions

After shoeing, hoof-surface interface interactions result in dynamic responses in the hoof promoting adaptation over time within the hoof's structural components, affecting linear and angular measurements. In the shod horse, the presence of the shoe prevents toe wear. Therefore, the adaptation which occurs over time will be influenced by the shoe. Even with shoeing intervals of four to six weeks, changes are observed in key parameters associated with foot balance. Our results suggest that, for the majority of horses, the weight bearing length of the foot increases (as the toe grows), causing a decrease in the heel angle and an increase in hoof angle displacement as the hoof pastern axis becomes more broken backwards, negatively influencing dorsopalmar balance. Changes also occur in the dorsal wall associated with loading during locomotion; in the shod horse, foot placement demonstrates a lateral-medial unrollment pattern. Therefore, increased loading may occur in the lateral hoof wall, which would result in lateral hoof wall length increasing and the lateral angle decreasing over time. In contrast, and in agreement with previous research [6], a four to six week interval retains consistency within fetlock joint angles ($-0.10° \pm 10.5°$) and vertical displacement (0.65 ± 2.6) of the HPA, positively influencing dorsopalmar balance, which should aid in the prevention of tendinopathies. Therefore, overall, we have to reject our original hypothesis that no changes would occur across HPA and hoof morphometric measurements during a four to six week shoeing interval. Further work is required to confirm these findings across more horses and with a comparison between different shoeing intervals, accompanied by an additional lameness and distal limb conformation evaluation. A comparison would also be worthwhile to evaluate whether similar changes are observed pre- and post-trimming within the unshod horse and with differing workloads and farriers. Horses within the current study were predominantly working on a soft surface, resulting in reduced loading forces on the hoof [1], and as such, the results from our cohort might underestimate the effect seen in horses working on more variable or harder terrain.

Caution is advised in the interpretation of these results, as a high degree of inter-subject variation was found across the measurements undertaken and as a number of variables could not be controlled due to the horses' working schedule. This variation could represent individual conformation differences in the hoof or distal limb, could be a cumulative result of previous farrier treatments [42], or may be a result of confounding variables. Based on our findings, we would recommend that horses are considered as individuals when determining their 'optimal' shoeing interval, but that the length of this period should not exceed six weeks. In addition, whilst we acknowledge that much published work still recommends that the 'perfect' foot should be symmetrical, it appears that this is not commonly observed within general riding horses, especially when they are shod. Therefore, we would respectfully suggest that the traditional aim of farriery to produce a balanced foot is adapted to a horse's specific functional requirements, in order to optimise performance and longevity. This can be achieved by shifting the focus to create a balanced foot with due consideration of the conformation of the individual's distal limb and the parallel alignment of the solar and weight bearing surfaces.

Author Contributions: Project design, planning, and data collection were undertaken by Kirsty Leśniak and Kerry Kuznik. Data analysis and the manuscript write up were performed by Kirsty Leśniak and Jane Williams. Peter Douglas provided valuable, practical industry interpretations of the results for the write up of the manuscript, in addition to editing the manuscript.

Conflicts of Interest: The authors declare no conflict of interest.

References

1. Oosterlinck, M.; Hardeman, L.C.; van der Meij, B.R.; Veraa, S.; van der Kolk, J.H.; Wijnberg, I.D.; Pille, F.; Back, W. Pressure plate analysis of toe-heel and medio-lateral hoof balance at the walk and trot in sound sport horses. *Vet. J.* **2013**, *198*, e9–e13. [CrossRef] [PubMed]

2. Dyson, S.J.; Tranquille, C.A.; Collins, S.N.; Parkin, T.D.H.; Murray, R.C. An investigation of the relationships between angles and shapes of the hoof capsule and the distal phalanx. *Equine Vet. J.* **2011**, *43*, 295–301. [CrossRef] [PubMed]

3. Baxter, G.M. *Adams and Stashak's Lameness in Horses*, 6th ed.; Baxter, G.M., Ed.; John Wiley & Sons: Oxford, UK, 2011.

4. Van Heel, M.C.V.; Moleman, M.; Barneveld, A.; Van Weeren, P.R.; Back, W. Changes in location of centre of pressure and hoof-unrollment pattern in relation to an 8-week shoeing interval in the horse. *Equine Vet. J.* **2005**, *37*, 536–540. [CrossRef] [PubMed]

5. Ducro, B.J.; Gorissen, B.; van Eldik, P.; Back, W. Influence of foot conformation on duration of competitive life in a Dutch Warmblood horse population. *Equine Vet. J.* **2009**, *41*, 144–148. [CrossRef] [PubMed]

6. Moleman, M.; van Heel, M.C.V.; van Weeren, P.R.; Back, W. Hoof growth between two shoeing sessions leads to a substantial increase of the moment about the distal, but not the proximal, interphalangeal joint. *Equine Vet. J.* **2006**, *38*, 170–174. [CrossRef] [PubMed]

7. Senden, A.I.P. A Comparison between Unshod and Shod Front Hooves of Thoroughbreds and the Effect of Trimming. Master's Thesis, Utrecht University, Utrecht, The Neherlands, 2009.

8. Kummer, M.; Geyer, H.; Imboden, I.; Auer, J.; Lischer, C. The effect of hoof trimming on radiographic measurements of the front feet of normal Warmblood horses. *Vet. J.* **2006**, *172*, 58–66. [CrossRef] [PubMed]

9. Van Heel, M.C.V.; Kroekenstoel, A.M.; van Dierendonck, M.C.; van Weeren, P.R.; Back, W. Uneven feet in a foal may develop as a consequence of lateral grazing behaviour induced by conformational traits. *Equine Vet. J.* **2006**, *38*, 646–651. [CrossRef] [PubMed]

10. Elishar, E.; McGuigan, M.P.; Wilson, A.M. Relationship of foot conformation and force applied to the navicular bone of sound horses at the trot. *Equine Vet. J.* **2004**, *36*, 431–435. [CrossRef]

11. Page, B.T.; Hagan, T.L. Breakover of the hoof and its effect on structures and forces within the foot. *J. Equine Vet. Sci.* **2002**, *22*, 258–264. [CrossRef]

12. Duberstein, K.J.; Johnson, E.L.; Whitehead, A. Effects of shortening breakover at the toe on gait kinematics at the walk and trot. *J. Equine Vet. Sci.* **2013**, *33*, 930–936. [CrossRef]

13. O'Grady, S.E. Therapeutic Shoes: Application of Principles. In *Equine Laminitis*; Belknap, J.K., Geor, R.J., Eds.; John Wiley & Sons, Inc.: Hoboken, NJ, USA, 2016; p. 343.

14. Parks, A. Foot balance and conformation: Clinical perspectives. *J. Equine Vet. Sci.* **2005**, *25*, 230. [CrossRef]

15. Johnston, C.; Back, W. Hoof ground interaction: When biomechanical stimuli challenge the tissues of the distal limb. *Equine Vet. J.* **2006**, *38*, 634–641. [CrossRef] [PubMed]

16. Floyd, A.; Mansmann, R. *Equine Podiatry*; Elsevier Health Sciences: Philidelphia, PA, USA, 2007; p. 480.

17. Van Heel, M.C.V.; Barneveld, A.; van Weeren, P.R.; Back, W. Dynamic pressure measurements for the detailed study of hoof balance: The effect of trimming. *Equine Vet. J.* **2004**, *36*, 778–782. [CrossRef] [PubMed]

18. Wilson, G.H.; McDonald, K.; O'Connell, M.J. Skeletal forelimb measurements and hoof spread in relation to asymmetry in the bilateral forelimb of horses. *Equine Vet. J.* **2009**, *41*, 238–241. [CrossRef] [PubMed]

19. Labens, R.; Redding, W.R.; Desai, K.K.; Vom Orde, K.; Mansmann, R.A.; Blikslager, A.T. Validation of a photogrammetric technique for computing equine hoof volume. *Vet. J.* **2013**, *197*, 625–630. [CrossRef] [PubMed]

20. Taylor, D.; Hood, D.M.; Wagner, I.P. Short-term effect of therapeutic shoeing on severity of lameness in horses with chronic laminitis. *Am. J. Vet. Res.* **2002**, *63*, 1629–1633. [CrossRef] [PubMed]

21. White, J.M.; Mellor, D.J.; Duz, M.; Lischer, C.J.; Voute, L.C. Diagnostic accuracy of digital photography and image analysis for the measurement of foot conformation in the horse. *Equine Vet. J.* **2008**, *40*, 623–628. [CrossRef] [PubMed]

22. Dyson, S.J.; Tranquille, C.A.; Collins, S.N.; Parkin, T.D.H.; Murray, R.C. External characteristics of the lateral aspect of the hoof differ between non-lame and lame horses. *Vet. J.* **2011**, *190*, 364–371. [CrossRef] [PubMed]

23. Clayton, H.M.; Gray, S.; Kaiser, L.J.; Bowker, R.M. Effects of barefoot trimming on hoof morphology. *Aust. Vet J.* **2011**, *89*, 305–311. [CrossRef] [PubMed]

24. Kroekenstoel, A.M.; Heel, M.C.V.; Weeren, P.R.; Back, W. Developmental aspects of distal limb conformation in the horse: The potential consequences of uneven feet in foals. *Equine Vet. J.* **2006**, *38*, 652–656. [CrossRef] [PubMed]

25. Wright, I.M. A study of 118 cases of navicular disease: Clinical features. *Equine Vet. J.* **1993**, *25*, 488–492. [CrossRef] [PubMed]

26. O'Grady, S.E.; Poupard, D.A. Physiological horseshoeing: An overview. *Equine Vet Educ.* **2001**, *13*, 330–334. [CrossRef]

27. Gill, D.W. *Farriery: The Whole Horse Concept: The Enigmas of Hoof Balance Made Clear*; Nottingham University Press: Notingham, UK, 2007.

28. Gordon, S.; Rogers, C.; Weston, J.; Bolwell, C.; Doloonjin, O. The Forelimb and Hoof Conformation in a Population of Mongolian Horses. *J. Equine Vet. Sci.* **2013**, *33*, 90–94. [CrossRef]

29. Hickman, J.; Humphrey, M. *Hickman's Farriery*, 2nd ed.; JA Allen: London, UK, 1988.

30. Cruz, C.; Thomason, J.; Faramarzi, B.; Bignell, W.; Sears, W.; Dobson, H.; Konyer, N.B. Changes in shape of the Standardbred distal phalanx and hoof capsule in response to exercise. *Equine Comp. Exerc. Physiol.* **2007**, *3*, 199. [CrossRef]

31. Thomason, J.J.; Biewener, A.A.; Bertram, J.E. Surface strain on the equine hoof wall in vivo: Implications for the material design and functional morphology of the wall. *J. Exp. Biol.* **1992**, *166*, 145–168.

32. Barrey, E. Investigation of the vertical hoof force distribution in the equine forelimb with an instrumented horseboot. *Equine Vet. J. Suppl.* **1990**, *9*, 35–38. [CrossRef]

33. O'Grady, S.E.; Poupard, D.A. Proper physiologic horseshoeing. *Vet. Clin. North Am. Equine Pract.* **2003**, *19*, 333–351. [CrossRef]

34. Holroyd, K.; Dixon, J.J.; Mair, T.; Bolas, N.; Bolt, D.M.; David, F.; Weller, R. Variation in foot conformation in lame horses with different foot lesions. *Vet. J.* **2013**, *195*, 361–365. [CrossRef] [PubMed]

35. Ovnicek, G.D.; Page, B.T.; Trotter, G.W. Natural balance trimming and shoeing: Its theory and application. *Vet. Clin. N. Am. Equine Pract.* **2003**, *19*, 353–377. [CrossRef]

36. Kane, A.J.; Stover, S.M.; Gardner, I.A.; Bock, K.B.; Case, J.T.; Johnson, B.J.; Anderson, M.L.; Barr, B.C.; Daft, B.M.; Kinde, H.; et al. Hoof size, shape, and balance as possible risk factors for catastrophic musculoskeletal injury of Thoroughbred racehorses. *Am. J. Vet. Res.* **1998**, *59*, 1545–1552. [PubMed]

37. Roland, E.; Stover, S.M.; Hull, M.L.; Dorsch, K. Geometric symmetry of the solar surface of hooves of Thoroughbred racehorses. *Am. Vet. Med. Assoc.* **2005**, *64*, 1030–1039. [CrossRef]

38. Pollitt, C.C. Clinical anatomy and physiology of the normal equine foot. *Equine Vet. Educ.* **1992**, *4*, 219–224. [CrossRef]

39. Reilly, P.T. In-Shoe Force Measurements and Hoof Balance. *J. Equine Vet. Sci.* **2010**, *30*, 475–478. [CrossRef]

40. Wilson, A.; Agass, R.; Vaux, S.; Sherlock, E.; Day, P.; Pfau, T.; Weller, R. Foot placement of the equine forelimb: Relationship between foot conformation, foot placement and movement asymmetry. *Equine Vet. J.* **2015**, *48*, 90–96. [CrossRef] [PubMed]
41. Egenvall, A.; Lönnell, C.; Roepstorff, L. Analysis of morbidity and mortality data in riding school horses, with special regard to locomotor problems. *Prev. Vet. Med.* **2009**, *88*, 193–204. [CrossRef] [PubMed]
42. Kummer, M.; Gygax, D.; Lischer, C.; Auer, J. Comparison of the trimming procedure of six different farriers by quantitative evaluation of hoof radiographs. *Vet. J.* **2009**, *179*, 401–406. [CrossRef] [PubMed]
43. Clayton, H. The effect of an acute hoof wall angulation on the stride kinematics of trotting horses. *Equine Vet. J.* **2010**, *22* (Suppl. S9), 86–90. [CrossRef]
44. Hood, D.M.; Taylor, D.; Wagner, I.P. Effects of ground surface deformability, trimming, and shoeing on quasistatic hoof loading patterns in horses. *Am. J. Vet. Res.* **2001**, *62*, 895–900. [CrossRef] [PubMed]

5

Was Jack the Ripper a Slaughterman? Human-Animal Violence and the World's Most Infamous Serial Killer

Andrew Knight [1,*] and Katherine D. Watson [2]

[1] Centre for Animal Welfare, Faculty of Humanities and Social Sciences, University of Winchester, Sparkford Road, Winchester SO22 4NR, UK

[2] School of History, Philosophy and Culture, Oxford Brookes University, Tonge Building, Gipsy Lane, Oxford OX3 0BP, UK; kwatson@brookes.ac.uk

[*] Correspondence: Andrew.Knight@winchester.ac.uk

Academic Editor: Clive J. C. Phillips

Simple Summary: The identity of Jack the Ripper remains one of the greatest unsolved crime mysteries in history. Jack was notorious both for the brutality of his murders and also for his habit of stealing organs from his victims. His speed and skill in doing so, in conditions of poor light and haste, fueled theories he was a surgeon. However, re-examination of a mortuary sketch from one of his victims has revealed several key aspects that strongly suggest he had no professional surgical training. Instead, the technique used was more consistent with that of a slaughterhouse worker. There were many small-scale slaughterhouses in East London in the 1880s, within which conditions were harsh for animals and workers alike. The brutalizing effects of such work only add to concerns highlighted by modern research that those who commit violence on animals are more likely to target people. Modern slaughterhouses are more humane in some ways but more desensitizing in others, and sociological research has indicated that communities with slaughterhouses are more likely to experience the most violent of crimes. The implications for modern animal slaughtering, and our social reliance on slaughterhouses, are explored.

Abstract: Hundreds of theories exist concerning the identity of "Jack the Ripper". His propensity for anatomical dissection with a knife—and in particular the rapid location and removal of specific organs—led some to speculate that he must have been surgically trained. However, re-examination of a mortuary sketch of one of his victims has revealed several aspects of incisional technique highly inconsistent with professional surgical training. Related discrepancies are also apparent in the language used within the only letter from Jack considered to be probably authentic. The techniques he used to dispatch his victims and retrieve their organs were, however, highly consistent with techniques used within the slaughterhouses of the day. East London in the 1880s had a large number of small-scale slaughterhouses, within which conditions for both animals and workers were exceedingly harsh. Modern sociological research has highlighted the clear links between the infliction of violence on animals and that inflicted on humans, as well as increased risks of violent crimes in communities surrounding slaughterhouses. Conditions within modern slaughterhouses are more humane in some ways but more desensitising in others. The implications for modern animal slaughtering, and our social reliance on slaughterhouses, are explored.

Keywords: serial murder; Jack the Ripper; slaughterman; slaughterhouse; abattoir; slaughter; human–animal violence; history of crime; forensic medicine; animal welfare

1. The World's Most Infamous Serial Killer

In 1888, the streets of London were rough and poorly lit. In Whitechapel and surrounding areas, times were hard, and work started early for some. Others worked throughout the night in trades licit—such as the meat industry—and illicit. At around 03:40 on 30 August, a cart driver named Charles Cross was on his way to work when he spied what appeared to be a body lying in front of a gated stable entrance [1] (p. 27). A surgeon subsequently summoned estimated that part-time prostitute Mary Ann "Polly" Nichols had died only some 10 minutes earlier. Her throat had been cut twice and her abdomen mutilated with a series of violent, jagged incisions [1] (pp. 35, 47). Although unaware of it at the time, those present were witnessing what would subsequently be considered the first known work of the world's most infamous serial killer—Jack the Ripper.

In the next 10 weeks, four other local women would share Polly's fate. All were prostitutes who lived and worked in the impoverished slums of East London, and all but one had their throats cut prior to abdominal mutilation. As police efforts to identify the killer(s) remained unsuccessful, a climate of fear descended upon the city. A vigilante committee was formed, whose efforts were similarly fruitless. The murderer was never identified, with four subsequent brutal killings in Whitechapel—ending in 1891—being attributed to others. Jack's final victim was considered to be Mary Jane Kelly, whose severely mutilated body was discovered on 9 November 1888 [2].

The extraordinary brutality of the murders, combined with the inability of the police or others to catch the perpetrator and consequent widespread media coverage, resulted in a fascination with the case that remains strong to this day. Hundreds of theories about Jack's identity now exist [3], ranging from the credible to the bizarre. One recent theory asserts that "Jack" may have, in fact, been a woman. DNA swabs from letters sent to police at the time, some of them believed to have been from the actual killer, were not conclusive, but nevertheless led Ian Findlay, an Australian professor of molecular and forensic diagnostics, to assert the possibility that the Ripper might have been female [4]. However, the victims were all physically overpowered, and swiftly had their throats cut, in populated areas, whilst making barely a sound, suggesting that Jack possessed considerable physical strength.

Another theory suggests that Jack was in fact the estranged husband of the fifth and final victim, Mary Jane Kelly, and that the first four victims were used as decoys. By day, Francis Spurzheim Craig was a courtroom reporter, and a contemporary sketch of an inquest into the Ripper's earlier murders is thought to show Craig sitting near the front of the court, reporting on a murder he himself might have committed. If true, it could be the only surviving image of the Ripper's face. In a final twist, Craig committed suicide by slashing his own throat with a blade—in a very similar manner to the style in which Jack dispatched his victims [5]. Suicide has always been a possible explanation for the sudden cessation of Jack's murders, along with other causes of death, unrelated imprisonment, institutionalization and emigration [6] (p. 371).

And yet, on several of his victims, Jack showed a particular propensity for anatomical dissection with a knife—and in particular, the rapid location and removal of specific organs. Only 14 minutes passed between successive patrols of Police Constable (PC) Watkins through Mitre Square after midnight on 30 September 1888. But within that short space of time, Jack was able to manoeuvre his fourth victim, Catherine Eddowes, into a darkened corner of the square, render her unconscious, cut her throat, pull up her clothing, and create a massive incision from groin to breastbone. Working in relative darkness, he then successfully located her uterus and left kidney and excised them. The difficulty of this task—even in good light, with a cadaver on a dissecting table at waist height—results from the location of the kidney, in particular. It lies buried within fat at the rear of the abdomen, beneath the stomach and other abdominal organs. And yet, in very poor light, and with the body awkwardly positioned at ground level, Jack nevertheless successfully completed this task with a speed that would have put most medical students to shame. He then created several relatively delicate cuts to her face, and had vanished into the night by the time PC Watkins reappeared.

Indeed, with the exception of the third victim, Elizabeth Stride, whose attacker may have been interrupted, only the first victim Mary Ann Nichols was *not* bereft of any organs. The second victim,

Annie Chapman, also had her uterus removed, and the final victim, Mary Jane Kelly, had her heart removed. Her body was also eviscerated, and her face severely mutilated.

Such obvious skills with the knife and, apparently, with anatomy, led commentators such as examining pathologist Phillips to conclude that "the murder could have been committed by a person who had been a hunter, a butcher, a slaughterman, as well as a student in surgery or a properly qualified surgeon" [6] (p. 246). Discomfiting though it is to one of us (AK) who is a member of the profession, he could even have been a veterinary surgeon. At least, in theory.

2. Not a Surgeon

However, examination of a mortuary sketch of the wounds inflicted on Catherine Eddowes' body (Figure 1) provides several strong indications that Jack was unlikely to have been a medically-trained professional, or a medical or veterinary student.

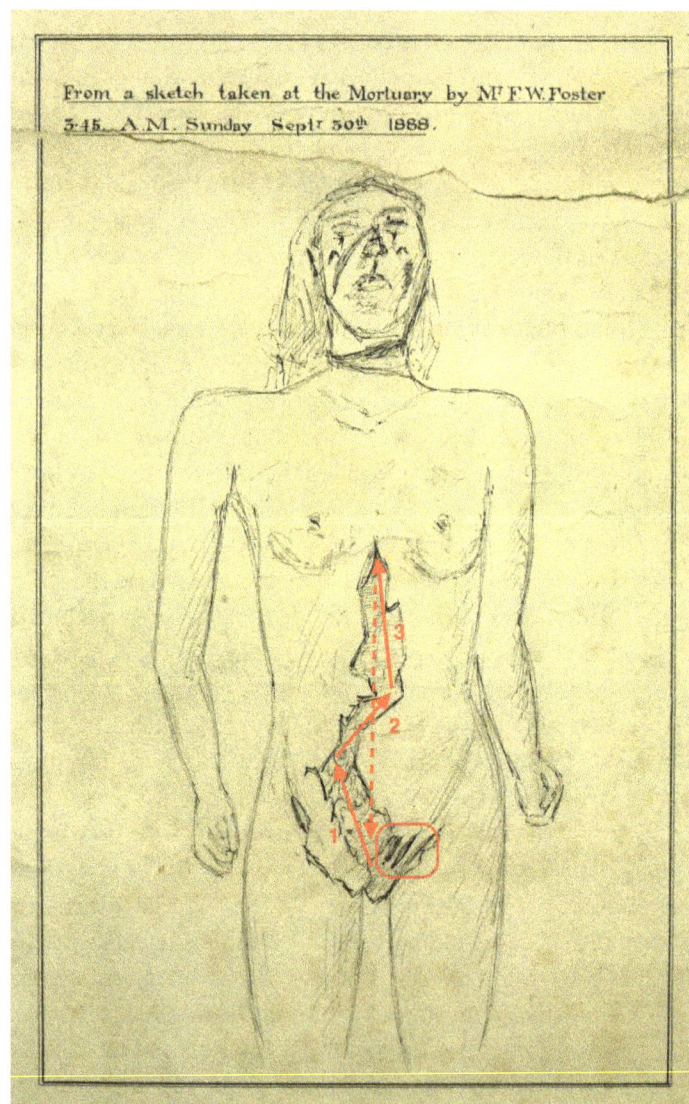

Figure 1. Analysis of wounds inflicted on Catherine Eddowes (From a sketch by Frederick William Foster, presented at the inquest held on 6 October 1888. Reproduced by permission of the Royal London Hospital Archives and Museum (Accession reference: RLHT1997/42). We have added locations of the exploratory incisions, along with the three primary incisions (solid) and the normal location and direction of the abdominal incision used for organ procurement (dashed) [7] (p. 21)).

It appears that Jack commenced by placing several exploratory incisions within Eddowes' lower abdominal region. These were displaced from the midline, and hence incorrectly located for opening the abdomen for general organ procurement, which normally utilises an abdominal midline approach [7] (p. 21).

Of course, it is possible that these "exploratory" incisions may have been placed after the main incision (Figure 1—three solid lines). However, the careful placement of these exploratory incisions makes this extremely unlikely. They are very close to each other, and are parallel. To place these incisions in such careful proximity in darkness and haste, it would have been necessary for the skin to remain very stable. This stability would have been provided by the normal tension of the skin, which would have been released as soon as the first major incision was made (Figure 2). Thereafter, it would have been difficult to place those small incisions with the deliberateness of location apparent in the sketch of Eddowes' body—and particularly in the case of one exploratory incision, directly next to the wound edge. Hence, it appears that these small incisions must have been placed prior to the main incision—i.e., they were indeed exploratory incisions which preceded the main incision.

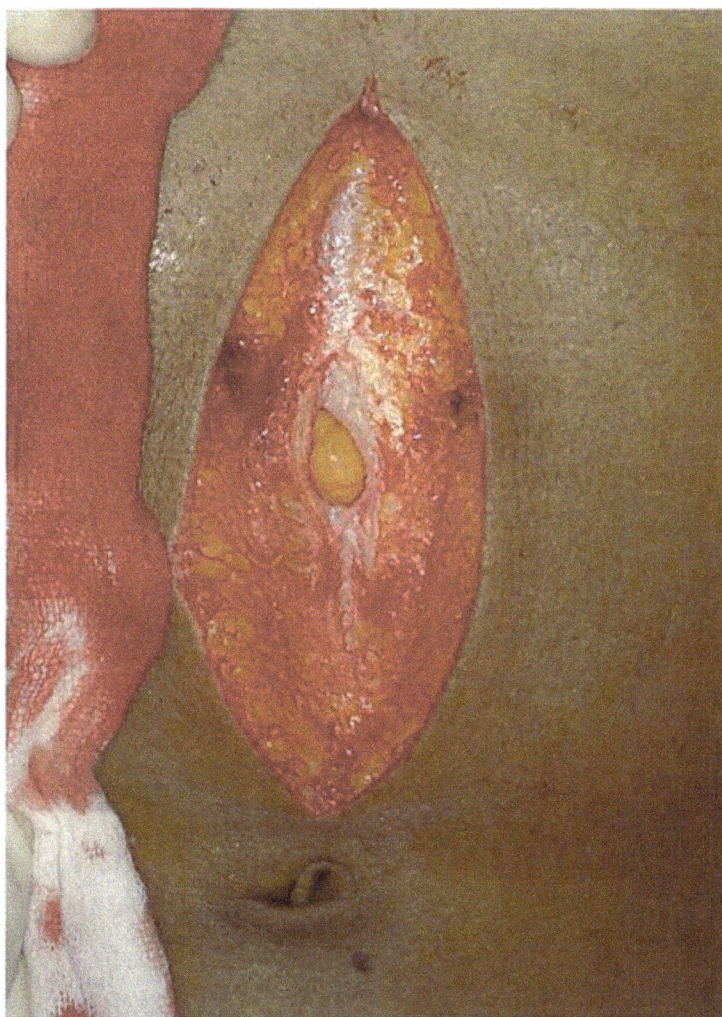

Figure 2. Normal abdominal surgical approach releasing skin tension following incision [8].

Having established that these were exploratory incisions, their location indicates the most likely point of origin of the main incision. All were in the region of the groin. It is most probable that the main incision started as an additional exploratory incision in the same region, which was then extended in three major cuts toward the sternum (Figure 1—solid lines).

However, when procuring organs, surgeons normally commence their abdominal incisions in the region of the sternum xiphoid process (i.e., the "head" end of the abdomen), and proceed toward the os pubis (i.e., the "feet" end) (Figure 1—dashed line) [7] (p. 21). Hence, it appears that the main incision to Eddowes' abdomen proceeded in the direction opposite to that used by trained surgeons.

Additionally, when performing a routine exploratory surgical approach to the abdomen, surgeons normally prefer the vertical midline approach, as it allows access via the *linea alba*—or "white line"—formed by the fusion of the aponeuroses (fibrous, fascial sheaths) surrounding the abdominal muscles—particularly the left and right rectus abdominis muscles (Figures 3 and 4).

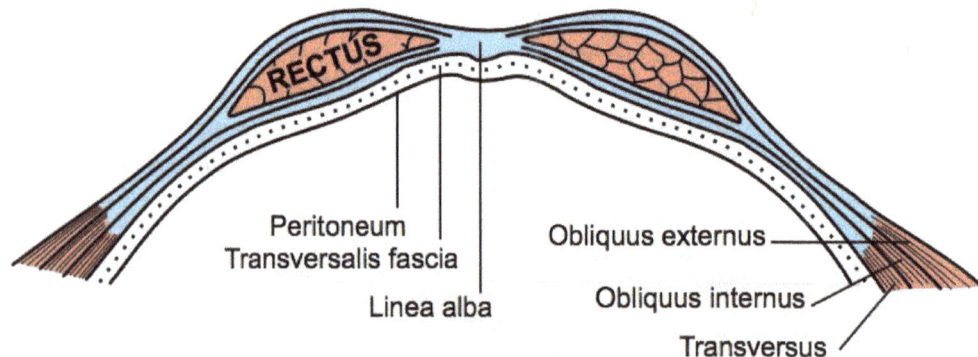

Figure 3. The linea alba is formed by the fusion of the aponeuroses surrounding the left and right rectus abdominis muscles [9].

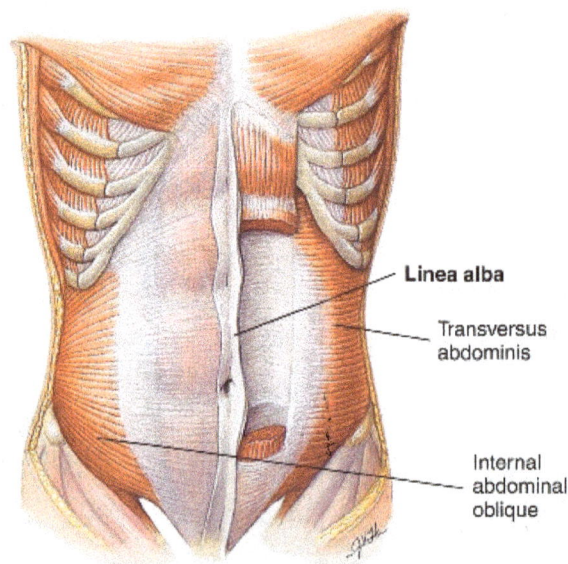

Figure 4. The linea alba runs the length of the abdominal midline from the xiphoid process to the pubic symphysis [10] (This article was published in Anatomy & Physiology, Thibodeau GA & Patton KT, p. 325.

An incision directly through this fascial line running vertically down the abdominal midline minimizes bleeding which would otherwise obscure the surgical field, and which could also potentially endanger the patient through blood loss. An incision in this location provides optimal exposure of the abdominal contents, and is preferred when abdominal exploration is desired. It also allows subsequent suture placement during wound closure within tough fibrous tissue, rather than within muscle. The latter is more fragile, and sutures are more likely to pull through under tension and the pressure applied by intra-abdominal contents, during the convalescent period [11] (p. 99).

For these reasons, correct placement of the primary abdominal incision directly through the linea alba, without deviation to either side, is so important that surgeons go to considerable effort to achieve it. The importance of this fundamental principle is deeply instilled within surgical students during basic training, to the point that it becomes automatic. Surgical texts from the 1880s do not provide the details of basic surgical principles commonplace within modern texts, but those historical texts consulted give no reason to believe this fundamental surgical principle would not have been similarly taught to the surgery students of the day [12–14]. Indeed, any deviation from the linea alba during routine abdominal surgical exploration in the 1880s would have immediately resulted in the same bleeding and other adverse consequences that would occur today, providing immediate feedback to the surgeon and a strong compulsion to return to the linea alba.

Admittedly, it is normal that the loss of skin tension and parting of the skin edges following commencement of any incision makes it difficult to keep to a straight line. Nevertheless, the degree of raggedness of the main incision apparent on Eddowes is quite severe. It exceeds that which would be probable in anyone possessed of even minimal surgical skill, and even when working under conditions of poor light and haste. The incorrect placement of the exploratory incisions, incorrect direction of the primary incision, and the degree of deviation from the abdominal midline—not to mention the raggedness of the primary incision—strongly suggest that it was highly unlikely that Jack possessed even minimal surgical training or experience.

3. Anatomical Skill Required

The mutilations inflicted on Eddowes were, however, consistent with someone familiar with more general principles of opening an abdomen, and—based on the organs subsequently removed in darkness and haste—familiar with rapid location and identification of certain desired organs, which would be difficult or impossible for the inexperienced to locate amongst the liver, pancreas, stomach, bladder, small bowel, colon, uterus, ovaries, mesenteries, ligaments, vessels, nerves, ureters, urethra and intraabdominal fat [7] (p. 33). Phillips opined that the weapon was very sharp, and the way it was used seemed to indicate great anatomical knowledge. Hence, Jack may well have been, as Phillips noted, a "hunter, butcher, a slaughterman", but most probably not "a student in surgery or a properly qualified surgeon" [15] (p. 109).

These sentiments were echoed by Frederick Gordon Brown (surgeon for the City Police) at the inquest on 5 October, 1888. Brown noted that certain organs were missing from the second and fourth victims, Annie Chapman and Catherine Eddowes, respectively. As reported in the *Denbighshire Free Press*, "Browne stated that the clever manner in which the left kidney and the other organ were removed betokened that the murderer was well versed in anatomy, but not necessarily in human anatomy, for he could have gained a certain amount of skill as a slaughterer of animals" [16].

However, the level of anatomical skill necessary for the excision of these organs was considered controversial by the experts of the day. At the autopsy of Catherine Eddowes, Phillips and Brown found that the injuries could have been inflicted by a person who had been a hunter, butcher, slaughterman, or a qualified or student surgeon [15] (p. 208). The mutilations were considered to have been inflicted by a sharp pointed knife, six inches in length. Some anatomical knowledge was considered necessary for removal of the left kidney, which can easily be overlooked. Such knowledge might have been possessed by someone in the habit of cutting up animals [15] (p. 229). However, the first doctor on the scene, George William Sequeira, did not think the perpetrator possessed any great anatomical skill, or that he had designs on any particular organ. City Public Analyst William Sedgwick Saunders was present at the autopsy and agreed with both of these points [15] (p. 232).

As reported in the *South Wales Echo* (27 September 1888), the coroner observed with respect to Annie Chapman, that, " . . . the uterus has been taken away. The body has not been dissected, but the injuries have been made by someone who had considerable anatomical knowledge and skill. There are no meaningless cuts. The organ has been taken away by one who knew where to find it, what difficulties he would have to contend against, and how he should use his knife so as to abstract the organ without injury to it. No unskilled person could have known where to find it, or have recognised it when it was found. For instance, no mere slaughterer of animals could have carried out these operations. It must have been someone accustomed to the post mortem room" [17].

As the coroner noted, a "mere slaughterer" might not have possessed the necessary dissection skills and anatomical knowledge. However, an abattoir worker experienced in both animal slaughter and butchery might well have done.

4. Could Jack Have Been a Slaughterman?

An intriguing array of other factors lend credence to the theory that Jack might have been a slaughterman. First, in 1888, there were many slaughterhouses in the Whitechapel area. Their presence stemmed from the appetite of the sizeable and growing London populace for meat, and from the lack of the modern refrigeration, transportation infrastructure and large-scale mechanization that characterize modern slaughtering and allow it to be conducted far removed from urban areas [18].

Indeed, the neighbouring borough of Islington was the centre of the live meat market in London at the time. As many as 10,000 cattle were on sale daily, and there was an account of 38,500 sheep being gathered for a single market. As reported in the *Birmingham Daily Post* in 1888, "In 1887, there were sold at Islington, for London consumption, 235,762 cattle, 809,914 sheep, 13,349 calves, and 1119 pigs". And yet, the 1887 market was recovering from a depression. In 1864, the even greater figure of 346,000 cattle were sold [19].

These enormous numbers of animals being consumed by the growing London population required a similarly sizeable slaughtering capacity. Victorian slaughterhouses were not the vast, industrialised killing and butchering factories of today, and workers were not assisted by machines. Instead, there were a very large number of small facilities.

Indeed, the body of Jack's first victim, Mary Ann Nichols, was discovered by a police constable (John Neil) in Buck's Row, very close to one of these establishments. As he reported in *The Flintshire Observer*, "The first to arrive on the scene after I had discovered the body were two men who work at a slaughterhouse opposite" [20]. Another then joined them. These men were reported as Henry Tomkin, horse slaughterer, and two companions, James Mumford and Charles Brittain, who worked for Messrs. Barker & Co. (Whitechapel, London, UK), Horse Slaughterers, in Winthrop Street, adjoining Buck's Row and only 150 yards from Nichols' body [21] (p. 102).

As noted by Odell, "Well practiced in the art of cutting throats, legitimately owning and carrying knives, working and probably living in or near Whitechapel and Spitalfields, the Ripper as a slaughterman made a great deal of sense. Moreover, he would have blended perfectly with the local colour and character of the streets … " [21] (pp. 102–103). This point is affirmed by Samuel Barnett in a letter published in *The Times* (19 September 1888): "At present animals are daily slaughtered in the midst of Whitechapel, the butchers with their blood stains are familiar among the street passengers, and sights are common which tend to brutalize ignorant natures" [22]. Working hours and conditions in 1888 were far removed from those of today, and animals were frequently slaughtered at night—facilitating the nocturnal presence—and indeed alibis—of any slaughtermen in the area.

Odell noted that such an assailant would have frequented "pubs and lodging houses and (was) probably known to the prostitutes. He would have many attributes that made him an accepted and unexceptional character, beyond suspicion and creating no fear" [21] (p. 103). The latter point in particular would have assisted a perpetrator to have approached these women without challenge, possibly entice them into quiet locations, and successfully overpower them, before any had the chance to raise an alarm. Most of these murders occurred nearby to other people, yet never a sound was heard.

In 1966, some sketches relating to the murder of Catherine Eddowes were discovered in a basement of the London Hospital. Professor Francis Camps, an eminent pathologist with an interest in the case, published the sketches with his analysis in *The London Hospital Gazette*. Commenting on the fact that the victims evidenced facial congestion, died without calling out, and with possibly less blood loss than might have been expected, he suggested that strangulation—"a common practice of sexual murderers"—might have been the real cause of death [23] (p. 27). However, this was contested by the doctors of the time. For Elizabeth Stride, the cause of death was given as a severed left carotid artery and division of the trachea (windpipe); for Catherine Eddowes, haemorrhage from the left carotid artery; and for Annie Chapman, also haemorrhage [21] (pp. 109–110).

Regardless of the degree to which strangulation was used, considerable physical strength would have been necessary, to so quietly and quickly overpower Jack's victims. Such strength would have been necessary for, and induced by, the very physical nature of the work in the slaughterhouses of this era. As described in the *Birmingham Daily Post*, " ... a slaughterhouse is at its best but a chamber of horrors ... in which oxen and sheep become beef and mutton under the hands of the brawny, half-naked pole-axing men" [19]. Half-naked, no doubt, because of the hard physical labour involved, and the exercise-induced body temperature rises and sweating.

Odell continues thus: "Added to this would be his knowledge of local geography ... It does not take much imagination to visualize a slaughterman killing his human prey and escaping to the blood-soaked sanctuary of the abattoir where he worked. Indeed, what better place could there be to hide the murderer and to conceal his murder weapon and visceral trophies" [21] (p. 103)?

The suspicion that Jack was intimately familiar with the local geography of the area was reinforced by a description of his likely movements, recited by Professor Camps in *The London Hospital Gazette* (1966). After murdering Catherine Eddowes in Mitre Square, Camps noted that Jack must have travelled across Houndsditch and Middlesex Street to Goulston Street where in a passage leading to a staircase of some flats, a blood-stained piece of Eddowes' apron was found by PC Alfred Long of H Division, Metropolitan Police, at 02:55, along with a message scrawled on a nearby doorway in chalk. Camps asserts that Jack would have then travelled north to Dorset Street, pausing there to wash blood off his hands at a public sink set back from the street. Camps asserted that Jack's knowledge of the sink location in particular suggested that he knew the neighbourhood [23].

5. Might Jack Have Been a Shochet?

Odell continued that, "If throat-cutting was Jack the Ripper's hallmark, there was one particular kind of slaughterman whose calling required perfection in this special skill. That was the Jewish ritual slaughterman, or shochet" [21] (p. 103).

And in fact, there was a significant need for Jewish ritual slaughter in nineteenth-century London. As Odell noted, there was a large Jewish population—estimated at 60,000—in the East End of London in 1889. Hence, there would have been a significant number of abattoirs conducting Jewish ritual slaughter (shechita), and a significant number of highly experienced Jewish ritual slaughtermen (shochetim) [21] (pp. 103, 105).

Shechita is the only method of producing meat and poultry allowed by Jewish law. Such meat is then designated as "kosher", signifying that it complies with the regulations of kashrut (Jewish dietary law). As described by Shechita UK, "Shechita is performed by a highly trained shochet. The procedure consists of a rapid and expert transverse incision with an instrument of surgical sharpness (a chalaf), which severs the major structures and vessels at the neck ... The frontal structures including the trachea, oesophagus, the carotid arteries and jugular veins are severed in a rapid and uninterrupted action" [24] (pp. 3, 5). Velarde et al. provided further details: "During religious slaughter, animals are killed ... by a transverse incision across the neck that is cutting the skin, muscles (brachiocephalic, sternocephalic, sternohyoid, and sternothyroid), trachea, esophagus, carotid arteries, jugular veins and the major, superficial and deep nerves of the cervical plexus" [25] (p. 278).

Such an incision is highly consistent with the neck incisions found on Jack's victims. Henry Llewellyn, the doctor called to examine the body of Mary Ann Nichols at the scene of her death, conducted a post-mortem examination later that morning. He reported that there was an incision about eight inches long running from a point below the left ear, rostrally (frontwards) around the neck, to a point below the right jaw, which had completely severed most of the tissues, including the large vessels (jugular veins and carotid arteries) on both sides of the neck. As he reported in *The Flintshire Observer*, "These cuts must have been caused with a long-bladed knife, moderately sharp, and used with great violence" [20].

Very similarly, when testifying at the inquest into the death of Catherine Eddowes, Dr Brown described her throat incision, thus: "The throat was cut across to the extent of about 6 or 7 inches. A superficial cut commenced about an inch and $\frac{1}{2}$ below the lobe about $2\frac{1}{2}$ inches behind the left ear and extended across the throat to about 3 inches below the lobe of the right ear. The big muscle across the throat was divided through on the left side—the large vessels on the left side of the neck were severed—the larynx was severed below the vocal chords (*sic*). All the deep structures were severed to the bone the knife marking intervertebral cartilages—the sheath of the vessels on the right side was just opened" [21] (p. 105).

Additionally, as reported by Shechita UK, the shochet's duties do not end there: "He examines the organs and vessels immediately after severance by the shechita incision, to ascertain that the shechita was properly performed, this examination is visual and tactile (b'dikath ha'simanim). This integral part of the shechita process is required by Halacha (Y.D. 25:1). The shochet also examines the internal organs and lungs (b'dikath ha'reyah) of an animal in order to ascertain whether there are any abnormalities or defects disqualifying the animal from being kosher (Y.D. 29-60)" [24] (p. 7). (Y.D. refers to the Yoreh Deah, or Codes of Jewish Law) (As reported by Shechita UK, "Jewish laws governing shechita and the animal welfare considerations are to be found in the Talmud (Oral Law of Judaism) Tractate Chullin, Mishneh Torah of Maimonides, the Shulchan Oruch: Yoreh Deah (Codes of Jewish Law) by Rabbi Joseph Karo . . . " Additionally, Halacha refers to Jewish law and jurisprudence, based on the Talmud [24] (p. 6)).

Hence, any experienced shochet is likely to be highly skilled at the type of neck incisions found on Jack's victims. They are also likely to be highly skilled at visual and tactile examination of internal organs. This familiarity—and in particular, tactile familiarity—would have been extremely helpful to an assailant seeking to rapidly locate and remove specific organs from the bodies of his victims, in poor lighting.

The names and details of licenced shochetim were held by the London Board of Shechita. Unfortunately, however, their records for the relevant time period were destroyed by the German bombing of London in 1940 [21] (p. 105).

But of course Jack was not necessarily a shochet. As Odell neatly surmised, "an ordinary slaughterman possessed all the skills demonstrated by the Ripper's knife work", although, "the Shochet had the edge when it came to throat-cutting" [21] (p. 106).

6. Analysing Jack's Words

Jack's crimes were the centre of public attention in nineteenth-century London, and many letters were received by the authorities purporting to be from the Ripper. Most are believed to have been hoaxes. However, a specimen accompanying one such letter (Figure 5) suggests authenticity.

On 16 October, 1888, Mr George Lusk, Chairman of the Whitechapel Vigilance Committee, received by post a cardboard box containing a portion of a human kidney preserved in ethanol ("spirits"). Openshaw, Pathological Curator of the London Hospital, subsequently examined it. He reportedly stated that it belonged to a woman of about 45 (Eddowes was 46), and had been removed within the preceding three weeks (Eddowes was killed a fortnight prior). This specimen reportedly matched Eddowes' missing left kidney, because two inches of renal artery remained in the victim's body, whilst the third inch was attached to the kidney, and because both the right kidney remaining in the body, and the left kidney received by post, showed signs of severe Bright's disease [23] (pp. 33–34). However, as with many historical details pertaining to the Ripper's murders, some of these details are contested. For example, police surgeon Dr Brown reportedly stated that the kidney had been trimmed up, and that the renal artery was entirely absent [1] (p. 189), [26] (p. 168).

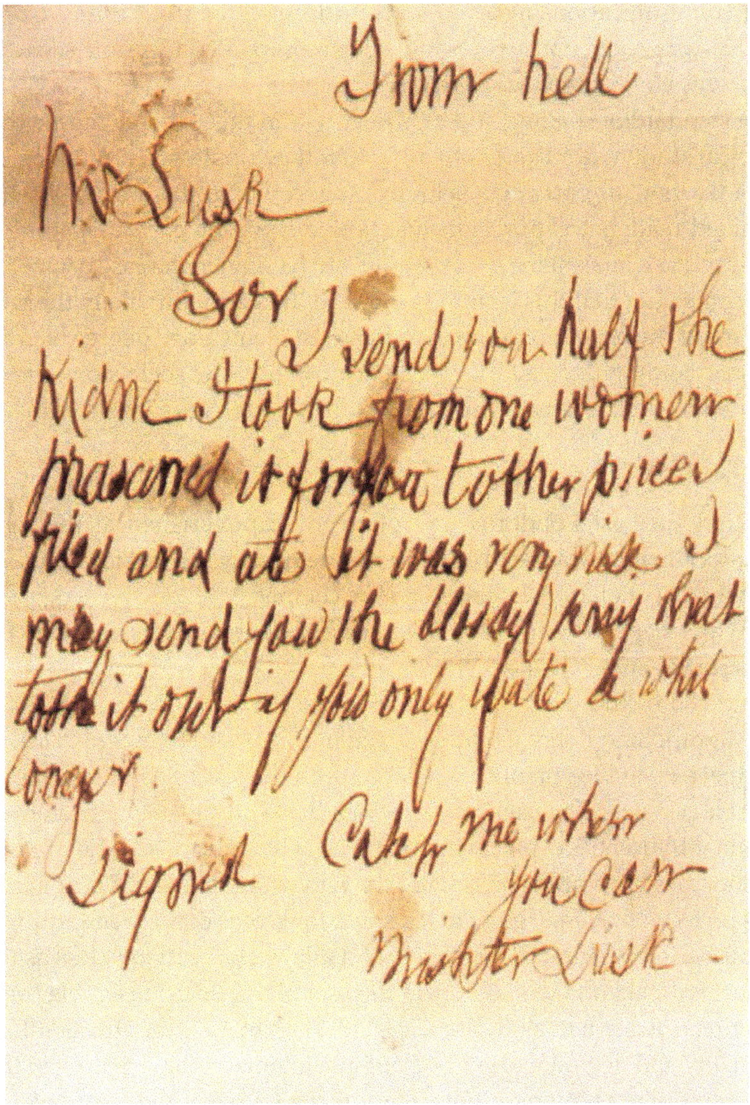
From hell
Mr Lusk
Sor
I send you half the
Kidne I took from one women
prasarved it for you tother piece
fried and ate it was very nise I
may send you the bloody knif that
took it out if you only wate a whil
longer
Signed Catch me when
you can
Mishter Lusk

Figure 5. Letter purportedly from Jack the Ripper (Anon. (n.d.). A photographic copy of the now lost "From Hell" letter, postmarked 15 October 1888 [27]).

Nevertheless, given the timing of the letter, and its accompanying specimen, this is the letter most likely to have been an authentic communication from Jack himself. Entitled "From hell", the letter stated,

> "Mr Lusk
> Sor
> I send you half the
> Kidne I took from one women
> prasarved it for you tother piece I
> fried and ate it was very nise. I
> may send you the bloody knif that
> took it out if you only wate a whil
> longer
> Signed Catch me when
> you can
> Mishter Lusk"

Several other communications received were addressed to "Dear Boss", or refer to the reader as "Boss" [23] (p. 33). However, none were similarly accompanied by crime scene artefacts, and it is unknown which, if any, were authentic.

The appalling standard of spelling and grammar within this letter suggest either that the author was neither a medical student nor professional, or that they possessed a rare degree of imagination. The misspelling of 'kidney' in particular is highly suggestive of the former. It may be difficult for non-medically trained readers to appreciate just how deeply the correct spelling of such words is ingrained in anyone with significant medical training, but having (in the case of one of us) been through such training, we can testify that this is indeed the case. It is far more likely the letter was authored by a person who lacked the benefit of more than the most elementary degree of education. Similarly, "Boss" is an honorific commonly used by people in jobs with low socioeconomic status—although, as stated, it is unknown whether any of the letters addressed to "Boss" were authentic.

7. Socioeconomic Factors

Living conditions in East London were relatively impoverished at the time, and as noted previously, the livestock market was recovering from a depression. It was far from a desirable locale in which to live and work. As noted by Superintendent Thomas Arnold: " . . . a considerable portion of the population of Whitechapel is composed of the low and dangerous classes, who frequently indulge in rowdyism and street offences" [15] (p. 314).

This was reinforced by the sentiments of Mr Samuel Barnett, Vicar of St Jude's, as paraphrased by James Monro, Metropolitan Police Commissioner, in Evans and Skinner: "Vice of a very low type exists in Whitechapel—such vice manifests itself in brawling and acts of violence which shock the feelings of respectable persons...The facility with which the Whitechapel murderer obtains victims has brought this prominently to notice, but to anyone who will take a walk late at night in the districts where the recent atrocities have been committed, the only wonder is that his operations have been so restricted. There is no lack of victims ready to his hand, for scores of these unfortunate women may be seen any night muddled with drink in the streets and alleys, perfectly reckless as to their safety, and only anxious to meet with anyone who will help them in plying their miserable trade" [15] (p. 495).

Barnett further reported in a letter to *The Times* (1889), that, " . . . the streets still offer almost every night scenes of brutality and degradation. A body of inhabitants . . . have patrolled the neighbourhood during the last nine months on many nights every week between the hours of 11 p.m. and 3 a.m. Their record tells of rows in which stabbing is common, but on which the police are able to get no charges; of fights between woman stripped to the waist, of which boys and children are spectators; of the protection afforded to thieves, and of such things as could only occur where opinion favours vice" [28].

However, it is not only humans that may fall victim to poor socioeconomic circumstances and any related tendencies toward violent behaviour. Animals may also be affected. In 2010, veterinarian Peter Wedderburn noted that times of economic hardship appear to result in greater numbers of companion animals being abandoned and mistreated, including within organized fights, and by drowning, stabbing, burning or neglect [29].

Prior to the implementation of modern worker protection laws and policies, and bereft of the benefits of modern machinery, slaughterhouse work would have been even harder and more dangerous than it is today, and the pay—particularly in the depressed boroughs of nineteenth-century East London—would have been low. Meat, milk and eggs were relatively more expensive than they have become today, with the benefits of modern industrialisation, mass production and market pressures [30].

Within the socioeconomically depressed environment of East London in the 1880s, it is easy to imagine workers appropriating small quantities of meats as they worked, to be taken home for later cooking and consumption. To a worker in the habit of regularly committing such petty thefts, taking home a kidney for cooking and consumption would have represented a far smaller step, that sprang to mind far more naturally, than might have occurred to a murderer from some other background.

8. Slaughterhouse Impacts on Workers

Even modern-day slaughterhouses are relatively dangerous places to work, with unusually high rates of injury and poor health. As Jacques (2015) put it, "The reality of slaughterhouse work is that this multi-billion dollar industry employs thousands of people who work for low wages in physically dangerous jobs" [31].

As reported by Cohidon et al. (2009) in a study of 3000 French meat industry employees: "Their risk of accidents is high, especially in slaughtering and cutting large animals; this is among the most dangerous of all French occupations. The use of knives and dangerous machines, the movements and postures required, and slips and falls cause most accidents" [32] (p. 808). They noted that "Other countries have made similar observations in the past several years". In a recent study of Estonian slaughterhouse workers, Kristina Mering confirmed this: "The workers are subject to rapid repetitive movements, incurring blisters and stiffness, having to work in heat and cold with really sharp knives which can cause accidents. All agreed that they were underpaid for the work that they do" [33].

Cohidon and colleagues also demonstrated poor perceived health among the meat industry employees studied. Working hours disrupting sleeping rhythms were perceived to be a contributing factor [32]. This would certainly have been a factor in the meat industry of East London in the 1880s, and indeed, Jack's murders all occurred during the small hours of the night.

9. Slaughterhouses and Violent Crime

Although conditions in modern slaughterhouses are usually better for both workers and animals, they are hardly conducive to the physical or psychological health of either. Unfortunately, it is not only the workers themselves that are affected. After analysing 1994–2002 data from 581 U.S. counties, Fitzgerald et al. (2009) reported that total arrest rates, and arrests for violent crimes, rape and other sex offenses were increased among slaughterhouse workers, when compared to those from other industries [34].

Comparative data were sourced for industries that were similar in the senses that they also had high immigrant worker concentrations, were also manufacturing industries (with the exception of one, which was included due to a high rate of immigrant concentration), and were similarly characterized by low pay, routinized labour, and dangerous conditions [35–38]. These were the iron and steel forging, truck trailer manufacturing, motor vehicle metal stamping, sign manufacturing, and industrial laundering industries.

After controlling for the number of young men in the county, population density, the total number of males, the number of people in poverty, international migration, internal migration, total non-White and/or Hispanic population, the unemployment rate, and the total county population, the authors found that slaughterhouse employment had significant positive (and "unique") effects on the arrest and report rate scales, as well as on rates of total arrests, arrests for violent crimes, arrests for rape, and arrests for other sex offences. In fact, the expected arrest and report values in counties with 7500 slaughterhouse employees were more than double the values where there were no such employees.

Of the comparison industries, only one (truck trailer manufacturing) had a significant effect on the total arrests variable, but it was a negative effect. Two of the comparison industries (truck trailer manufacturing and motor vehicle metal stamping) had significant effects on violent arrests, but both were negative effects. Similarly, only one comparison industry (iron and steel forging) demonstrated a significant effect on arrests for rape, but once again, it was a negative effect [34].

The authors noted that, although "employment in the manufacturing sector in general has suppressant effects on crime (e.g., Lee and Ousey, 2001); this is clearly not the case for the slaughterhouse subsector of manufacturing" [34] (p. 175).

Similarly, Jacques analysed 2000 data from 248 U.S. counties in states chosen for their concentrations of cattle slaughterhouses and employment within them. After controlling for key variables in the social disorganization literature, she found that slaughterhouse presence in the counties studied corresponded with a 22% increase in total arrests, a 90% increase in offenses against the family, increased aggravated assaults, and a 166% increase in arrests for rape [31].

Particularly noteworthy was the significant positive effect of slaughterhouse employment on sexual assault rates, revealed by Fitzgerald et al. (2009). Offences within this category included sexual attacks on males, incest, indecent exposure, statutory rape, and "crimes against nature". As these authors revealed, "Increases in slaughterhouse employment had a significant positive effect on rape arrests across the entire time period under study" [34] (p. 174).

10. Human-Animal Violence Links

Fitzgerald et al. (2009) observed that, "Many of these offenses are perpetrated against those with less power, and we interpret this as evidence that the work done within slaughterhouses might spillover (sic) to violence against other less powerful groups, such as women and children" [34] (p. 174). Indeed, most of the increases in violent crime rates surrounding slaughterhouses have been attributed to increases in domestic violence and child abuse [39,40] (p. 40), [41] (p. 103).

Links between the commission of violence toward vulnerable groups, including women, children and the elderly, and the commission of violence toward animals, have been extensively documented since the first case report published in 1806, describing an adult male who was violent toward both animals and humans [42].

One of the first researchers in this area was MacDonald, who in 1961 became the first to explore the links between childhood animal cruelty and later violence toward humans. By sampling 48 psychotic patients and 52 nonpsychotic patients, he identified three characteristics consistently found among the most sadistic individuals: enuresis, fire setting, and childhood cruelty toward animals. He subsequently concluded that this "triad" of behaviours could be a strong predictor of homicidal behaviour [43].

Three years later, Mead similarly noted that childhood animal cruelty could indicate the formation of a spontaneous, assaultive character disorder. Animal cruelty "could prove a diagnostic sign" and " . . . such children, diagnosed early, could be helped instead of being allowed to embark on a long career of episodic violence and murder" [44] (p. 22).

Since the late 1970s, behavioural specialists at the Federal Bureau of Investigation's Behavioural Science Unit have suspected that animal cruelty may be involved in the development of serial killers [45], and in 1988, an FBI study implicated animal cruelty as a possible early warning sign of serial murder [46].

In 1987, the American Psychiatric Association (APA) continued in this vein, adding animal cruelty as a symptom of childhood conduct disorders to the third (revised) edition of its *Diagnostic and Statistical Manual of Mental Disorders* [47]. The *DSM-IV* defined conduct disorder as "a repetitive and persistent pattern of behaviour in which the basic rights of others or major age-appropriate societal norms or rules are violated" [48] (p. 90). The APA suggested that many of these same children would progress to show similar symptoms during adulthood, and that some of these would meet the criteria for anti-social personality disorder. This has been continued within recent editions *DSM-IV* [49], and *DSM-5* [50].

A series of studies examining the relationship between childhood animal cruelty and later violence against humans have occurred in the last two decades. A number demonstrated such an association [45,51–57]. Ressler et al. (1998), for example, studied 36 male sexual murderers, 29 of whom were serial murderers. Of the 28 subjects for whom childhood background data were available, 36% had committed animal cruelty as children, 46% had committed animal cruelty as adolescents, and 36% had committed animal cruelty as adults. The authors concluded not only that cruelty to animals might predispose toward violence against humans later in life, but that it might also predict the most extreme forms of violence [55].

Merz-Perez et al. (2001) interviewed 45 violent and 45 nonviolent offenders incarcerated in a Florida maximum-security prison. Violent offenders were significantly more likely than nonviolent offenders (56% vs. 20%) to have committed acts of animal cruelty as children. Particularly significant, given the way in which Jack killed his victims, and the similarity to Jewish ritual slaughter, they discovered that the way in which violent offenders abused animals resembled the methods they subsequently used to commit crimes against their human victims [53].

Wright and Hensley (2003) investigated 354 cases of serial murder, finding that 21% of these murderers had engaged in animal cruelty. They also described, in chilling detail, five cases in which children suffering humiliation or abuse vented their repressed frustration and aggression on animals, and later "graduated" to become the well-known serial killers Carroll Cole, Jeffrey Dahmer, Edmund Kemper, Henry Lee Lucas, and Arthur Shawcross [45].

These cases were consistent with the so-called 'violence graduation hypothesis', which holds that early animal cruelty provides the individual with the opportunity to learn first-hand about violence, practice violence on available targets (animals), and be desensitized to the consequences of violent behaviour [58].

A number of studies have specifically focused on the commission of violence towards women, usually by surveying female victims of intimate partner violence during their visits to secure shelters. Overall, around 50% of women in violent relationships reported that their partner had hurt or killed one of their pets (e.g., 46% in Faver and Strand, 2003; 52.9% in Volant et al., 2008; 53% in Carlisle-Frank et al., 2004; 54% in Ascione et al., 2007; 57% in Ascione, 1998) [59–63]. Somewhat divergently, Flynn (2000) reported a comparatively lower figure of 26% [64].

Furthermore, batterers who also abuse pets appear to differ from those who do not in other ways as well. One study found that batterers who abused pets were more dangerous, and used more controlling behaviours, than men who had not abused pets [65]. Batterers who had committed pet abuse also exhibited higher rates of sexual violence, marital rape, emotional violence, and stalking.

On the other hand, one-fifth of children are believed to have participated in some form of animal cruelty [66], and the vast majority do not "graduate" to become serial killers. Unsurprisingly, therefore, other studies have shown no relationship between childhood animal cruelty and later violence against humans, or have refuted the notion that one comes before the other, i.e., a time order relationship [67,68].

In 1987, Felthous and Kellert published a meta-analysis of 15 studies from the 1970s and 1980s to examine the link between childhood animal cruelty and later violence toward humans. They found that most studies failed to indicate a relationship between childhood animal cruelty and later violence toward humans, and they described data which supported this association as being "soft and of dubious reliability" [69] (p. 69).

However, nine of the ten studies that failed to find a clear link between childhood animal cruelty and later violence against humans analysed single acts of violence directed toward humans rather than recurrent violence—which limits their applicability to serial killers such as Jack the Ripper. In their survey of 180 inmates from one medium-security and one maximum security prison in 2007, Hensley et al. (2009) found that repeated acts of animal abuse in earlier life were significantly related to later repeated acts of interpersonal violence as an adult [52].

Other limitations of these 10 studies included lack of clear definitions of the behaviours being defined, and reliance on case records, rather than face to face interviews. Accordingly, significant concerns persist about the possibility that the commission of violence towards animals may predispose to similar behaviour towards humans.

As Flynn (2011) put it, "animal abuse and interpersonal violence do often go together. Animal abuse can be a risk factor, a marker, and sometimes a precursor of other forms of violence, and vice versa. . . . it is still important for judges, juries, prosecutors, clinicians, child protective workers, shelter workers, veterinarians, police, and legislators to take animal abuse seriously" [66] (p. 461).

11. Slaughterhouse Work: Predisposing Toward Violence

There appears to be something about slaughterhouse work in particular, that predisposes toward violent crime. This was observed and documented as early as the turn of the twentieth century in his book *The Jungle* by Upton Sinclair, as recounted by Fitzgerald et al. (2009): "(Sinclair) exposed the devastating work conditions and living environments of those who toiled in Chicago's stockyard slaughterhouses. In *The Jungle*, he made a connection between the numerous after-work fights instigated by slaughterhouse workers and the killing and dismembering of animals all day at work: "He (the police officer) has to be prompt—for these two-o'clock-in-the-morning fights, if they once get out of hand, are like a forest fire, and may mean the whole reserves at the station. The thing to do is to crack every fighting head that you can see, before there are so many fighting heads that you cannot crack any of them. There is but scant account kept of cracked heads in back of the (stock) yards, *for men who have to crack the heads of animals all day seem to get into the habit, and to practice on their friends, and even on their families, between times* (Sinclair, 1905/1946, pp. 18–19 emphasis added)"" [34] (p. 158).

The other manufacturing industries studied by Fitzgerald et al. were similar in labour force composition, injury and illness rates, but different in one crucial way: the materials of production are inanimate objects, rather than living animals. As the authors noted, " . . . Rémy (2003) and Smith (2002) have demonstrated that the slaughterhouse occupies a contradictory position within society. Formal rules about requiring humane slaughter acknowledge that sentient creatures are being killed. Yet those who are engaged in the work of the slaughterhouse also develop constructions that allow them to carry out this work" [34] (p. 159). As Jacques (2015) put it, "The setting of slaughterhouse work promotes a disconnection between humans and nonhuman animals, one in which nonhuman animals are treated as "products" and the act of slaughtering a nonhuman animal is compartmentalized into separate tasks from the kill floor to the fabrication room" [31] (p. 3).

Animals killed in slaughterhouses are objectified to some degree as 'things' that may be killed, dismembered, repackaged and otherwise used for human purposes. Such constructions would have been even more easily acquired prior to the development of modern legislation requiring more humane slaughter, and that accordingly encouraged specific consideration of the need for humane treatment of animals.

The objectification of animals in these environments facilitates the suppression of the sympathy for animals, and concern for their interests, that would otherwise manifest more strongly. Such sympathy and concern would create greater psychological stress for slaughterhouse workers who are required to treat animals in ways very contrary to that morally compelled by their true status as sentient beings who have done us no wrong, and as creatures who are commonly fearful and stressed in these environments, and who do not wish to die.

In her recent study of Estonian slaughterhouse workers, Kristina Mering confirmed this suppression of natural sympathy: "In order for them to be able to do their work, they need to block out all emotions. Since they understand that they are taking the life of an animal, they need a strong blocking mechanism to keep thoughts like this out. They build a routine that numbs the emotions and lets them do their work without thinking about the killing. When I asked one person about the stabbing, they put it like this: "If we would think about it, it would be the wrong place to work". They wear earphones and listen to music or the radio" [33].

Sociologist Erika Cudworth also confirmed this during her interviews with local authority inspectors and slaughterhouse workers in London from 1994 to 1995. She reported that, "According to those who teach the skill at Smithfield market (*sic*), the largest meat market in London, it takes a "certain kind of person" to slaughter, one who has "disregard for the lives of animals" and has "got to be callous" (interview, butcher and tutor, Smithfield Meat Market, November 1993)" [70] (p. 13).

If slaughterhouse workers allowed themselves to feel appropriate sympathy and concern for the animals, given their status as sentient beings who do experience fear, pain, stress and other forms of suffering, it could interfere with their abilities to fulfil the roles required of them, and hence, their economic survival. Given the low socioeconomic status of most slaughterhouse workers, and the limited employment prospects in many of the rural locations where abattoirs are located, this is no small matter today. However, in the depressed environment of nineteenth-century East London, where social security was almost non-existent, it could have significantly impacted chances of literal survival. Hence, the workplace pressures in these nineteenth-century slaughterhouses likely to result in objectification of, and decreased empathy for, the animals that were killed in them, were most probably even stronger than they are today.

The suppression of natural sympathy that might otherwise manifest affects both animals and workers. As noted by Dillard (2008), "By habitually violating one's natural preference against killing, the worker very likely is adversely psychologically impacted" [71] (p. 401).

The rapid pace of many modern slaughterhouse production lines also places considerable pressure on workers, increasing rates of worker injury [72]. Pachirat (2011) exemplified the pressures in a description of the work in the liver-packer room of a beef slaughterhouse: "At the rate of one cow, steer, or heifer slaughtered every twelve seconds per nine-hour working day, the reality that the work of the slaughterhouse centers around killing evaporates into a routinized, almost hallucinatory blur. By the end of the day, by liver number 2394 or foot number 9576, it hardly matters what is being cut, shorn, sliced, shredded, hung, or washed: all that matters is that the day is once again, finally coming to a close" [73] (p. 138).

It is understandable (if not excusable), that the rapid pace of slaughtering and processing required by high volume production processes, combined with the necessity of a callous mind-set toward the animals, and the minimal training, difficult conditions and low pay rates provided to workers, create conditions in which workers might vent their frustrations on the animals—when they baulk at strange or disturbing sounds, smells, environments, or at rapid, forceful handling, which cause delays and require physically tired workers to exert extra effort. Burt (2006) asserted that increasingly detached forms of the dispatching of animals are prompted more by concern for speed and thus profit, than for welfare [74]. In her study of London slaughterhouse workers, Cudworth (2015) reported verbal abuse of animals, and the use of electric goads used to hurry them. She stated that "violence towards domesticated animals is routinized, systemic and legitimated" [70] (p. 14).

Given such circumstances, it is perhaps unsurprising that Gail Eisenitz's (1997) extensive study of U.S. slaughterhouses revealed alarming tales of systematic and normative cruelty against animals [75]. And indeed, despite commitments to humane practices and applicable legislation, abuses of animals within slaughterhouses remain prevalent even today.

12. Implications for Modern Slaughterhouses

Socioeconomic conditions in East London in the 1880s were dire, and the harsh realities of the time were reflected in the slaughterhouses that were so numerous within its crowded and squalid streets [18]. As noted previously, Barnett (1888, p. 3) described the resultant deplorable scenes in *The Times*, concluding that "For the sake of both health and morals the slaughtering should be done outside the town" [22].

More than 125 years later, Barnett's wishes have come true. Slaughtering is no longer conducted within urban centres, and has generally been removed to rural locations far less visible. The numerous small operations of the 1880s have been amalgamated into larger corporate enterprises. However, these have become vaster, more impersonal, industrialised systems of killing, within which animal abuse continues.

Modern standards for humane slaughter do exist [76–78]. They acknowledge that after traveling what may be considerable distances to these much larger, modern, slaughterhouses, animals often arrive hungry, thirsty and exhausted. Significant social stress may result from mixing with unfamiliar animals. They prescribe that when lairaged in pens at the slaughterhouse, animals should be watered, fed, and protected from environmental extremes. Those that arrive ill should be treated or slaughtered without delay. Too often, however, this does not occur [79].

The races and approaches to the killing area should be designed to minimise fear and distress, animals should always be handled humanely, and the killing process should be conducted using humane restraint and effective stunning. Different species are killed using a variety of methods determined partly by their physical size and the mechanisation of the slaughter process, but to eliminate pain and suffering associated with the killing method, animals should always be unconscious at the time of slaughter.

In reality however, slaughterhouse designs are often suboptimal, stunning equipment is used at insufficient voltages, or is poorly maintained, resulting in ineffective stunning, and high line speeds and time constraints continue to place slaughterhouse staff under considerable pressure. Within such systems, animal stress, fear, pain and suffering is inevitable.

Various undercover investigations have revealed inhumane treatment, and even blatant abuse, of animals, in slaughterhouses. Since 2009, British animal advocacy organization Animal Aid has covertly filmed from within ten randomly chosen British slaughterhouses. They found evidence of cruelty and law breaking in nine of them. Their footage reveals animals being kicked, slapped, stamped on, picked up by fleeces and ears, and thrown into stunning pens. Animals are improperly stunned and killed, including by throat-cutting, while still conscious. Some are deliberately beaten, and pigs were filmed being burned with cigarettes [80].

The effects for both humans and animals caught up within these systems are deeply disturbing. Significant empirical evidence indicates that ongoing involvement in the commission of violent acts—particularly when required for economic or literal survival (as in the case of warfare [81,82])—can result in desensitisation toward violence in general, and increases in rates of the most violent crimes within surrounding communities. As noted by Kristina Mering in her study of Estonian slaughterhouse workers, "The core problem is the animal-industrial complex, the system of exploiting animals which also has negative effects on the workers in the system ... " [33]. Today, such exploitative systems undoubtedly contribute to the disturbing rates of animal welfare abuses reported within modern slaughterhouses. In East London in the 1880s, they may well have contributed to the development of the world's most infamous serial killer.

Stimulated by the disturbing slaughterhouse practices of the day, a broad urban-based animal welfare and slaughterhouse reform movement emerged in nineteenth-century Britain. Contemporary techniques based on the pole-axe, nape-stab, and Jewish ritual slaughter were too unreliable or too slow to ensure insensibility prior to exsanguination. And so stunning technologies such as captive bolt pistols were developed and tested throughout the nineteenth century. Humanitarian groups advocated the humane slaughter principle—that no animal should be slaughtered without first being stunned into insensibility. However, they were successfully opposed by the butchers' trade organization, so the humane slaughter principle did not receive legislative sanction until the 1930s [83].

This old struggle between proponents and opponents of animal slaughtering reforms continues with similar vigour today. Within the UK, recent animal welfare abuses have led to the installation of CCTV, to monitor and improve animal welfare. According to the Food Standards Agency, 90% of British slaughterhouses now have CCTV installed. However, the footage is not monitored independently of the slaughterhouse business operator, and even the official veterinarians required to oversee the slaughtering and processing process are commonly refused access to it. As of January 2017, this deplorable situation persists, despite the serious objections of the British Veterinary Association (BVA) and the Veterinary Public Health Association (VPHA). BVA President Sean Wensley stated, "It is unacceptable that there are slaughterhouses that are not willing to share CCTV footage with official veterinarians. We are lobbying for CCTV to be mandatory in all slaughterhouses and for legislation to ensure that footage is readily available to vets" [84].

13. Conclusions

The brutality with which Jack the Ripper despatched and subsequently mutilated his victims in the 1880s was unprecedented within modern history, and plunged East London into a climate of fear. Widespread media reporting of Jack's crimes, combined with the inability of the police to catch him, resulted in a fascination with the case that remains strong to this day.

Jack's ability to rapidly locate and remove specific organs from several of his victims, in conditions of haste and very poor light, led to theories that he must have been surgically trained. However, re-examination of a mortuary sketch of one of his victims has revealed key aspects of the incisional technique used that are highly inconsistent with professional surgical training. Related discrepancies are also apparent in the language used within the only letter from Jack considered probably authentic.

Furthermore, the throat-cutting technique used to kill his victims, combined with Jack's undoubted propensity for anatomical dissection with a knife, were highly consistent with the skillset of slaughterers of the times. And indeed, a very large number of small-scale slaughterhouses existed within the districts in which the murders occurred. The harsh socioeconomic conditions of the times may have influenced how the animals and their body parts were treated, as well as the subsequent behaviour of the murderer. We will never know for certain, but it is highly likely that Jack the Ripper honed the physical skills, and the psychological and behavioural attributes employed on his victims to such devastating effect, during his employment as a slaughterhouse worker.

These insights should stimulate a fundamental re-examination of the acceptability of animal slaughter today. Modern slaughterhouses are more humane in some ways than those of nineteenth-century East London; however, the vast, impersonal, mechanized killing operations of the twenty-first century are more desensitizing in others. With more than 70 billion terrestrial animals slaughtered annually in slaughterhouses of varying standards internationally by 2013 (The most recently reported year, by April 2017) [85], this represents one of the greatest animal welfare issues today.

Additionally, a considerable weight of recent sociological evidence indicates that those who commit violence towards animals are more likely to target people, and that rates of the most violent crimes are increased in communities surrounding slaughterhouses. Accordingly, the acceptability of animal slaughter should also be profoundly questioned on the basis of its potential human and societal impacts.

Acknowledgments: Open access publication costs were covered by the University of Winchester.

Author Contributions: Andrew Knight conceived the study, researched the aspects relating to the technical skills and language exhibited by the murderer, and the aspects relating to animal welfare and human–animal violence links, and authored the paper. Katherine D. Watson researched the historical aspects including those relating to the case of Jack the Ripper, and the social demographics and slaughterhouses in nineteenth-century London, and co-authored the paper.

Conflicts of Interest: The authors declare no conflict of interest.

References

1. Evans, S.P.; Skinner, K. *The Ultimate Jack the Ripper Sourcebook: An Illustrated Encyclopedia*; Constable and Robinson: London, UK, 2000.
2. Bond, T. *Notes of Examination of Body of Woman Found Murdered & Mutilated in Dorset Street*; MEPO 3/3153, ff. 12–14; The National Archives: Kew, UK, 1888.
3. Ryder, S.P. Casebook: Jack the Ripper, 1996–2013. Available online: http://www.casebook.org (accessed on 26 September 2016).
4. Marks, K. Was Jack the Ripper a woman? *The Independent.* 18 May 2006. Available online: http://www.independent.co.uk/news/science/was-jack-the-ripper-a-woman-478597.html (accessed on 28 August 2015).
5. Weston-Davies, W. *The Real Mary Kelly: Jack the Ripper's Fifth Victim and the Identity of the Man that Killed Her*; Blink: London, UK, 2016.
6. Sugden, P. *The Complete History of Jack the Ripper*; Robinson: London, UK, 2002.
7. Baranski, A. *Surgical Technique of Abdominal Organ Procurement*; Springer: London, UK, 2009.

8.   Vikram, K.; Maroju, N.K. Exploratory Laparotomy. 2015. Available online: http://emedicine.medscape. com/article/1829835-overview (accessed on 5 February 2017).

9.   Carter, H.V. Diagram of sheath of Rectus above the arcuate line. In *Anatomy of the Human Body*; Gray, H., Ed.; Lea & Febinger: Philadelphia, PA, USA; New York, NY, USA, 1918; Available online: https://commons. wikimedia.org/w/index.php?curid=4735337 (accessed on 5 February 2017).

10. Thibodeau, G.A.; Patton, K.T. Linea alba. In *Mosby's Medical Dictionary*, 9th ed.; Elsevier: Amsterdam, The Netherlands, 2009; Available online: http://medical-dictionary.thefreedictionary.com/linea+alba (accessed on 5 February 2017).

11. Roses, R.E.; Morris, J.B. Incisions, closures and management of the abdominal wound. In *Maingot's Abdominal Operation*, 12th ed.; Zinner, M.J., Ashley, S.W., Eds.; McGraw Hill Medical: New York, NY, USA, 2013; pp. 99–122.

12. Hamilton, F.H. *Principles and Practice of Surgery*, 3rd ed.; William Wood & Co.: New York, NY, USA, 1886.

13. Holme, T. *A Treatise on Surgery: Its Principles and Practice*, 5th ed.; Smith, Elder & Co.: London, UK, 1888.

14. Williams, W. *The Principles and Practice of Veterinary Surgery*; John Menzies & Co.: Edinburgh, UK, 1893.

15. Evans, S.P.; Skinner, K. *Jack the Ripper and the Whitechapel Murders*; Document Pack; PRO Publications: Kew, UK, 2002.

16. Anonymous. The London murders. *Denbighshire Free Press*, 6 October 1888; 6.

17. Anonymous. The murder of Annie J. Chapman. *South Wales Echo*, 27 September 1888; 4.

18. MacLachlan, I. A bloody offal nuisance: The persistence of private slaughter-houses in nineteenth-century London. *Urban History* **2007**, *34*, 227–254. [CrossRef]

19. Anonymous. The meat supply of London. *Birmingham Daily Post*, 24 December 1888; 7.

20. Anonymous. Horrible murder in Whitechapel. *The Flintshire Observer*, 6 September 1888; 2.

21. Odell, R. *Ripperology: A Study of the World's First Serial Killer and a Literary Phenomenon*; The Kent State University Press: Kent, OH, USA, 2006.

22. Barnett, S.A. At last (letter). *The Times*, 19 September 1888; 3.

23. Camps, F.E. More about "Jack the Ripper". *Lond. Hosp. Gaz.* **1966**, *69*, 27–35.

24. Shechita UK. *A Guide to Shechita*; Shechita UK: London, UK, 2009; Available online: http://www.shechitauk. org/publications (accessed on 9 January 2016).

25. Velarde, A.; Rodriguez, P.; Dalmau, A.; Fuentes, C.; Llonch, P.; von Holleben, K.V.; Anil, M.H.; Lambooij, J.B.; Pleiter, H.; Yesildere, T.; et al. Religious slaughter: Evaluation of current practices in selected countries. *Meat Sci.* **2014**, *96*, 278–287. [CrossRef] [PubMed]

26. Evans, S.P.; Rumbelow, D. *Jack the Ripper: Scotland Yard Investigates*; Sutton Publishing: Stroud, UK, 2006.

27. Image in the Public Domain. Available online: https://en.wikipedia.org/wiki/From_Hell_letter#/media/ File:FromHellLetter.jpg (accessed on 5 February 2017).

28. Barnett, S.A. Whitechapel horrors (letter). *The Times*, 23 July 1889; 10.

29. Wedderburn, P. Dangerous dogs: Time for a new approach. *Daily Telegraph*, 5 July 2010.

30. Seng, P.M.; Laporte, R. Animal welfare: The role and perspectives of the meat and livestock sector. *Rev. Sci. Tech.* **2005**, *24*, 613–623. [PubMed]

31. Jacques, J.R. The slaughterhouse, social disorganization, and violent crime in rural communities. *Soc. Anim.* **2015**, *23*, 594–612. [CrossRef]

32. Cohidon, C.; Morisseau, P.; Derriennic, F.; Goldberg, M.; Imbernon, E. Psychosocial factors at work and perceived health among agricultural meat industry workers in France. *Int. Arch. Occup. Environ. Health* **2009**, *82*, 807–818. [CrossRef] [PubMed]

33. Leenaert, T. Slaughterhouse Workers: The Meat Industry's Other Victims. 2016. Available online: http://veganstrategist.org/2016/08/05/slaughterhouse-workers-the-meat-industrys-other-victims/ (accessed on 29 January 2017).

34. Fitzgerald, A.J.; Kalof, L.; Dietz, T. Slaughterhouses and increased crime rates: An empirical analysis of the spillover from "The Jungle" into the surrounding community. *Organ. Environ.* **2009**, *22*, 158–184. [CrossRef]

35. U.S. Bureau of Labor Statistics. *Table SNR01: Highest Incidence Rates of Total Nonfatal Occupational Injury and Illness Cases, Private Industry, 2003*; U.S. Department of Labor, Bureau of Labor Statistics: Washington, DC, USA, 2005. Available online: https://www.bls.gov/iif/oshsum.htm#03Summary_News_Release (accessed on 11 February 2017).

36. U.S. Bureau of Labor Statistics. *Table SNR06: Highest Incidence Rates of Total Nonfatal Occupational Injury Cases, Private Industry, 2003*; U.S. Department of Labor, Bureau of Labor Statistics: Washington, DC, USA, 2005. Available online: https://www.bls.gov/iif/oshsum.htm#03Summary_News_Release (accessed on 11 February 2017).

37. Cortes, K. *Do Immigrants Benefit from An Increase in the Minimum Wage Rate? An Analysis by Immigrant Industry Concentration*; University of California Press: Berkeley, CA, USA, 2005.

38. U.S. Census Bureau, Economic Planning and Coordination Division. *County Business Patterns*; U.S. Census Bureau: Washington, DC, USA, 2006; Volume 2006.

39. Broadway, M.J. Meatpacking and its social and economic consequences for Garden City, Kansas in the 1980s. *Urban Anthropol.* **1990**, *19*, 321–344.

40. Broadway, M.J. Planning for change in small towns or trying to avoid the slaughterhouse blues. *J. Rural Stud.* **2000**, *16*, 37–46. [CrossRef]

41. Stull, D.; Broadway, M. *Slaughterhouse Blues: The Meat and Poultry Industry in North America*; Wadsworth: Toronto, ON, Canada, 2004.

42. Pinel, P. *Treatise on Insanity*; Hafner: New York, NY, USA, 1962; (Original Work Published 1806).

43. Macdonald, J.M. *The Murderer and His Victim*; Charles C. Thomas: Springfield, IL, USA, 1961.

44. Mead, M. Cultural factors in the cause and prevention of pathological homicide. *Bull. Menn. Clin.* **1964**, *28*, 11–22.

45. Wright, J.; Hensley, C. From animal cruelty to serial murder: Applying the graduation hypothesis. *Int. J. Offender Ther. Comp. Criminol.* **2003**, *47*, 72–89. [CrossRef] [PubMed]

46. Ressler, R.; Burgess, A.; Douglas, J. *Sexual Homicides: Patterns and Motives*; Lexington Books: Lexington, MA, USA, 1988.

47. American Psychological Association. *Diagnostic and Statistical Manual of Mental Disorders*, 3rd ed.; American Psychological Association: Washington, DC, USA, 1987.

48. American Psychological Association. *Diagnostic and Statistical Manual of Mental Disorders*, 4th ed.; American Psychiatric Association: Washington, DC, USA, 1994.

49. American Psychological Association. *Diagnostic and Statistical Manual of Mental Disorders*, 4th ed.; Text Revision; American Psychiatric Association: Washington, DC, USA, 2000.

50. American Psychological Association. *Diagnostic and Statistical Manual of Mental Disorders*, 5th ed.; American Psychiatric Association: Washington, DC, USA, 2013.

51. Gleyzer, R.; Felthous, A.R.; Holzer, C.E. Animal cruelty and psychiatric disorders. *J. Am. Acad. Psych. Law* **2002**, *30*, 257–265.

52. Hensley, C.; Tallichet, S.E.; Dutkiewicz, E.L. Recurrent childhood animal cruelty: Is there a relationship to adult recurrent interpersonal violence? *Crim. Justice Rev.* **2009**, *34*, 248–257. [CrossRef]

53. Merz-Perez, L.; Heide, K.M.; Silverman, I.J. Childhood cruelty and subsequent violence against humans. *Int. J. Offender Ther. Comp. Criminol.* **2001**, *45*, 556–573. [CrossRef]

54. Merz-Perez, L.; Heide, K.M. *Animal Cruelty: Pathway to Violence Against People*; Rowman & Littlefield: Lanham, MD, USA, 2004.

55. Ressler, R.K.; Burgess, A.W.; Hartman, C.R.; Douglas, J.E.; McCormack, A. Murderers who rape and mutilate. *J. Interpers. Violence* **1998**, *1*, 273–287. [CrossRef]

56. Tallichet, S.E.; Hensley, C. Exploring the link between recurrent acts of childhood and adolescent animal cruelty and subsequent violent crime. *Crim. Justice Rev.* **2004**, *29*, 304–316. [CrossRef]

57. Verlinden, S. Risk Factors in School Shootings. Ph.D. Thesis, Pacific University, Forest Grove, OR, USA, 2000.

58. Walters, G.D. Testing the specificity postulate of the violence graduation hypothesis: Meta-analyses of the animal cruelty-offending relationship. *Aggress. Violent Behav.* **2013**, *18*, 797–802. [CrossRef]

59. Faver, C.A.; Strand, E.B. To leave or to stay? Battered women's concern for vulnerable pets. *J. Interpers. Violence* **2003**, *18*, 1367–1377. [CrossRef] [PubMed]

60. Volant, A.M.; Johnson, J.A.; Gullone, E.; Coleman, G.J. The relationship between domestic violence and animal abuse: An Australian study. *J. Interpers. Violence* **2008**, *23*, 1277–1295. [CrossRef] [PubMed]

61. Carlisle-Frank, P.; Frank, J.M.; Nielsen, L. Selective battering of the family pet. *Anthrozoos* **2004**, *17*, 26–42. [CrossRef]

62. Ascione, F.R.; Weber, C.V.; Thompson, T.M.; Heath, J.; Maruyama, M.; Hayashi, K. Battered pets and domestic violence: Animal abuse reported by women experiencing intimate violence and by nonabused women. *Violence Against Women* **2007**, *13*, 354–373. [CrossRef] [PubMed]

63. Ascione, F.R. Battered women's reports of their partners' and their children's cruelty to animals. *J. Emot. Abuse* **1998**, *1*, 119–133. [CrossRef]

64. Flynn, C.P. Woman's best friend: Pet abuse and the role of companion animals in the lives of battered women. *Violence Against Women* **2000**, *6*, 162–177. [CrossRef]

65. Simmons, C.A.; Lehmann, P. Exploring the link between pet abuse and controlling behaviors in violent relationships. *J. Interpers. Violence* **2007**, *22*, 1211–1222. [CrossRef] [PubMed]

66. Flynn, C.P. Examining the links between animal abuse and human violence. *Crime Law Soc. Change* **2011**, *55*, 453–468. [CrossRef]

67. Arluke, A.; Levin, J.; Luke, C.; Ascione, F.R. The relationship of animal abuse to violence and other forms of antisocial behavior. *J. Interpers. Violence* **1999**, *14*, 963–976. [CrossRef]

68. Miller, K.S.; Knutson, J.F. Reports of severe physical punishment and exposure to animal cruelty by inmates convicted of felonies and by university students. *Child Abuse Negl.* **1997**, *21*, 59–82. [CrossRef]

69. Felthous, A.R.; Kellert, S.R. Childhood cruelty to animals and later aggression against people: A review. *Am. J. Psychiatry* **1987**, *144*, 710–717. [PubMed]

70. Cudworth, E. Killing animals: Sociology, species relations and institutionalized violence. *Sociol. Rev.* **2015**, *63*, 1–18. [CrossRef]

71. Dillard, J. A slaughterhouse nightmare: Psychological harm suffered by slaughterhouse employees and the possibility of redress through legal reform. *Georget. J. Poverty Law Policy* **2008**, *15*, 391–408.

72. Winders, B.; Nibert, D. Consuming the surplus: Expanding "meat" consumption and animal oppression. *Int. J. Sociol. Soc. Policy* **2004**, *24*, 76–96. [CrossRef]

73. Pachirat, T. *Every Twelve Seconds: Industrialized Slaughter and the Politics of Sight*; Yale University Press: New Haven, CT, USA, 2011.

74. Burt, J. Conflicts around slaughter in modernity. In *Killing Animals*; The Animal Studies Group; University of Illinois Press: Urbana, IL, USA, 2006; pp. 120–144.

75. Eisenitz, G. *Slaughterhouse: The Shocking Tales of Greed, Neglect and Inhumane Treatment inside the U.S. Meat Industry*; Prometheus Books: New York, NY, USA, 1997.

76. Shimshony, A.; Chaudry, M.M. Slaughter of animals for human consumption. *Rev. Sci. Tech.* **2005**, *24*, 693–710. [PubMed]

77. American Veterinary Medical Association. *AVMA Guidelines for the Humane Slaughter of Animals: 2016 Edition*; American Veterinary Medical Association: Schaumburg, IL, USA, 2016. Available online: https://www.avma.org/KB/Resources/Reference/AnimalWelfare/Documents/Humane-Slaughter-Guidelines.pdf (accessed on 6 April 2017).

78. World Organisation for Animal Health (OIE). Chapter 7.5. Slaughter of Animals. 2016. Available online: http://www.oie.int/international-standard-setting/terrestrial-code/access-online/ (accessed on 14 June 2016).

79. Farm Animal Welfare Council. *Report on the Welfare of Farmed Animals at Slaughter or Killing Part 1: Red Meat Animals*; Defra Publications: London, UK, 2003.

80. Animal Aid. The "Humane Slaughter" Myth. 2016. Available online: http://www.animalaid.org.uk/h/n/CAMPAIGNS/slaughter/ALL/// (accessed on 6 August 2016).

81. Sanday, P.R. The socio-cultural context of rape: A cross-cultural study. *J. Soc. Issues* **1981**, *37*, 5–27. [CrossRef]

82. Archer, D.; Gartner, R. *Violence and Crime in Cross-National Perspective*; Yale University Press: New Haven, CT, USA, 1987.

83. MacLachlan, I. Coup de grâce: Humane cattle slaughter in nineteenth-century Britain. *Food Hist.* **2005**, *3*, 145–171. [CrossRef]

84. Anon. Vets Call for Unrestricted Access to Slaughterhouse CCTV. 2016. Available online: https://www.bva.co.uk/News-campaigns-and-policy/Newsroom/News-releases/Vets-call-unrestricted-access-slaughterhouse-CCTV/ (accessed on 6 August 2016).

85. Food and Agriculture of the United Nations. FAOSTAT (Database): Livestock Primary (2017). Available online: http://www.fao.org/faostat/en/#data/QL (accessed on 3 April 2017).

6

Exploration Feeding and Higher Space Allocation Improve Welfare of Growing-Finishing Pigs

Herman M. Vermeer *, **Nienke C. P. M. M. Dirx-Kuijken and Marc B. M. Bracke**

Wageningen Livestock Research, P.O. Box 338, Wageningen 6700 AH, The Netherlands; nienke.dirx@wur.nl (N.C.P.M.M.D.-K.); marc.bracke@wur.nl (M.B.M.B.)
* Correspondence: herman.vermeer@wur.nl

Academic Editor: Clive J. C. Phillips

Simple Summary: A lack of exploration materials in pig pens can result in damaging behavior towards pen mates. The objective of our study was to reduce skin and tail lesions by frequently providing small amounts of feed on the floor and by providing more space per pig. Both the so-called "exploration feeding" and the additional space resulted in fewer skin lesions. Finally, this can lead to a more welfare-friendly pig husbandry.

Abstract: Lack of environmental enrichment and high stocking densities in growing-finishing pigs can lead to adverse social behaviors directed to pen mates, resulting in skin lesions, lameness, and tail biting. The objective of the study was to improve animal welfare and prevent biting behavior in an experiment with a $2 \times 2 \times 2$ factorial design on exploration feeding, stocking density, and sex. We kept 550 pigs in 69 pens from 63 days to 171 days of life. Pigs were supplemented with or without exploration feeding, kept in groups of seven (1.0 m^2/pig) or nine animals (0.8 m^2/pig) and separated per sex. Exploration feeding provided small amounts of feed periodically on the solid floor. Skin lesion scores were significantly lower in pens with exploration feeding ($p = 0.028$, $p < 0.001$, $p < 0.001$ for front, middle, and hind body), in pens with high compared to low space allowance ($p = 0.005$, $p = 0.006$, $p < 0.001$ for front, middle and hind body), and in pens with females compared to males ($p < 0.001$, $p = 0.005$, $p < 0.001$ for front, middle and hind body). Males with exploration feeding had fewer front skin lesions than females with exploration feeding ($p = 0.022$). Pigs with 1.0 m^2 compared to 0.8 m^2 per pig had a higher daily gain of 27 g per pig per day ($p = 0.04$) and males compared to females had a higher daily gain of 39 g per pig per day ($p = 0.01$). These results indicate that exploration feeding might contribute to the development of a more welfare-friendly pig husbandry with intact tails in the near future.

Keywords: animal welfare; environmental enrichment; feeding method; pig; stocking density

---

1. Introduction

The Dutch Ministry of Economic Affairs would like to see an increased number of pig production chains addressing improved pig welfare. The sustainable pork chain called "De Hoeve" wants to be at the forefront in taking the next step in the area of animal welfare. This step consists of no longer docking the tails of the piglets. Up to now, not docking in conventional pig husbandry increases the risk of tail biting [1,2]. More enrichment, space (low stocking density), stable social groups, and improved management may contribute significantly to healthy curly tails of slaughter pigs [1,3,4].

Enrichment was identified as the main risk factor [5], but also fully and partially slatted floors, more than five animals per feeding space and less than 1 m^2 per animal may increase the risk of tail biting. The European Union welfare regulations require 0.65 m^2 per pig and in The Netherlands 0.80 m^2 per pig up to 110 kg. This project examined how tail and skin damage can be prevented with exploration feeding, a lower stocking density, and separate sexes (males and females). The study was conducted at the demonstration farm of the Dutch sustainable pork chain "De Hoeve". The proximate aim of this project was to reduce biting wounds on the skin and tails by periodically providing small amounts of food on the floor as environmental enrichment.

The objective was to produce slaughter pigs without tail biting in docked tails, skin without lesions, and sound legs, including good performance as a step on the route towards no tail biting in pigs with intact tails.

2. Materials and Methods

2.1. Animals

In total 550 pigs in nine batches were followed during the growing finishing period. These were crossbred German Pietrain terminal boar × Topigs20 sow. Half of the pigs were males ($n = 275$) and half were females ($n = 275$). The animals entered the growing finishing unit at nine weeks of age. After 108 (89–133) days on average they were ready for slaughter at 116 (91–140) kg body weight. The animals were born and finished at the same farm. At weaning, the littermates were kept together as much as possible, and groups contained both males and females. Weaners were kept in stable groups of 15–20 animals. Mixing happened when the pigs entered the finishing house at 63 days of age, where males and females were raised in separate pens. The animals had a tail of medium length, which was about 8 cm long at the time of slaughter. Tails were docked using electric cauterization at three to four days after birth, combined with an iron injection and receiving an ear tag. The tails were left slightly longer than was routine practice at the farm and males were not castrated.

2.2. Ethical Statement

The study was conducted in accordance with the Declaration of Helsinki, and the protocol was considered not harmful for the animals. The treatments were additional environmental enrichment and regarded as beneficial for animal welfare and the observations were all non-invasive.

2.3. Housing

The animals were housed in a finishing house in nine identical rooms with eight pens of 6.9 m^2 each (Figure 1). Each pen contained either seven or nine animals, resulting in space allowances of 1.0 m^2/pig or 0.8 m^2/pig respectively. The pens were equipped with a chain and plastic ball combination as enrichment material. Starting from the inspection alley, pens had concrete slats (1.20 m), a solid convex lying area (1.40 m), and metal slats (1.05 m). The pens were 1.90 m wide with a total area of 6.94 m^2. Fresh air entered through the ceiling and was discharged via a fan in the back of the unit. Artificial light was on from 6 a.m. to 10 p.m.

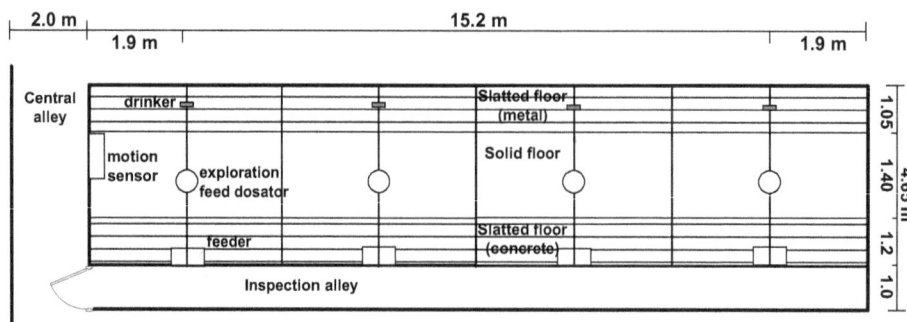

Figure 1. Layout of one of the nine rooms with eight pens with motion sensors and dosators.

The animals were all fed ad libitum using dry pelleted feed. Feed was provided in a dry-wet feeder with one feeding space per pen. Several times a day the feeder was replenished by an automatic feeding system. Drinking water was presented ad libitum in a water bowl in the back of the pen.

2.4. Design

The study had a 2 × 2 × 2 factorial design. The three factors were:

(1)   Exploration feeding: present or absent.
(2)   Space allowance/group size: nine pigs at 0.8 m² per pig or seven pigs at 1.0 m²/pig.
(3)   Sex: males (entire males) or females.

Nine identical rooms were used and each room had eight pens. Pens were randomly assigned to treatment combinations, and every combination was allocated to one pen per room. Males and females were kept in alternate pens. Due to a lack of sufficient animals, 3 pens of the potential 72 pens remained empty, resulting in a total of 69 pens in the dataset.

2.5. Exploration Feeding

In the pens with exploration feeding, the animals received additional small amounts of pelleted feed on the solid floor 25 to 30 times a day during the light period. The feed was provided via a volume dispenser containing several litres of feed (dosator) with an auger. Per two pens, one dosator was mounted with two outflow openings, one per pen (Figure 1). In the pens without exploration feeding the outflow opening was closed. The system was specially designed for this experiment (Coppens Constructie en Stalinrichtingen BV, Westerhoven, The Netherlands).

Provision of the feed was only possible during the light period between 6 a.m. and 10 p.m. The number of seconds that the auger turned determined the amount of feed provided. Times were set using a central process computer in the central corridor, where provided portions were recorded as "pulses". The quantity of feed provided each time was dependent on the age of the animals. During the first three weeks in the finishing house the pigs received feed for 3 s per portion, which resulted in the distribution of 27 g of feed on average. After three weeks, feed was provided for just one second per portion, which resulted in 12 g each time. Supply frequencies depended on the activity of a single pig or group(s) of pigs as registered with a motion sensor. The maximum number of portions was 42 in the first period and 29 in the last period. This infrared sensitive motion sensor was mounted at the front wall of the room where it detected activity especially in the first pens. When activity was registered for three minutes exploration feed was provided; but when within this period a period of more than 15 s of inactivity was registered, the timer was restarted. The minimum waiting time between bouts of exploration feeding was set at 20 min (during the first three weeks) or 30 min (after three weeks).

The first three weeks in the finishing house up to 42 portions per day could be provided (between 6 a.m. and 10 p.m. = 16 h divided by 23 min (20 min + 3 min activity). After three weeks until 100 days after start of the finishing period the maximum number of portions per day was 29 (16 h divided by 33 min). More details are available in the Dutch research report [6].

2.6. Data Collection

All data was collected on the animal level, but for analysis the pen averages per observation were used. From the second week on lesions of the skin, legs, and tails were scored using existing protocols every four to five weeks. Some batches were scored three, others four times, depending on how soon the first pigs were ready for slaughter in the fourth month and the observations stopped.

For skin lesions, separate scores were given for the front, middle, and hind parts of the pigs on a scale from 0 to 5 with increasing level of lesions (where 0 = none, 1 = low, 2 = mild, 3 = moderate, 4 = severe, 5 = very severe). In this visual score fresh, red lesions have a higher weight than older, black scars (crusts). With this protocol, it is not possible to discriminate between lesions caused by aggression due to the initial mixing of the pigs and by competition for resources like feed.

For scoring legs the Welfare Quality®, lameness protocol was used [7], using a scale from 0 to 2 (where 0 = not lame; 1 = non symmetrical walking but using all feet; 2 = not using one of the legs).

Tails were scored according to the protocol of Zonderland [8], where tail length related to starting length is scored in five classes (1: complete tail; 2: three quarters left; 3: half left; 4: one quarter left; 5: less than a quarter of the tail left), tail lesions in three classes (1: no injury; 2: bite marks; 3: one or more wounds), and blood on the tail in four classes (1: no blood; 2: dark brown/black, i.e., dry crust; 3: dark red/brown, i.e., older blood; 4: red, i.e., fresh blood and wet tail tips).

The following production and slaughter parameters were recorded per pig: mortality, starting weight, starting date, slaughter date, cold carcass weight (from which mean end weights and growth rates per pen were calculated), meat percentage, muscle, and fat thickness. We used the Dutch equation live weight = carcass weight × (1.3 + (83 − carcass weight) × 0.0025) to calculate live weight from cold carcass weight [9].

2.7. Statistical Analysis

Skin, leg, and tail scores were analyzed with a generalized linear mixed model for ordinal data in Genstat 18th Edition (VSN International, Hemel Hempstead, UK) [10]. Fixed effects were month after start of batch, exploration feeding, group size, and sex (including two way interactions). Random effects were room, pen number, starting date, and the interaction between starting date and month. The hypotheses were all tested with a significance level of 0.05.

In the ordinal model the K-1 intercept terms or thresholds (αn) are estimated, where K is the number of classes in the class-score, using the equation Logit (γn (x)) = αn + βTx, where βTx is a short notation of all model terms. Thresholds, averages for the underlying distribution Z, and variance components for all the terms in the random model were estimated using the method as described in [11], using the procedure IRCLASS [12].

Growth rates were calculated—using the starting weight, number of days in the room, and the calculated live weight—and analyzed using REML (REsidual Maximum Likelihood) in Genstat 18th Edition [10] with exploration feeding, group size, and sex as fixed effects and room and pen as random effects.

3. Results

3.1. Usage of Exploration Feeding

Growing pigs (until three weeks in the finishing house) realized about 30 portions per day, which was 75% of the maximum number of portions. During the rest of the finishing period the pigs realized 23 portions, which was 80% of the maximum portions. Over time, the number of portions slightly decreased, but this is partly caused by the extension of the intervals between the portions. On average, pig pens with exploration feeding received 1250 g of additional feed per animal during the growing-finishing period, this was 12 g per animal per day. Assuming that all the exploration feed was consumed, this implied that exploration feeding contributed about 0.5% to the overall feed intake (which was 2.6 kg/day).

3.2. Skin, Leg, and Tail Scores

In Table 1, the results of the skin scores are summarized for the main factors (exploration feeding, space allowance, and sex). All factors had significant effects on the skin lesion scores. Over time, the skin lesion scores on the front body declined ($p = 0.03$). The skin lesion scores on the middle and hind body were not affected by month (Table 2).

Table 1. Mean skin lesion scores (0–5) at the front, middle and back of the pigs related to the main treatment factors with SEM (Standard Error of the Mean) and p value for 64 pens in total.

Lesion Score	Exploration Feeding	No Exploration Feeding	SEM	p Value
Front	1.66	1.77	0.039	0.028
Middle	1.34	1.58	0.040	<0.001
Back	1.26	1.5	0.036	<0.001
n pens	33	36		
	1.0 m²/pig	**0.8 m²/pig**	**SEM**	**p Value**
Front	1.66	1.78	0.039	0.005
Middle	1.39	1.53	0.040	0.006
Back	1.30	1.46	0.036	<0.001
n pens	33	36		
	Males	**Females**	**SEM**	**p Value**
Front	1.86	1.57	0.039	<0.001
Middle	1.54	1.38	0.040	0.005
Back	1.48	1.28	0.036	<0.001
n pens	36	33		

Table 2. Mean skin lesion scores (0–5) at the front, middle and back of the pigs related to month (age) with SEM and p value for 64 pens in total; different superscripts within a row indicate a statistical difference ($p < 0.05$).

Lesion Score	Month 1	Month 2	Month 3	Month 4	SEM	p Value
Front	1.92 [a]	1.89 [a]	1.56 [b]	1.48 [b]	0.034	0.03
Middle	1.64	1.68	1.3	1.22	0.033	0.123
Back	1.32	1.55	1.29	1.42	0.033	0.675
n pens	69	53	63	53		

An interaction was found between exploration feeding and sex ($p = 0.022$) for the skin lesion score on the front of the pig. Males had higher skin lesion scores at the front than females, and this difference is smaller with exploration feeding compared to no exploration feeding ($p = 0.022$; Figure 2). Another significant interaction was found between space allowance and month for the skin lesions scores at the hind body part ($p = 0.042$; Figure 3). A higher stocking density resulted in more skin lesions at the hind body part and the difference increased over time.

Of the 2178 observed legs, only 33 (1.5%) scored a 1 or 2 for lameness, with no effect of treatments. Initial tail lengths varied considerably, and the experimental treatments had no effect on the scores for tail length, tail lesion, and blood score. During the trial, hardly any tail was shortened due to tail biting. Occasionally tail biting was observed. The level of tail wounds and blood scores decreased from the first to the third month (Table 3).

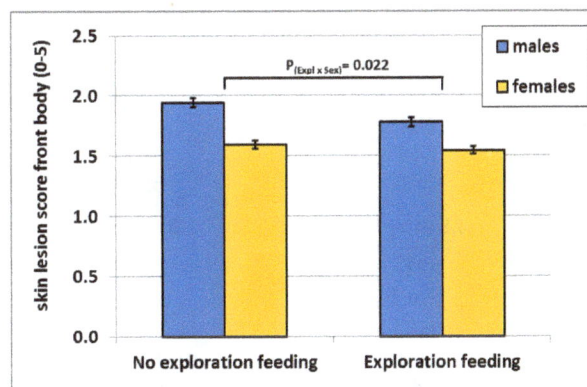

Figure 2. Mean front skin lesion score per treatment (exploration feeding) and sex with SEM.

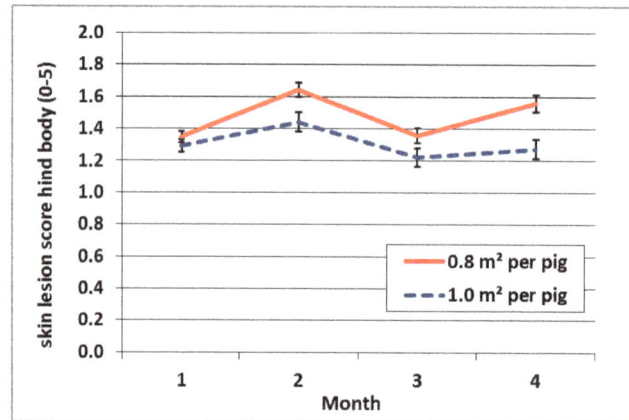

Figure 3. Mean skin lesion scores at the hind body part with SEM in error bars per month for high and low space allowance.

Table 3. Mean tail length, lesions, and blood scores over time with SEM and p value; different superscripts within a row indicate a statistical difference ($p < 0.05$).

Month	1	2	3	4	SEM	p Value
Tail length	1.028	1.000	1.000	1.002	0.007	no analysis possible *
Tail lesions	1.34 [a]	1.24 [b]	1.10 [c]	1.13 [c]	0.015	0.010
Blood scores	1.20 [a]	1.13 [b]	1.06 [c]	1.09 [b,c]	0.013	0.004

* Too many treatment combinations with only score 1.

3.3. Performance

Table 4 shows the effects per treatment on performance. Exploration feeding had no effect on performance. Males had a 39 g/d ($p = 0.01$) higher daily gain and a 2 mm ($p = 0.02$) lower muscle thickness than females. A space allowance of 0.8 m^2/pig had a 27 g/d ($p = 0.04$) lower daily gain than 1.0 m^2/pig.

Table 4. Mean performance data per main treatment factor with SEM and p value.

Variable	No Exploration Feeding	Exploration Feeding	SEM	p Value
Number of pens	24	21		
Growth (g/pig/d)	808.9	810.1	9.2	0.75
Muscle thickness (mm)	61.3	60.6	0.38	0.42
Fat thickness (mm)	14.3	14.0	0.13	0.29
Lean meat (%)	58.4	58.6	0.11	0.49
	Males	**Females**	**SEM**	**p Value**
Number of pens	24	21		
Growth (g/pig/d)	828.9	790.1	9.2	0.01
Muscle thickness (mm)	60.0	62.0	0.38	0.02
Fat thickness (mm)	14.1	14.2	0.13	0.76
Lean meat (%)	58.4	58.6	0.11	0.43
	0.8 m^2/pig	**1.0 m^2/pig**	**SEM**	**p Value**
Number of pens	21	24		
Growth (g/pig/d)	796.1	822.9	9.2	0.04
Muscle thickness (mm)	60.7	61.1	0.38	0.60
Fat thickness (mm)	13.9	14.3	0.13	0.21
Lean meat (%)	58.6	58.4	0.11	0.49

4. Discussion

Exploration feeding offers the pigs the opportunity to perform elements of species specific foraging behavior. In this experiment, we measured not the behavior around exploration feeding itself, but features related with health and behavior—like skin lesions, lameness, and tail biting. In this way, the effect of aggression and damaging behavior during the previous weeks is measured with a limited number of observations like described in the Welfare Quality® Pig Protocol [8].

Exploration feeding reduces aggression as measured by the number of scratches (lesions) at the front, middle, and hind body part of the pigs. Although the original objective of reducing tail biting by applying exploration feeding was not achieved in this experiment, the overall skin condition was better in pigs with exploration feeding, implying a reduction of unwanted behavior towards penmates by providing additional nutritional enrichment. In a situation with intact tails, the effect of exploration feeding on tail biting might have been more pronounced. Despite exploration feeding, the pigs in some pens nevertheless showed tail biting. This indicates that tail biting is multifactorial and that exploration feeding alone may not be sufficient to prevent it [1,4,13].

Beattie [14] concluded that pen enrichment is more important than lowering the stocking density to prevent skin damage. In the present study, both exploration feeding and pens with increased space allowance reduced skin lesion scores.

Floor feeding will only work in pens with partly slatted floors, to prevent loss of feed. The pen floors in this study had a 40% convex solid floor measuring 1.4×1.9 m. This floor was used both as lying area and for exploration feeding. The convex floor had a downward slope to the slatted floor on both sides, increasing the risk of feed losses. A better design would be a slightly sloping floor with provision of the exploration feed at the highest point reducing the risk of feed loss. The solid floors in pens with exploration feeding remained clean. The pigs clearly separated the functional areas for foraging/lying on one side and excretion on the other side. However, more fouling of the solid floor was (occasionally) observed at the lower stocking densities.

Exploration feeding was controlled by a sensor registering general activity in the front pens in each unit. The pigs received 75%–80% of the maximum number of servings recorded by the process computer. Occasional visual observations showed that the pigs did not react very quickly on a new portion, however hardly any feed was left on the floor at the start of the next serving. The motion sensor only reacted on activity in the first pens of a unit with eight pens on a row, so the sensor was not selective. Providing a sensor in each pen would probably be too costly. However, pig activity within a room is often strongly synchronized [15]. The question remains which moments or types of activity stimulates the sensor the most. Alternatively, the system could work effectively without motion sensors as well, possibly with a limited number of portions with fixed intervals during the light (active) period.

In this experiment, feed was provided ad libitum and exploration feed was the same as the feed provided in the feed trough. Exploration feed might be more interesting when the pigs would be feed restricted or when another type of feed was provided. However, floor feeding as only feeding system is also known to have a higher risk on increased levels of aggression [16], and this would be counterproductive.

Increased space allowance (1.0 versus 0.8 m^2/pig) improved both production and welfare as measured by better skin scores and elevated growth rates. This study does not allow a conclusion as to whether this effect was due to increased space allowance only or also due to reduced group size. The review of D'Eath et al. [2] and the analysis of Gonyou et al. [17] both reported a reducing effect of a lower space allowance on daily gain, especially below 0.8 m^2 per pig. Vermeer et al. [16] even found an improved daily gain with increased space allowances above 1.0 m^2 per pig. This could have an effect through the number of pigs per feeding space. However, both D'Eath et al. [2] and Gonyou et al. [17] considered feeder space allowance as less important. This is supported by our study where feeder space was not limiting with less than 10 pigs per ad libitum feeder. Moinard [5] found similar effects on tail biting of the combined effect of increased space allowances per pig and reduced numbers per feeding space. For an unbiased comparison of stocking densities, the group sizes should be constant and pen sizes could be varied in a future study.

Males generally exhibit more aggression than females. Aggression leads to higher front skin lesion scores. In this experiment, exploration feeding reduced skin scores more in males compared to females. This reduction in male aggression by exploration feeding at the standard space allowance of 0.8 m^2 per pig was not evident at the lower stocking density of 1.0 m^2 per pig. As a consequence, in addition to reducing stocking density, exploration feeding can provide another possible strategy to reduce aggression in the growing EU tendency of raising non-castrated males.

The motion sensor ensured that feed was distributed only when there was activity in the pens. However, only one motion sensor was used for the entire unit with eight pens. The synchronicity of activity in pig rooms ensures that control on a room level will be sufficient. However, there is a possibility that exploration feed was provided in pens where the pigs were not active and as occasionally observed the pigs were not immediately activated by the falling exploration feed. Only when a stockman entered the unit or when the pigs became active at a later moment, they will be focused on the previously spread feed on the floor. This suggests that the pigs were not activated by the servings of exploration feed per se that was also available ad libitum from a dry-wet feeder.

Exploration feeding will be more easily adopted by pig farmers when it is economically beneficial. In this experiment, exploration feeding showed no clear advantage or disadvantage for the performance of the pigs. However, the real advantage should come from a higher financial return in a market concept without castration and tail docking. Exploration feeding could contribute to a conversion towards such a market concept. Detailed costings of the dosage system for large scale application are difficult to make, but a rough estimation is possible. An investment of €10 per pig place with 10% annual costs and three batches per year the costs per pig would be estimated at €0.33. The estimated food spillage is €0.10 to €0.20 per pig, resulting in estimated costs for exploration feeding per pig between €0.45 and €0.50. This implies that a higher welfare level can be reached for €0.005 per kg of carcass weight.

Animal Welfare Implications

The pig welfare in the exploration feed treatment was improved as concluded from the reduced skin lesion scores and no negative effects compared to the control treatment. Similar welfare and health improvements were found for pigs with a higher space allowance.

5. Conclusions

From this study on intensively reared, growing-finishing pigs we conclude that:

- Exploration feeding, reduced stocking density, and a lower group size all improved skin lesion scores.
- Males showed more skin lesions than females.
- Exploration feeding reduced the difference between males and females in skin lesion scores at the front of the pigs.
- The difference of skin lesion scores at the hind of the pigs between high and low stocking densities/group sizes increased during the finishing period, with the lowest skin lesion score for the lowest stocking density.
- Tail scores were not affected by one of the treatments, but declined in the course of time.
- The daily gain of the males is higher than the females.
- The daily gain in the low stocking density is higher than in the high stocking density.
- At the low stocking density, the difference in daily gain between males and females is smaller than in high stocking density.
- Exploration feeding has no effect on performance.
- Both exploration feeding and lowering stocking density improve animal welfare.

Acknowledgments: This project was funded by the Dutch Ministry of Economic Affairs and in kind supported by sustainable pork chain "De Hoeve BV".

Author Contributions: Herman M. Vermeer and Nienke C. P. M. M. Dirx-Kuijken conceived and designed the experiments; Nienke C. P. M. M. Dirx-Kuijken performed the experiments. Herman M. Vermeer analyzed the data; Herman M. Vermeer and Marc B. M. Bracke wrote the paper.

Conflicts of Interest: The authors declare no conflict of interest.

References

1. European Food Safety Authority. Scientific opinion of the Panel on Animal Health and Welfare on a request from commission on the risks associated with tail biting in pigs and possible means to reduce the need for tail docking considering the different housing and husbandry systems. *EFSA J.* **2007**, *611*, 1–13.

2. D'Eath, R.B.; Arnott, G.; Turner, S.P.; Jensen, T.; Lahrmann, H.P.; Busch, M.E.; Niemi, J.K.; Lawrence, A.B.; Sandøe, P. Injurious tail biting in pigs: How can it be controlled in existing systems without tail docking? *Animal* **2014**, *8*, 1479–1497. [CrossRef] [PubMed]

3. Petherick, J.C.; Blackshaw, J.K. A review of the factors influencing the aggressive and agonistic behavior of the domestic pig. *Aust. J. Exp. Agric.* **1987**, *27*, 605–611. [CrossRef]

4. Zonderland, J.J. Talking Tails-Quantifying the Development of Tail Biting in Pigs. Ph.D. Thesis, Wageningen University, Wageningen, The Netherlands, 2010.

5. Moinard, C.; Mendl, M.; Nicol, C.J.; Green, L.E. A case control study of on-farm risk factors for tail biting in pigs. *Appl. Anim. Behav. Sci.* **2003**, *81*, 333–355. [CrossRef]

6. Vermeer, H.M.; Dirx-Kuijken, N.; Wisman, A.; Bikker, A. *Effect Van Exploratie Voedering en Hokbezetting op Welzijn van Vleesvarkens (Effect of Exploration Feeding and Space on Welfare of Growing Finishing Pigs)*; Report 546; Wageningen UR Livestock Research: Lelystad, The Netherlands, 2011.

7. Welfare Quality®. *Welfare Quality® Assessment Protocol for Pigs (Sows and Piglets, Growing and Finishing Pigs)*; Welfare Quality®Consortium: Lelystad, The Netherlands, 2009.

8. Zonderland, J.J.; Fillerup, M.; Van Reenen, C.G.; Hopster, H.; Spoolder, H.A.M. *Preventie en Behandeling van Staartbijten Bij Gespeende Biggen. (Prevention and Treatment of Tail Biting in Weaned Pigs)*; RIAH Report 18; Praktijkonderzoek: Lelystad, The Netherlands, 2003.

9. Wageningen UR Livestock Research. *Handboek Varkenshouderij-Praktisch Naslagwerk Voor de Nederlandse Varkenshouderij (Handbook Pig Husbandry)*; Wageningen UR Livestock Research: Wageningen, The Netherlands, 2015; pp. 380–381.

10. Genstat. *Reference Manual*; Release 6.1; VSN International: Oxford, UK, 2002.

11. Keen, A.; Engel, B. Analysis of a mixed model for ordinal data by iterative re-weighted REML. *Stat. Neerl.* **1997**, *51*, 129–144. [CrossRef]

12. Keen, A. Procedure IRCLASS. In *Biometris GenStat Procedure Library Manual*, 12th ed.; Goedhard, P.W., Thissen, J.T.N.M., Eds.; Biometris: Wageningen, The Netherlands, 2009; Available online: http://edepot.wur.nl/50492 (accessed on 1 April 2015).

13. Bracke, M.B.M.; Hulsegge, B.; Keeling, L.; Blokhuis, H.J. Decision support system with semantic model to assess the risk of tail biting in pigs: 1. Modelling. *Appl. Anim. Behav. Sci.* **2004**, *87*, 31–44. [CrossRef]

14. Beattie, V.E.; Walker, N.; Sneddon, I.A. An investigation of the effect of environmental enrichment and space allowance on the behavior and production of growing pigs. *Appl. Anim. Behav. Sci.* **1996**, *48*, 151–158. [CrossRef]

15. Vermeer, H.M.; De Greef, K.H.; Houwers, H.W.J. Space allowance and pen size affect welfare indicators and performance of growing pigs under comfort class conditions. *Livest. Sci.* **2014**, *159*, 79–86. [CrossRef]

16. Czermely, D.; Wood-Gush, D.G.M. Agonistic behavior in grouped sows. *Biol. Behav.* **1986**, *11*, 244–252.

17. Gonyou, H.W.; Brumm, M.C.; Bush, E.; Deen, J.; Edwards, S.A.; Fangman, R.; McGlone, J.J.; Meunier-Salaun, M.; Morrison, R.B.; Spoolder, H.; et al. Application of broken-line analysis to assess floor space requirements of nursery and grower-finisher pigs expressed on an allometric basis. *J. Anim. Sci.* **2006**, *84*, 229–235. [CrossRef] [PubMed]

7

A Survey of Public Opinion on Cat (*Felis catus*) Predation and the Future Direction of Cat Management in New Zealand

Jessica K. Walker [1,*], Stephanie J. Bruce [2] and Arnja R. Dale [3]

[1] New Zealand Companion Animal Council, P.O. Box 4, Waiuku, Auckland 2341, New Zealand
[2] Environmental and Animal Sciences Network, Unitec Institute of Technology, Auckland 1025, New Zealand; stephaniejean.bruce@gmail.com
[3] Royal New Zealand Society for the Prevention of Cruelty to Animals, 3047 Great North Road, New Lynn, Auckland 0610, New Zealand; arnja.dale@spca.nz

* Correspondence: manager@nzcac.org.nz

Simple Summary: The need to balance the benefits of cat ownership with the prevention of wildlife predation in New Zealand evokes strong and opposing views. This paper evaluates public concern for wildlife predation by four categories of cats; owned cats, managed-stray cats, unmanaged-stray cats, and feral cats. In addition, public support for a National Cat Management Strategy and a range of management techniques are investigated. Although the participants expressed concern regarding wildlife predation by all four categories of cats, the highest levels of concern were predation by feral cats, followed by unmanaged stray cats, then managed stray cats, and finally owned cats. The large majority of participants were found to support the implementation of a National Cat Management Strategy. Management techniques for owned cats that obtained public support included; cat exclusion zones, limits on ownership numbers, microchipping, Council registration, and de-sexing. Trap-Neuter-Return (TNR) was the favoured management technique for managed stray cats, while TNR and lethal management techniques were equally favoured for unmanaged stray cats. Lethal control methods were favoured for feral cats. The findings presented in this paper will be useful to consider during the development of legislation relating to cat management and predation in New Zealand.

Abstract: Cat predation is a prominent issue in New Zealand that provokes strong and opposing views. We explored, via 1011 face-to-face questionnaires, public opinion on (a) support for a National Cat Management Strategy (78% support); (b) concern regarding predation of wildlife by owned and un-owned cats (managed stray, unmanaged stray, and feral cats); (c) the acceptability of management techniques for owned cats; and (d) the acceptability of population management techniques for un-owned cats. The highest concern was expressed regarding the predation of non-native and native wildlife by feral cats (60 and 86% repectively), followed by unmanaged stray cats (59 and 86% respectively), managed stray cats (54 and 82% respectively), and finally owned cats (38 and 69% repectively). Limits to the number of cats owned and cat restriction zones received high levels of support (>65%), and compulsory microchipping, Council registration, and de-sexing were supported by the majority (>58%). Public support of population control methods for unowned cats was explored, and the influence of participant demographic variables on responses is described. These findings provide insight into public opinion regarding the management of cats in New Zealand, which should be considered during the development of legislation in this area.

Keywords: companion cat; cat management; cat predation; feral cat; stray cat; National Cat Management Strategy; New Zealand; public opinion

1. Introduction

Cats are widely kept and popular companion animals that offer significant benefits to their human owners while simultaneously having the potential to have a negative impact on society in general, as a result of a lack of legislation regarding their management. In New Zealand, 35–44% of households have at least one companion cat, making them the country's most popular companion animal [1,2]. The presence of, and interaction with, companion cats is well documented to enhance the health and wellbeing of humans (e.g., [3–6]). Conversely, unregulated cat management is associated with negative societal effects, including the predation of wildlife and a reduction in the abundance of native species [2,7,8] of high cultural value, disease transmission [9], interbreeding and contribution to stray cat populations [10], nuisance behaviours (including fouling, fighting, and spraying) [11,12], and a risk of injury and death as a result of fighting, dog attacks, and traffic accidents [12,13]. In New Zealand, cats are legislatively categorised into three groups; companion cats, stray cats, and feral cats [14], and for the purposes of this study these are defined as follows:

1. Companion cats: domestic cats that live with humans and are dependent on humans for their welfare [14].
2. Stray cats: companion cats that are lost or abandoned and are living as an individual or in a group. Stray cats live around centres of human habitation and have their needs provided by for, either directly or indirectly, by humans.
3. Feral cats: not stray or owned and have none of their needs provided for by humans. Feral cats generally do not live around centres of human habitation [14].

Currently there are an estimated 1.134 million owned companion cats in New Zealand [1]. One study by Mahlow and Slater [15] has suggested that stray cat populations equate to 14% of the owned companion cat population, and this calculation has been used on a single occasion to estimate the stray cat population numbers in New Zealand to be 196,000 [16]. Feral cat population numbers have not been accurately quantified as feral cat densities vary widely across New Zealand.

Predation by cats is a prominent issue in New Zealand that evokes strong and opposing views. The number of prey items killed annually by New Zealand's companion cat population has been approximated to be between 18 and 44 million, which has been calculated based on 35% of the companion cat population being active hunters [16]. Other studies suggest the rate is higher with between 44 and 70% of companion cats thought to be active hunters [2,8]. It is suggested that between 14 and 33 million prey are killed by stray cats annually [16]. Feral cat data is not reported as a result of the difficulties of accurately quantifying their population numbers. Although these estimated predation levels have not been validated in New Zealand, international predation levels have been demonstrated to affect the abundance of prey species [17,18]. Cats are opportunistic predators capable of killing a wide range of species [8]. While it is suggested that mammal species such as mice and rats account for the majority of cat prey items, avian, reptilian, amphibian, and invertebrate species can also be the targets of cat predation, making cats generalist predators as well as opportunists [19–21]. Their generalist nature means that cats are not limited by the abundance of one prey species, allowing them to drive populations and in some cases entire species, to extinction [20,22]. This is of particular importance in New Zealand, where many native fauna species are vulnerable to predation as a result of their evolving in environments without mammalian predators [22,23].

Cats' abilities to predate and the negative impacts that this can have on New Zealand's native fauna may be ameliorated by the implementation of a National Cat Management Strategy that includes regulatory management methods which aim to reduce the predation of wildlife. One such method is the employment of cat exclusion zones, areas that surround ecologically sensitive locations where residents are prohibited from owning cats [23,24] or where residents are required to keep cats indoors at all times. By reducing the number of cats in these areas, it is hoped that the negative impact they have on wildlife will also be reduced [24]. Research has documented that cats living near native populations hunt these species in larger quantities than cats that do not [12,24]. Restricting the number of cats allowed per household is another possible management technique, as fewer cats should theoretically equate to reduced predation impacts [24,25]. Cat curfews require owners to confine their cats indoors, whether it be during the day or night or continuously. In addition to reducing the risk of injury or death resulting from road accidents [13], confinement reduces the number of interactions between cats and prey species, potentially reducing predation levels [26]. Mandatory de-sexing, micro-chipping, and registration of cats are suggested key components of responsible companion cat ownership [27,28]. While these methods do not directly reduce predation levels, they do reduce the chance that companion cats will contribute to stray and feral populations through breeding, abandonment, or becoming lost [8,29,30]. Trap-Neuter-Return (TNR) programmes capture stray cats, de-sex and vaccinate them, and then return them to their capture site. Often these programmes will be carried out in conjunction with the adoption of socialised individuals [31,32]. Using cat exclusion zones, compulsory micro-chipping, and de-sexing in conjunction has been suggested to be the most effective way to manage cat populations in terms of reducing predation levels [8,25].

A National Cat Management Strategy may achieve a balance between the significant benefits of cat ownership with the aforementioned negative societal and environmental impacts of cats [26]. Understanding public concern regarding cat predation and attitudes towards management techniques is an important consideration when creating a management strategy [25]. Studies conducted internationally suggest that public opinion regarding cat predation and possible management techniques differ based upon a number of demographic variables including; knowledge and experience, employment status, beliefs and values and in some cases gender [12,25,33,34]. While little research in this area had been conducted in New Zealand, one notable exception is a recent study by Hall et al. [35], in which 347 New Zealand participants contributed to an online survey which aimed to elucidate attitudes towards companion cat predation across six countries. The results suggested that in New Zealand non-cat owners were more supportive of the need for cat legislation than cat owners.

Given the limited research investigating the palatability of national legislation surrounding the management of cats in New Zealand, we aimed, through the administration of a face-to-face questionnaire, to explore public opinion on:

1.   A range of management measures thought to contribute to the reduction of risk to wildlife, and;
2.   Demographic variables that influence these opinions.

2. Materials and Methods

2.1. Participants

Public opinion on cat predation and management was explored via 1016 face-to-face interviews in three central Auckland locations and two upper North Island rural towns. The surveying took place in central shopping areas. A team of 14 research assistants approached 8485 (12% response rate) members of the general public using simple random sampling [36] and asked them to participate in a 10-minute "social attitudinal survey". Further details about the study were not provided to avoid the potential bias of attracting participants with a greater empathy or interest in cats. Before commencing the survey, the participants were provided with an information sheet outlining the length of the survey, the anonymity and confidentiality of the information they provided, and their right to withdraw from the survey at any time including up to four months after completion of the survey. After completing the survey participants were provided with a take home information sheet which included a unique number identifier that participants could use if they wished to withdraw their responses to the survey at a subsequent date. All aspects of the research were provided by the Unitec Research Ethics Committee, Auckland, New Zealand (2015–1083). A written script was followed during questioning to ensure the accurate and standardised delivery of the questions. Five questionnaires were discarded due to partial completion.

2.2. Questionnaire Design

A pilot study was conducted using five randomly selected participants in central Auckland. Based on this, some questions were altered for ease of understanding. The final questionnaire consisted of 62 questions that were separated into three sections, namely, (a) cat predation and management, (b) cat ownership; and (c) participant demographics, and were asked in that order to reduce bias from questions about cat ownership influencing answers to subsequent questions about cat management. Cats were categorised into one of four sub-groups to allow information pertaining to methods of population management to be differentiated for each.

"A companion cat (1) is a common domestic cat that lives with humans and is dependent on humans for its welfare" [14].

"A stray cat is a companion cat that is lost or abandoned and that is living as an individual or in a group. Stray cats live around centres of human habitation. There are two categories of stray cat, colony and unmanaged. Colony cats (2) have many of their needs, such as food and shelter, directly supplied by humans. Unmanaged stray cats (3) have their needs supplied indirectly by humans by scavenging etc."

"A feral cat (4) is a cat that is not stray or owned and that has none of its needs provided for by humans. Feral cats generally do not live around centres of human habitation" [14].

The questions in section (a) related to the perceived impact of predation by each different cat sub-group and the use of different techniques to manage New Zealand's populations of these cat sub-groups in turn. Firstly, the participants were asked if they thought New Zealand should have a National Strategy in place to manage cat populations. No information was provided regarding what a National Cat Management Strategy might include. Participants were then asked whether they were concerned about the predation of both native and non-native wildlife by each of the four sub-groups of cats. For the companion cat sub-group, participants were asked an additional 11 questions relating to their management. These included whether there should be a limit to the number of cats one household can own at one time and what the limit should be; whether de-sexing, microchipping, and registration should each be compulsory; whether cats should be confined to their owners' property or inside their owners home and at what times (options: always, day, night, other); and whether there should be certain areas that companion cats should not be allowed to be owned and where these areas should be. For the colony, unmanaged stray, and feral cat subgroups, three additional questions were asked about their management. These included whether action should be taken to control each subgroups population numbers and, if so, who should be responsible for controlling these populations (options: Government, Council, Society for the Prevention of Cruelty to Animals (SPCA), other).

The participants were asked how each group of cats should be controlled. This question was open-ended and the responses were categorised following data collection into one of the following five categories: (1) lethal methods (e.g., shooting); (2) Trap-Neuter-Return (TNR); (3) "non-killing" methods (e.g., de-sexing, socialising, and rehoming); (4) other (do nothing, leave cats alone); and (5) don't know.

After the respondents described their chosen method of population control, they were read a definition developed by the research team for lethal methods of population control and TNR. Following this, they were given the opportunity to change their chosen population control method to one of three posited options ("lethal methods", "TNR", or "nothing"). The definitions were as follows:

"Lethal methods can be employed to kill cats and reduce population numbers. These methods may include poisoning and kill trapping".

"Trap-Neuter-Return is a program through which stray and feral cats are trapped humanely; de-sexed and medically treated; and then returned to the location where they were found".

"Nothing—leave the cat populations as they are".

The categories, "other" and "nothing" were combined into one category, "other", for comparative data analysis due to the small number of respondents selecting "nothing" and because "leave the cats alone" and "do nothing" were common responses observed in the "other" category.

The questions in section (b) covered demographic information about the number of participants that owned companion cats (32%; n = 326), including the total number of cats each participant owned (median = 1), the length of ownership (the median was seven years), the reasons for ownership (companionship 54%; pest control 4%; other 42%), how the cats were housed (indoor 13%; outdoor 7%; both 80%), the number that wore collars (35%), the number that were de-sexed (94%), the number that were microchipped (37%), and the number of microchips that were registered (81%). The participants were also asked if they owned other companion animals (yes = 26%) or had owned companion animals during the previous five years (yes = 39%) or during childhood (yes = 85%). The respondents who did not own a cat were asked to elucidate as to why. This question was open-ended and responses were categorised following (living situation not suitable 26%; allergies 4%; lifestyle 19%; don't want/like 11%; have other animals 6%; last one passed away 6%; other 28%).

The third and final section of the questionnaire collected demographic information about each participant. All age categories were well represented, with a slightly higher representation of 18–35 year olds. Male and female participants were equally represented. The majority of participants were New Zealand European and 45% were single, with an equal number either married or in de facto relationships. Over 70% of participants lived in urban/suburban locations with 14% living rurally. Most earned over $50,000 per annum and 70% were employed. The majority were well educated, with over 75% having attained tertiary qualifications. Taken together, these demographic data indicate that our sample population showed similar trends to the most recent New Zealand census data (see Table 1).

Table 1. Participant demographics (n = 1011) showing a comparison of survey sample sizes with New Zealand national statistics.

Demographic	Demographic Categories	N	Survey Sample %	New Zealand Census 2013%
Age	18–25 years	253	25%	14%
	26–35 year	217	21%	16%
	36–45 years	132	13%	18%
	46–55 years	134	13%	19%
	56–65 years	135	13%	15%
	65+ years	138	14%	18%
Gender	Male	497	49%	49%
	Female	494	49%	51%
Ethnicity	New Zealand European	515	51%	64%
	Māori	70	7%	15%
	Asian/Indian	124	12%	12%
	European	188	19%	8%
	Pacific Cook Island	25	2%	7%
	Other	79	8%	2%
Marital Status	Single	457	45%	35%
	Married	327	32%	48%
	Divorced	52	5%	11%
	De facto	140	14%	-
	Widowed	33	3%	6%
Residential Location	Urban	332	32%	72% #
	Suburban	427	42%	-
	Rural	145	14%	14% #
Income	<$50,000 per annum	277	27%	6%
	$50,000–$100,000 per annum	262	26%	21%
	>$100,000	117	12%	6%
	No answer	52	5%	10%

Table 1. *Cont.*

Demographic	Demographic Categories	N	Survey Sample %	New Zealand Census 2013%
Income	<$50,000 per annum	277	27%	6%
	$50,000–$100,000 per annum	262	26%	21%
	>$100,000	117	12%	6%
	No answer	52	5%	10%
Education	No formal education/Primary	19	2%	21%
	Secondary	224	22%	33%
	Certificate/Diploma	230	23%	29%
	Undergraduate	296	29%	14%
	Postgraduate	229	23%	6%
Employed	Yes	708	70%	61%
	No	301	30%	39%
Cat Owner *	Yes	326	32%	44%
	No	684	68%	56%

Total *n* for each demographic differs from the total survey population as a result of non-response from participants. %'s are calculated based on the total number of respondents (*n* = 1011). Source: [37]; * Source: [1]; # Based on 2006 census data.

The questions used in this research were based upon those of similar studies (e.g., [25,38]) and were written in a neutral manner so as not to influence participants' answers with negative or positive wording [34]. Unless otherwise stated, respondents were asked to answer "yes", "no", or "don't know" to all posited questions. Three versions of the questionnaire were developed so that the cat categories in section (a) were rotated between participants to prevent delivery fatigue. In an effort to reduce participant confusion, the definition of each of the cat sub-groups was repeated before the questions were asked.

2.3. Statistical Analysis

All questionnaire data was entered into Microsoft Excel and then exported into Minitab Statistical Software (version 17, Minitab Pty Ltd, Sydney, Australia). Cross-tabulation with a Chi-Squared (χ^2) test of association was used to investigate the differences in participant concern regarding the predation by each of the cat groups.

Nominal logistic regression was used to investigate associations between demographic variables and each question about the management of cats in New Zealand. Unanswered questions were coded as missing data. The regression model was refined using a backwards stepwise technique, sequentially removing non-significant predictors and refitting to identify which predictors were important. The final model was as follows:

$$Z = b_0 + b_1X_1 + b_2X_2 + b_3X_3 + b_4X_4 + b_5X_5 + b_6X_6 + b_7X_7 + b_8X_8$$

where Z is the log odds of the dependent variable; b_0 is a constant; b_1 is the coefficient for companion cat ownership (X_1); b_2 is the coefficient for age (X_2); b_3 is the coefficient for gender (X_3); b_4 is the coefficient for ethnicity (X_4); b_5 is the coefficient for marital status (X_5); b_6 is the coefficient for residential location (X_6); b_7 is the coefficient for income (X_7); and b_8 is the coefficient for education (X_8).

The above regression model was used for each of the questions of interest in the survey. For all models, validity was assumed with a log-likelihood *p* value of <0.05 and Goodness of Fit Pearson and Deviance chi-squared *p* values of >0.05. The results are presented as odds ratios (OR) and *p* values. Only significant results are presented.

3. Results

3.1. A National Cat Management Strategy

When asked whether New Zealand should have a National Cat Management Strategy, 78% of participants responded "yes" ("no" = 12%; "don't know" = 9%). The participant responses were found to be influenced by several demographic variables, including annual income, ethnicity, and residential location. Participants earning in excess of $100,000 per annum were more likely to respond "no" ($Z = 2.51$, OR = 2.84, $p = 0.012$, CI = 1.26–6.39) than participants earning less than $50,000 per annum. Participants of Pacific/Cook Island ethnicity were more likely than NZ Europeans to respond "don't know" ($Z = 2.03$, OR = 4.09, $p = 0.042$, CI = 1.05–15.92), and participants residing in urban locations were less likely to respond 'yes' than suburban respondents ($Z = -1.49$, OR = 0.49, $p = 0.028$, CI = 0.25–0.93).

3.2. Cat Predation

The participants were asked whether they were concerned about the predation of non-native and native wildlife by each of the four categories of cat. The participants expressed greater concern about the predation of native wildlife than non-native wildlife by all four cat groups ($\chi^2 = 792.4$, df = 1, $p < 0.0001$). In the case of non-native wildlife, the participants were more concerned about predation by colony cats (54%; $\chi^2 = 51.6$, df = 1, $p < 0.0001$), unmanaged stray cats (59%; $\chi^2 = 91.5$, df = 1, $p < 0.0001$), and feral cats (60%; $\chi^2 = 98$, df = 1, $p < 0.0001$) than predation by companion cats (38%) and more concerned about predation by unmanaged stray cats ($\chi^2 = 5.9$, df = 1, $p = 0.015$) and feral cats ($\chi^2 = 7.8$, df = 1, $p = 0.005$) than by colony cats (Figure 1). With regard to native wildlife, participants were more concerned about the predation of native wildlife by colony cats (82%; $\chi^2 = 42.8$, df = 1, $p < 0.0001$), unmanaged stray cats (86%; $\chi^2 = 83.8$, df = 1, $p < 0.0001$), and feral cats (86%; $\chi^2 = 89.4$ df = 1, $p < 0.0001$) than predation by companion cats (69%) and more concerned about native wildlife predation by unmanaged stray cats ($\chi^2 = 7.4$, df = 1, $p = 0.007$) and feral cats ($\chi^2 = 9.2$, df = 1, $p = 0.002$) than by colony cats (Figure 1).

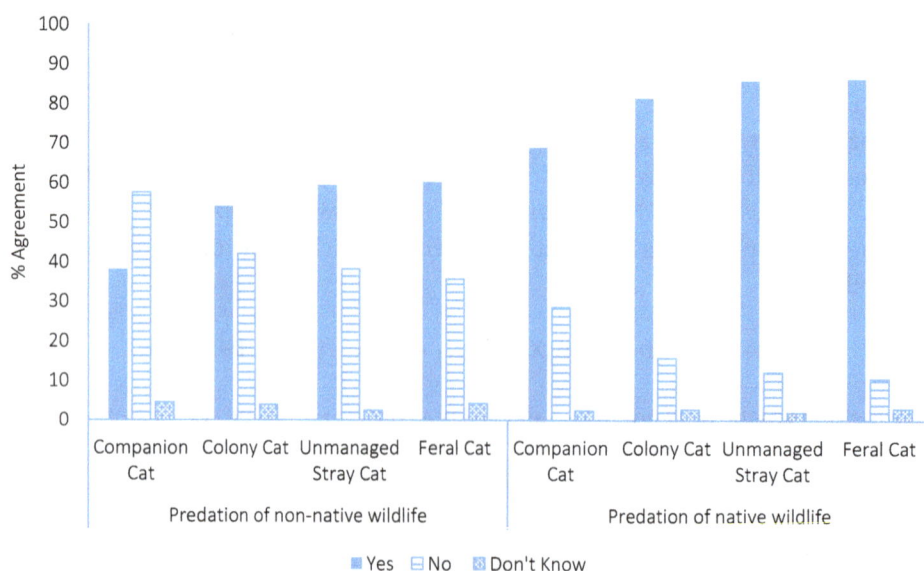

Figure 1. Participant concern about the predation of non-native and native wildlife by each sub group of cat in New Zealand.

Concern regarding the predation of both non-native and native wildlife by each of the different categories of cat was found to be influenced by age, gender, ethnicity, income, residential location, marital status, and education (Supplementary Materials Table S1). Younger respondents were less likely to be concerned about predation by companion cats ($p < 0.0001$; $p < 0.0001$, respectively); colony cats ($p < 0.0001$; $p = 0.004$, respectively); unmanaged stray cats ($p = 0.001$; $p = 0.001$, respectively); and predation solely of non-native wildlife by feral cats ($p = 0.002$). Males are more likely to express concern about the predation of native wildlife by companion cats than are females ($p = 0.038$). Participants of NZ European ethnicity were less likely than those of Asian/Indian ethnicity to be concerned about the predation of non-native wildlife by companion cats ($p < 0.0001$), colony cats $p = 0.001$), unmanaged stray cats ($p = 0.001$), and feral cats ($p = 0.010$) and more likely to be concerned about the predation of native wildlife by colony cats ($p = 0.030$) than participants identifying as "other" ethnicities. Participants earning greater than \$100,000 per annum were more likely than those earning less than \$50,000 per annum to be concerned about the predation of native wildlife by unmanaged stray cats ($p = 0.016$), while those who elected not to disclose their annual income were more likely than those earning less than \$50,000 per annum to be unsure whether they were concerned about non-native ($p = 0.02$) and native ($p = 0.014$) predation by colony cats. Rural participants were more likely to be concerned about the predation of non-native wildlife by unmanaged stray cats ($p = 0.047$) than were urban participants. Married participants were more likely than single participants to be concerned about the predation of non-native wildlife by colony cats ($p = 0.004$) and unmanaged stray cats ($p = 0.05$), and participants with primary or no formal education were less likely than participants with a certificate/diploma ($p = 0.039$), undergraduate ($p = 0.021$), or postgraduate ($p = 0.017$) qualification to be concerned about the predation of native wildlife by colony cats. These participants were also more likely than participants with secondary education ($p = 0.046$) and postgraduate education ($p = 0.038$) to respond "don't know" when asked if they were concerned about the predation of non-native wildlife by feral cats.

3.3. Management of Companion Cats

The participants were asked three questions regarding the responsible management and identification of companion cats. Fifty-eight percent ($n = 584$) of participants responded "yes", it should be compulsory for companion cats to be de-sexed, while 66% ($n = 667$) responded "yes", it should be compulsory for companion cats to be microchipped, and 61% ($n = 616$) responded "yes", it should be compulsory for companion cats to be registered with the Council.

Demographic variables (Supplementary Materials Table S2) were found to influence the responses. Support for compulsory de-sexing was influenced by gender, with male participants being less supportive than females ($p = 0.031$). Age influenced agreement with compulsory de-sexing, with increasing support observed as age reduced ($p < 0.0001$), and compulsory microchipping, with increasing age corresponding to increased uncertainty ($p = 0.019$). Support for compulsory microchipping was also influenced by residential location, with suburban residents more likely to be uncertain ($p = 0.018$), and marital status, with married participants demonstrating less support than single participants ($p = 0.024$). Mandatory Council registration was influenced by cat ownership, with owners demonstrating less support ($p < 0.0001$); ethnicity, with NZ Europeans being less supportive than participants of Asian/Indian ethnicity ($p = 0.002$); and age, with older participants demonstrating more support ($p < 0.0001$).

The participants were asked a further four questions relating to restrictions on cat ownership (Figure 2). Seventy percent ($n = 706$) agreed that there should be a limit to the number of cats per household.

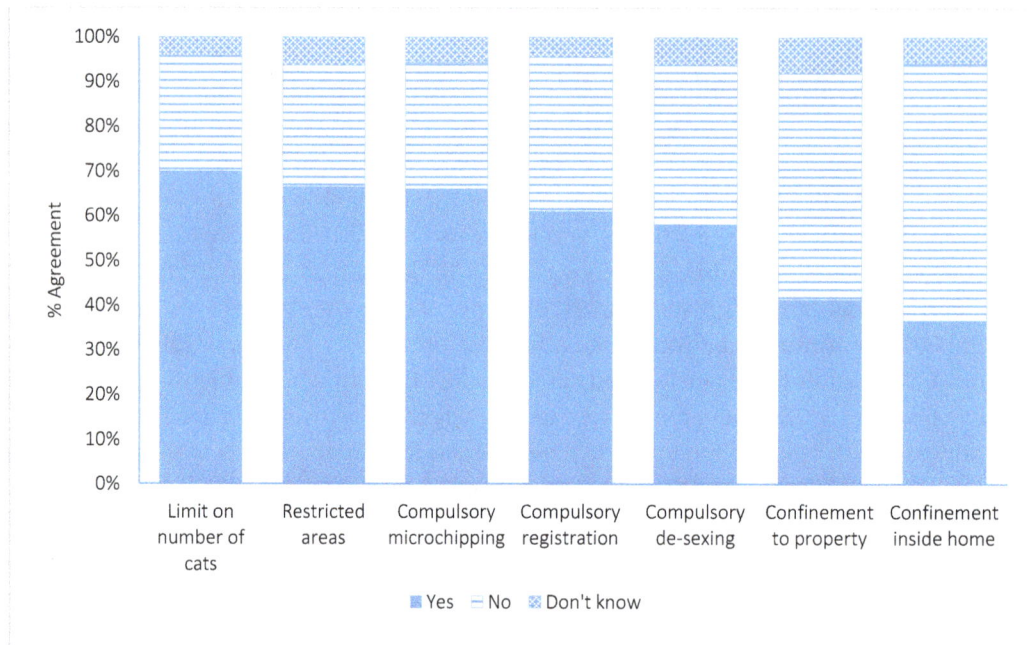

Figure 2. Participant agreement to seven posited restrictions regarding companion cat ownership in New Zealand.

Forty-one percent ($n = 417$) agreed there should be times when cats must be confined to their owner's property, of which 8% believed this should occur during the day, 45% at night, 19% at all times, 25% at other times, and 3% did not respond. Thirty-six percent ($n = 368$) agreed there should be times when cats must be confined inside their owner's homes, of which 27% agreed this should occur at all times, 6% during the day, 54% at night, 11% at other times, and 1% did not respond. The majority of participants (66%; $n = 671$) agreed there should be areas that companion cats are not allowed to be owned, of which 70% suggested this should be in areas near endangered/protected species, 5% near human habitation (e.g., apartments, urban areas), 15% other, and 10% did not answer.

The responses to these questions were influenced by a number of demographic variables (Supplementary Materials Table S2). Support for a restriction on the number of cats each household could own was influenced by age, with decreased support observed as age reduced ($p = 0.047$); marital status, with single participants less supportive than married participants ($p = 0.009$); education, with participants that had only primary or no formal education demonstrating less support than those with a certificate or diploma ($p = 0.030$); and ethnicity, with NZ Europeans being more supportive ($p = 0.026$) than Europeans. Support for the confinement of cats to their owner's property was influenced by ownership, with owners being less supportive ($p = 0.008$), and ethnicity, with NZ Europeans less supportive than Māori ($p = 0.039$), Asian/Indian ($p < 0.001$), and Pacific/Cook Islanders ($p = 0.028$). On the other hand, the confinement of cats inside their owners' homes was influenced by age, with decreased support observed as age reduced ($p < 0.0001$); income, with those earning more than $100,000 per annum demonstrating more support ($p = 0.019$); and ethnicity, with NZ Europeans being less supportive than Asian/Indian ($p < 0.0001$) and Pacific/Cook Islanders ($p = 0.004$). Support for areas of exclusion of companion cat ownership was influenced by cat ownership, with cat owners demonstrating less support ($p < 0.0001$); ethnicity, with NZ Europeans being more supportive than Asian/Indian ($p = 0.021$) and Europeans ($p = 1.71$); and income, with those earning between $50,000–$100,000 per annum ($p = 0.008$) or greater than $100,000 per annum ($p = 0.033$) being less likely to be unsure than participants earning less than $50,000 per annum.

3.4. Management of Colony Cats

The participants were asked three questions regarding the management of each of the three categories of un-owned cats. In the case of colony cats, 83% ($n = 825$) of the participants agreed that action should be taken towards controlling colony cat populations (Figure 3). Of these, 13% believed the Government should be responsible for controlling these populations, 34% local Councils, 10% SPCA, 33% a combination of all three, and 10% selected "other" (Figure 4). When asked what action should be taken towards controlling colony cats, 20% agreed that lethal methods should be engaged, 7% selected TNR, 28% selected non-killing methods (e.g., rehoming), 32% selected "other", and 13% selected "don't know". Following the explanation of lethal methods and TNR, 33% ($n = 336$) indicated that they would like to change their answer, resulting in 23% agreement with lethal methods, 38% agreement with TNR, 16% agreement with "non-killing" methods, 20% agreement with "other" methods, and 3% selecting "don't know" (Figure 5).

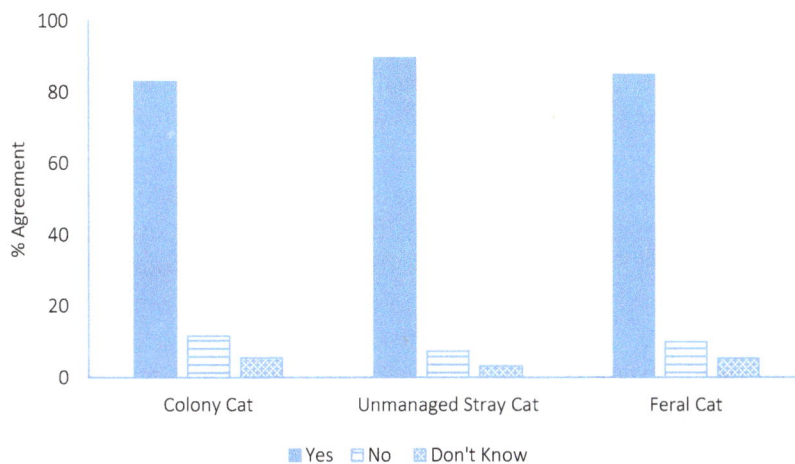

Figure 3. Participant agreement that action should be taken toward controlling each of the un-owned subgroups of cats in New Zealand.

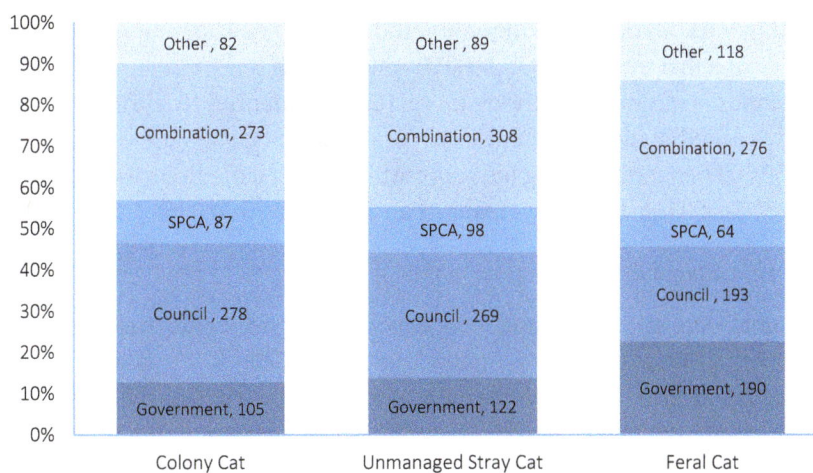

Figure 4. Participant opinion as to which organisation should be responsible for the control of each subgroup of un-owned cats in New Zealand.

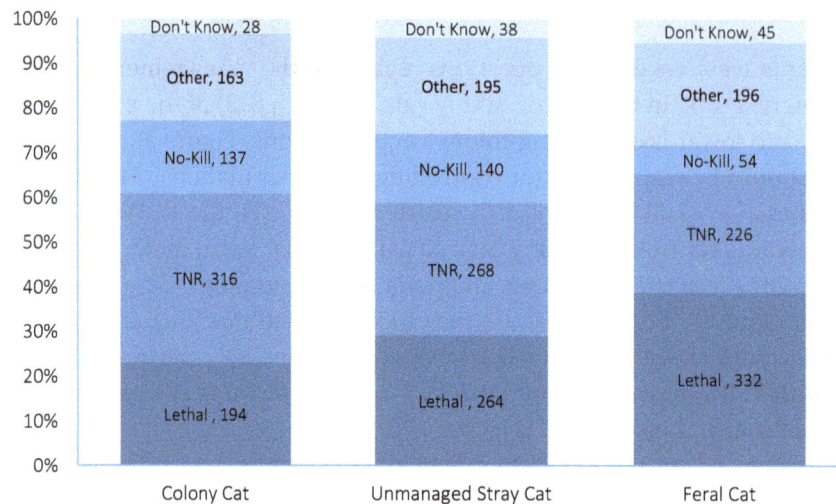

Figure 5. Participant opinion on the action that should be taken to control each subgroup of un-owned cats in New Zealand.

Responses regarding responsibility for colony cat control were found to be influenced by a number of demographic variables (Supplementary Materials Table S3), including ownership, with non-owners being more likely to agree that the SPCA should be the organisation responsible ($p = 0.048$); ethnicity, with NZ Europeans less likely than Asian/Indian ($p = 0.022$), European ($p = 0.033$), and "other" ethnicities ($p = 0.02$) to agree that the Government should be responsible; residential location, with suburban participants being more likely than urban participants to agree that a combination (i.e., SPCA, local Council, and Government) ($p = 0.012$), the SPCA ($p = 0.012$), or the Council ($p = 0.04$) should be responsible; and income, with those earning less than \$50,000 per annum being less likely than those with an income bracket of \$50,000–\$100,000 or greater than \$100,000 to agree that the Government ($p = 0.03$; $p = 0.022$, respectively) should be responsible. Demographic variables also influenced participant opinion on the type of control method that should be utilised for colony cats (Supplementary Materials Table S3), including ownership, with owners being less supportive of lethal methods than TNR ($p = 0.032$) or "non-killing" methods ($p = 0.025$); age, with younger participants being less supportive of lethal methods ($p < 0.0001$); gender, with females demonstrating more support for non-killing methods over lethal methods ($p = 0.026$); residential location, with urban residents being less supportive of lethal methods than were rural residents ($p = 0.001$); and income, with those earning less than \$50,000 per annum being less supportive of lethal methods than those with an income bracket of \$50,000–\$100,000 ($p = 0.006$) or greater than \$100,000 ($p = 0.006$).

3.5. Management of Unmanaged Stray Cats

When participants were asked the same three questions regarding the management of unmanaged stray cats, 90% ($n = 905$) of participants agreed that action should be taken towards controlling populations (Figure 2). Of these, 14% believed that the Government should be responsible for their management, 30% local Councils, 11% the SPCA, 35% a combination of all three, and 10% selected "other" (Figure 3). When asked what action should be taken towards controlling unmanaged stray cats, 27% agreed that lethal methods should be engaged, 17% selected TNR, 19% selected non-killing methods, 25% selected "other", and 12% selected "don't know". Following the explanation of lethal methods and TNR, 16% ($n = 163$) indicated that they would like to change their answer, resulting in 26% agreement with lethal methods, 26% agreement with TNR, 14% agreement with "non-killing" methods, 19% agreement with "other" methods, and 4% ($n = 38$) of participants selecting "don't know" (Figure 4).

Demographic variables were found to influence responses (Supplementary Materials Table S3), including age, with younger participants being less likely to agree that the control of unmanaged stray cat populations should occur ($p = 0.014$); ethnicity, with NZ Europeans being less likely than participants identifying with "other" ethnicities to agree that control should occur ($p = 0.004$); and income, with participants earning less than \$50,000 per annum, compared to those earning greater than \$100,000 per annum, being more likely to agree control should occur ($p = 0.001$). The organisation believed by participants to be responsible for the control of unmanaged stray cat populations was influenced by gender, with males being less likely to agree that control should be provided by a combination of organisations ($p = 0.025$); ethnicity, with NZ Europeans being less likely than Asian/Indian participants to agree that the Government should provide control ($p = 0.008$); income, with those earning more than \$100,000 per annum being less likely to agree that the SPCA should provide control ($p = 0.007$); and residential location, with suburban residents being more likely than urban residents to agree that a combination of organisations should provide control ($p = 0.022$). The selected method of control was influenced by age, with younger participants being less likely to select lethal methods over TNR ($p < 0.0001$), "non-killing" methods ($p < 0.0001$), "other" methods ($p < 0.0001$), or "don't know" ($p = 0.001$); ethnicity, with Asian/Indian respondents being more likely than NZ Europeans to select "non-killing" methods ($p = 0.049$), and "other" methods ($p = 0.017$) over lethal methods and Europeans being more likely to select "non-killing" methods over lethal methods ($p = 0.045$) than were NZ Europeans; income, with those earning between \$50,000 and \$100,000 per annum ($p = 0.003$) and those earning greater than \$100,000 per annum ($p = 0.002$) being less likely than those earning less than \$50,000 to select lethal methods over TNR; marital status, with single participants being less likely than those in de facto relationships to select lethal methods over TNR ($p = 0.007$) or "non-killing" methods ($p = 0.002$); and residential location, with urban participants being less likely than rural participants to select lethal methods over "other" methods ($p = 0.05$) of control.

3.6. Management of Feral Cats

Eighty-five percent of participants ($n = 857$) agreed that action should be taken towards controlling feral cats. Of these, 22% believed that the Government should be responsible for their management, 23% local Councils, 8% the SPCA, 33% a combination of all three, and 14% selected "other". When asked what action should be taken towards controlling feral cats, 39% agreed that lethal methods should be engaged, 9% selected TNR, 8% selected non-killing methods, 17% selected "other", and 11% selected "don't know". Following the explanation of lethal methods and TNR, 22% ($n = 222$) of participants indicated that they would like to change their answer, resulting in 33% agreement with lethal methods, 22% agreement with TNR, 5% agreement with "non-killing" methods, 19% agreement with "other" methods, and 4% selecting "don't know" (Figure 4).

The responses to these questions were found to be influenced by a number of demographic variables (Supplementary Materials Table S3), including; age, with younger participants being less likely to agree that action should be taken towards controlling feral cats ($p < 0.0001$); and ethnicity, with Asian/Indian ethnicity ($p = 0.044$) and "other" ethnicities ($p = 0.011$) being more in agreement that action should be taken than were NZ Europeans. In addition, NZ Europeans were less likely than Asian/Indian participants to agree that the Government, rather than "other" organisations, should be responsible for controlling feral cats ($p = 0.033$). Ethnicity also influenced participants' preferred method of control for feral cats, with Europeans ($p = 0.001$), Asian/Indians ($p = 0.020$), and Pacific/Cook Islanders ($p = 0.015$) all being more likely than NZ Europeans to select "non-killing" methods over lethal methods, while Māori participants ($p = 0.020$), Asian/Indian participants ($p = 0.006$) and Pacific/Cook Island participants ($p = 0.029$) were more likely than NZ Europeans to select "other" methods of control over lethal methods. Marital status also influenced control methods, with single participants being less likely than those that were married to select lethal methods over non-killing methods ($p = 0.003$) and less likely than participants in de facto relationships to select lethal methods over TNR ($p = 0.014$).

4. Discussion

The main aim of this study was to explore public support for a National Cat Management Strategy and opinions on posited cat management techniques. Our survey demonstrated strong public agreement (78%) that New Zealand should have a National Strategy in place to manage cat populations. Support for cat legislation has been similarly favoured in a number of Australian public opinion surveys [11,25,35,39], yet public support in New Zealand has recently been documented at only 55% [35]. This discrepancy might be explained by the small sample size ($n = 347$) and the middle class demographic of the participants involved in the recent study by Hall et al. [35].

4.1. Cat Predation

Our participants were concerned about the predation of both non-native and native wildlife, with the greatest level of concern expressed towards native wildlife. Concern regarding the predation of both non-native and native wildlife was highest for feral cats, followed by unmanged stray cats, then colony cats, and finally companion cats. Lower levels of concern regarding companion cat predation have been reported in previous studies (e.g., [25]) and appear to reflect a common misconception that companion cats have less or no impact upon wildlife populations [24]. This idea has been evidenced to be largely misguided, with well fed companion cats being just as likely to predate as other cat types [24,40].

The importance of preserving New Zealand's native fauna species is evident on both a national and individual level and may explain the high levels of concern expressed regarding cat predation. In New Zealand many native fauna species are vulnerable to predation as a result of their evolving in environments without mammalian predators [20,23]. Native fauna preservation efforts are important for the culture and identity of many New Zealanders, with species such as the kiwi (*Apteryx* spp.) considered to be *tāonga* (treasure; something of value) to Māori and of significant national importance to all cultures within New Zealand [41]. Furthermore, the abundance of native fauna species is linked to the New Zealand economy through tourism, with approximately 90% of international visitors to New Zealand experiencing the natural surroundings [42,43]. Degradation of the country's natural environments and a loss of iconic fauna species would result in an estimated loss of 4.9% GDP per annum received from the tourism sector [44].

Sixty-six percent of our participants supported the idea of cat ownership exclusion zones, a higher figure than has been reported in international studies [25,26]. New Zealand Europeans were more supportive of cat exclusion zones than participants of other ethnicities and demonstrated less concern regarding the predation of non-native wildlife. These results reflect the cultural importance of endemic species preservation within New Zealand.

We also found that male participants were more likely to demonstrate concern regarding the predation of native wildlife by companion cats. Gender is a well-established variable of influence when it comes to attitudes towards animals [45], with females frequently being reported to show more positive attitudes toward individual animals [46–50], while, on the other hand, males are reported to maintain a more utilitarian view of animals, expressing greater concern for species preservation and habitat conservation [45,51–53].

4.2. Management of Companion Cats

We observed only 58% public support for mandatory de-sexing. This was surprising as voluntary de-sexing levels for companion cats were reported at 94% in the present study and greater than 93% in previous New Zealand studies [1,35], 88–93% in Australia [11,25], and 86% in Singapore [54]. High levels (>70%) of support for mandatory de-sexing have also been observed for both owners and non-owners of companion cats in public opinion research internationally [25]. We found that males demonstrated less support for mandatory de-sexing, which is not surprising as females are frequently reported to be more in favour of de-sexing as a mechanism to control cat populations [25,39,54].

However, our almost equal proportions of male and female participants might go some way to explaining our seemingly low level of public support for mandatory de-sexing overall, as research investigating similar trends often describes female participant rates of 60–80% [25,54], which is likely to equate to higher levels of support for mandatory de-sexing.

Public agreement that microchipping should be compulsory in the present study was more than double (66%) the current 31% of companion cats microchipped within New Zealand [1] and much higher than the 37% of cats in the current study that were reported as microchipped. Unlike other methods of identification (e.g., collars and tags), microchipping is the only permanent and unalterable form of identification currently available for cats and gives cats a greater degree of protection and a much higher chance of being returned to their home when lost. Research has indicated that return-to-owner rates for cats that are microchipped is 20 times higher than for cats that are not microchipped [27]. Our results suggest that although participants were in favour of compulsory microchipping this was not being translated into practice. We found that older participants were more inclined to be unsure about compulsory microchipping which may be a reflection of a lack of understanding around the technology associated with microchipping. Further investigation is required to elucidate the discrepancy between public support for compulsory microchipping and the practice of microchipping.

Over 60% of respondents agreed that cats should be registered with local Councils. However this figure is lower than international levels of support for Council registration, which have been reported to be as high as 80% [25]. We found that non-owners were more likely to support the practice of registering cats with Councils. Likewise, ownership has been found to influence agreement regarding the control of cats in Australia, with non-owners demonstrating higher levels of support for mandatory registration with the Councils [25]. If mandatory Council registration of cats was to be included in a National Strategy within New Zealand, a demonstration of the benefits to cat owners might encourage compliance.

We asked participants whether there should be a limit to the number of cats per household and what that limit should be. There was 70% agreement with a limit on ownership numbers, with a median number of a two cat limit observed. This finding supports current cat ownership behaviour in New Zealand, where the average number of cats per household is 1.5 [1,35], and the median in the current study was one cat per household.

We observed low levels of public agreement regarding cat confinement. Less than half of the participants agreed that cats should be confined to their owner's property, and only 36% agreed that cats should be confined inside the owner's home. These findings are consistent with other studies in which constant indoor confinement has been found to be less widely accepted [25,35]. In one New Zealand study, the percentage of owned cats constantly confined was reported to be as low as 3% [55]. Of the participants that did agree with cat confinement, both to the owner's property and inside the owner's home, 45% and 54%, respectively, believed this should occur during the night. This finding parallels a recent study by Harrod et al. [56], who found that 48% of respondents agreed with the confinement of cats indoors overnight. Keeping companion cats continuously confined, as they are in some countries (50–60% in North America), should reduce their ability to hunt in comparison to that of unowned cats [57], yet keeping cats confined only at night may contribute little to reducing predation behaviour as research suggests that companion cats largely hunt during the day [24]. Unlike in other countries that are home to native nocturnal mammals vulnerable to predation by cats (e.g., Australia), introducing mandatory confinement overnight could result in a reduction of the number of rodent predations, which pose a significant threat to New Zealand native wildlife. Furthermore, compliance levels relating to the confinement of cats at night have been reported to vary between 32–80% in Australia [12,13]. Conversely, keeping cats confined at night would be beneficial for cat welfare as cat curfews have been documented to reduce the injury rates associated with road accidents, encounters with other cats, and dog attacks [12,13]. Our results suggest that age and ownership status are demographic variables that impact upon support for cat confinement, with older participants and non-owners being more likely to support mandatory confinement to the owner's property. Both national [36,55] and international [12,25,39] research document non-owner support of the confinement of cats to their owner's property, with the underlying motivation suggested to be based on the belief that containment is important to protect neighbours from nuisance behaviour [12]. If cat confinement or curfews are introduced in New Zealand as part of a National Cat Management Strategy, the benefits for both owners (i.e., reduced injury rates) and non-owners (i.e., reduced nusiance behaviour) would need to be illuminated in order to promote support and compliance.

4.3. Management of Unowned Cats

We found high levels of public agreement that action should be taken to control colony (83%), unmanaged stray (90%), and feral (85%) cat populations within New Zealand. A National Cat Management Strategy would likely need to be governed and enforced, and therefore participant opinion regarding which organisation(s) should be responsible for each subgroup of cats is an important part of the determination process. We found that participants were most likely to select the Council as the organisation that should be responsible for controlling colony cats, while all three organisations combined (Government, Council, and the SPCA) were favoured for controlling both unmanaged stray cats and feral cats. These results indicate that participants viewed unmanaged stray and feral cat population control on more of a nationwide basis, hence the multi-organisation seletion, but colony cat populations on an area by area basis, hence the Council control. New Zealand Europeans were less likely to believe that the Government should be responsible for colony cats and more likely to agree that lethal methods should be used to control feral cat populations, which might reflect the Department of Conservation's (a Government department) historical and ongoing role in feral cat control within New Zealand.

After participants were read our definitions of lethal methods and TNR, they were asked if they would like to replace their free-answer to the question of how each group of unowned cats should be controlled. Overall we observed low levels of agreement amongst participants. TNR was the favoured population control method for colony cats, obtaining 31% support, while TNR and lethal methods were equally favoured for unmanaged stray cats at 26%, and lethal methods were favoured for feral cats at 33%. As much less than half of the study population was in agreement regarding control methods. Further research should be carried out to investigate public support for alternative methods. In New Zealand, feral cats are classified as pests; consequently lethal methods of control such as kill trapping and poisoning are employed to manage population numbers [33], which may explain the higher level of support for the use of lethal methods with feral cats. Similarly, it has been suggested that lethal methods may be used to control stray cat populations unless evidence of their "ownership" can be provided [33]. This may in part explain the division of favour between TNR and lethal methods in the case of unmanaged stray cats. We found that females were more likely to select TNR over lethal methods of control for all sub-groups of unowned cats. Similar findings have been found in previous studies where females have been reported to be less supportive of lethal control methods for both stray and feral cats [58] and more supportive of TNR as a management technique [59–61]. In order to gain the greatest level of support for the management techniques posited in a National Strategy, the techniques must be demonstrated to not only positively impact wildlife through reduced predation but do so in a manner that is considerate of the welfare of individual cats and their humane treatment. Similar to the demographic variables of influence reported in other research [58], we found that older participants and those living in rural locations were more accepting of lethal control methods. This could be a reflection of increased interaction with wildlife in rural areas or increased exposure to unowned cats in rural areas.

Furthermore, it is important to point out that based on our definition, TNR may have been interpreted by participants as a robust mechanism of population control for all categories of cats specified in our study that does not involve euthanasia. Consequently, participants may have favoured TNR when it was considered alongside lethal methods, which suggests a possible bias in our results.

Although TNR programmes aim to create a stable population in which cats can no longer reproduce and natural attrition eventually results in decreased numbers [62], in reality, the effectiveness of TNR at reducing the population numbers of cats within a colony depends on a number of variables. These include the prevention of immigration of cats from outside of the colony, maintaining ongoing high levels of de-sexing of the individuals within the colony and any new immigrants, the ongoing removal of a maximum number of cats for adoption, and the allowance of time for natural attrition to occur. Successful TNR programmes have been reported in a limited number of studies where the programme has been targeted and managed closely. For example Levy, et al. [63] reported that over an 11 year period a colony population was successfully reduced by 66%, but this successfulness included the removal and adoption of 47% of the original population and the continual de-sexing of new arrivals to the colony before breeding could occur. In a further study by Stoskopf and Nutter [64], six de-sexed colonies showed a mean decrease in population of 36% during the first two years of study. Conversely, other examples of TNR reported in the scientific literature suggest that TNR is an ineffective mechanism for the population control of stray cats, in particular those that are unmanaged. For example Foley, et al. [65] reported that TNR was not successful at reducing the population numbers of stray cats in San Diego County, California and Alachua County, Florida and concluded that a reduction in growth per capita did not occur because the critical value of a 71–94% de-sexing rate was not achieved. Other research has used modeling to come up with similar figures of 75% or greater proportions of stray cats requiring de-sexing for population control to be effective [66]. In Rome, over the course of a decade, a 32% decrease in the population size over 103 colonies was observed, but the effectiveness of the TNR effort was substantially reduced by a 21% immigration rate of cats into these colonies from the companion cat population [67]. Furthermore, the successes of TNR programmes based on the impact on wildlife have not be reported. The successfulness of TNR would therefore seem to depend on how the programme is applied and managed, with scientific literature suggesting that TNR would likely be unsuccessful for cats categorised as unmanaged or feral in the present study. Consequently, we may have observed differing levels of support for TNR in the present study if it had been presented as a management strategy that requires intensive management and effort to remove and adopt cats as part of the TNR programme, and our results relating to TNR should be interpreted with caution.

4.4. Limitations

Aside from the limitations previously mentioned, it is important to point out that the majority of our participants were well educated. The proportion of participants with tertiary education was much higher than that represented in the most recent New Zealand census, potentially biasing our results. Additionally, although we gained participation from individuals living in locations in similar proportions to the recent New Zealand census (e.g., urban, suburban, and rural), the locations in which we collected responses were restricted to cities and towns in the upper North Island. Furthermore, although we utilised a standardised sampling method [36], we had no control over participants who independently chose to approach and participate. Consequently, the representative nature of our findings to the New Zealand population as a whole must be considered with caution. On the other hand, as discussed, our findings often parallel public opinion expressed regarding cat management both nationally and internationally, and therefore it is likely that similar trends would be observed in the lower North Island and throughout the South Island of New Zealand. Further research in these geographical areas is needed to confirm this.

5. Conclusions

To conclude, the results of this study indicate that the New Zealand public is largely in favour of a National Cat Management Strategy to control both owned and unowned cats and to aid in the reduction of cat predation, with high levels of concern expressed regarding the predation of both non-native and native wildlife. The findings of this research provide useful insights into public acceptance of a range of management strategies and the demographic variables that influence these. In particular, older participants expressed increased concern regarding the predation of wildlife by cats and were generally more in favour of the management techniques for owned cats and lethal methods of control for unowned cats. This suggests that older individuals may be more willing to comply with a National Cat Management Strategy, while younger indivdiuals may benefit from educational drives that detail the benefits for both wildlife populations and cat populations.

The differences observed between males and females suggests that females are more concerned about the humane treatment of individual animals as opposed to overall species conservation. Consequently, to increase female buy-in, the management techniques posited within a National Strategy must be demonstrated to be humane and considerate of individual animal welfare. Finally, the benefits of a National Cat Management Strategy must illuminate the differing benefits of cat manangement for both owners and non owners.

Acknowledgments: We are grateful to the participants who gave their time to complete the questionnaire. We would like to thank the Research Assistants who collected the data. We would like to thank the New Zealand Companion Animal Trust for funding this research and its publication in open access.

Author Contributions: Arnja Dale conceived the research idea and provided feedback on the manuscript. Arnja Dale and Stephanie Bruce designed the questionnaire. Stephanie Bruce facilitated data collection, input data, compiled literature, and provided feedback on the manuscript. Jessica Walker achieved funding, supervised the project, conducted statistical analysis, and wrote the manuscript.

Conflicts of Interest: Jessica Walker is currently an employee of the New Zealand Companion Animal Council, which is a subsidiary of the New Zealand Companion Animal Trust. Jessica was not employed by the New Zealand Companion Animal Council when this research was conceived, funded, and conducted, and the funding body had no role in any aspects of the study design, data collection, analysis, interpretation of the data, the writing of the manuscript, or in the decision to publish the results. Arnja Dale and Stephanie Bruce declare no conflicts of interest.

References

1.   New Zealand Companion Animal Council Inc. *Companion Animals in New Zealand*; New Zealand Companion Animal Council Inc.: Auckland, New Zealand, 2016.

2.   van Heezik, Y.; Smyth, A.; Adams, A.; Gordon, J. Do domestic cats impose an unsustainable harvest on urban bird populations? *Biol. Conserv.* **2010**, *143*, 121–130. [CrossRef]

3.   Bernstein, P.L. The human-cat relationship. In *The Welfare of Cats*; Springer: Berlin, Germany, 2007; pp. 47–89.

4.   Friedmann, E.; Son, H. The human-companion animal bond: How humans benefit. *Vet. Clin. N. Am. Small.* **2009**, *39*, 293–326. [CrossRef] [PubMed]

5.   Serpell, J. Beneficial effects of pet ownership on some aspects of human health and behaviour. *J. R. Soc. Med.* **1991**, *84*, 717–720. [PubMed]

6.   Wells, D.L. The effects of animals on human health and well-being. *J. Soc. Issues* **2009**, *65*, 523–543. [CrossRef]

7.   Gillies, C.; Clout, M. The prey of domestic cats (*Felis catus*) in two suburbs of Auckland city, New Zealand. *J. Zool.* **2003**, *259*, 309–315. [CrossRef]

8.   Loyd, K.A.T.; Hernandez, S.M.; Carroll, J.P.; Abernathy, K.J.; Marshall, G.J. Quantifying free-roaming domestic cat predation using animal-borne video cameras. *Biol. Conserv.* **2013**, *160*, 183–189. [CrossRef]

9.   Dabritz, H.; Conrad, P.A. Cats and toxoplasma: Implications for public health. *Biol. Conserv.* **2010**, *57*, 34–52.

10.   Nutter, F.B.; Levine, J.F.; Stoskopf, M.K. Reproductive capacity of free-roaming domestic cats`and kitten survival rate. *J. Am. Vet. Med. Assoc.* **2004**, *225*, 1399–1402. [CrossRef] [PubMed]

11.   Perry, G. Cats-perceptions and misconceptions: Two recent studies about cats and how people see them. In Proceedings of the Eight National Conference on Urban Animal Management in Australia, Gold Coast, Brisbane, Australia, 12–13 August 1999; pp. 127–130.

12.   Toukhsati, S.R.; Young, E.; Bennett, P.C.; Coleman, G.J. Wandering cats: Attitudes and behaviors towards cat containment in Australia. *Anthrozoös* **2012**, *25*, 61–74. [CrossRef]

13. Loyd, K.; Hernandez, S.; Abernathy, K.; Shock, B.; Marshall, G. Risk behaviours exhibited by free roaming cats in a suburban US town. *Vet. Rec.* **2013**, *173*, 295. [CrossRef] [PubMed]

14. National Animal Welfare Advisory Committee. *Animal Welfare (Companion Cats) Code of Welfare*; Ministry of Primary Industries: Wellington, New Zealand, 2007.

15. Mahlow, J.C.; Slater, M.R. Current issues in the control of stray and feral cats. *J. Am. Vet. Med. Assoc.* **1996**, *209*, 2016–2020. [PubMed]

16. Farnworth, M.J.; Muellner, P.; Benschop, J. *A Systematic Review of the Impacts of Feral, Stray and Companion Domestic Cats (Felis Catus) on Wildlife in New Zealand and Options for Their Management*; New Zealand Veterinary Association: Wellington, New Zealand, 2013.

17. Baker, P.; Bentley, A.J.; Ansell, R.J.; Harris, S. Impact of predation by domestic cats (*Felis catus*) in an urban area. *Mamm. Rev.* **2005**, *35*, 302–312. [CrossRef]

18. Lepczyk, C.A.; Mertig, A.G.; Liu, J. Landowners and cat predation across rural-to-urban landscapes. *Biol. Conserv.* **2004**, *115*, 191–201. [CrossRef]

19. Courchamp, F.; Langlais, M.; Sugihara, G. Cats protecting birds: Modelling the mesopredator release effect. *J. Anim. Ecol.* **1999**, *68*, 282–292. [CrossRef]

20. Norbury, G.; Heyward, R. Predictors of clutch predation of a globally significant avifauna in New Zealand's braided river ecosystems. *Anim. Conserv.* **2008**, *11*, 17–25. [CrossRef]

21. Woods, M.; McDonald, R.A.; Harris, S. Predation of wildlife by domestic cats (*Felis catus*) in Great Britain. *Mamm. Rev.* **2003**, *33*, 174–188. [CrossRef]

22. Dowding, J.E.; Murphy, E.C. The impact of predation by introduced mammals on endemic shorebirds in New Zealand: A conservation perspective. *Biol. Conserv.* **2001**, *99*, 47–64. [CrossRef]

23. Aguilar, G.D.; Farnworth, M.J. Stray cats in Auckland, New Zealand: Discovering geographic information for exploratory spatial analysis. *Appl. Geogr.* **2012**, *34*, 230–238. [CrossRef]

24. Metsers, E.M.; Seddon, P.J.; van Heezik, Y.M. Cat-exclusion zones in rural and urban-fringe landscapes: How large would they have to be? *Wildl. Res.* **2010**, *37*, 47–56. [CrossRef]

25. Lilith, M.; Calver, M.; Styles, I.; Garkaklis, M. Protecting wildlife from predation by owned domestic cats: Application of a precautionary approach to the acceptability of proposed cat regulations. *Austral Ecol.* **2006**, *31*, 176–189. [CrossRef]

26. Gordon, J.; Matthaei, C.; Van Heezik, Y. Belled collars reduce catch of domestic cats in New Zealand by half. *Wildl. Res.* **2010**, *37*, 372–378. [CrossRef]

27. Lord, L.K.; Griffin, B.; Slater, M.R.; Levy, J.K. Evaluation of collars and microchips for visual and permanent identification of pet cats. *J. Am. Vet. Med. Assoc.* **2010**, *237*, 387–394. [CrossRef] [PubMed]

28. Lord, L.K.; Wittum, T.E.; Ferketich, A.K.; Funk, J.A.; Rajala-Schultz, P.J. Search and identification methods that owners use to find a lost cat. *J. Am. Vet. Med. Assoc.* **2007**, *230*, 217–220. [CrossRef] [PubMed]

29. Aguilar, G.D.; Farnworth, M.J. Distribution characteristics of unmanaged cat colonies over a 20 year period in Auckland, New Zealand. *Appl. Geogr.* **2013**, *37*, 160–167. [CrossRef]

30. Jones, C. Microchipping and its importance in dogs. *Companion Anim.* **2013**, *18*, 468–473. [CrossRef]

31. Levy, J.; Isaza, N.; Scott, K. Effect of high-impact targeted trap-neuter-return and adoption of community cats on cat intake to a shelter. *Vet. J.* **2014**, *201*, 269–274. [CrossRef] [PubMed]

32. Spotte, S. Foraging. In *Free-Ranging Cats*; John Wiley & Sons Ltd.: Hoboken, NJ, USA, 2014; pp. 181–213.

33. Farnworth, M.; Campbell, J.; Adams, N. Public awareness in New Zealand of animal welfare legislation relating to cats. *N. Z. Vet. J.* **2010**, *58*, 213–217. [CrossRef] [PubMed]

34. Wald, D.M.; Jacobson, S.K.; Levy, J.K. Outdoor cats: Identifying differences between stakeholder beliefs, perceived impacts, risk and management. *Biol. Conserv.* **2013**, *167*, 414–424. [CrossRef]

35. Hall, C.M.; Adams, N.A.; Bradley, J.S.; Bryant, K.A.; Davis, A.A.; Dickman, C.R.; Fujita, T.; Kobayashi, S.; Lepczyk, C.A.; McBride, E.A. Community attitudes and practices of urban residents regarding predation by pet cats on wildlife: An international comparison. *PLoS ONE* **2016**, *11*, e0151962. [CrossRef] [PubMed]

36. De Vaus, D.A. *Surveys in Social Research*; Allen and Unwim: Sydney, Australia, 2002.

37. Statistics New Zealand. The New Zealand Census of Population and Dwellings. Available online: http://www.stats.govt.nz/Census/2013-census/data-tables/total-by-topic.aspx (accessed on 21 November 2016).

38. McGrath, N.; Walker, J.; Nilsson, D.; Phillips, C. Public attitudes towards grief in animals. *Anim. Welf.* **2013**, *22*, 33–47. [CrossRef]

39. Grayson, J.; Calver, M.; Styles, I. Attitudes of suburban Western Australians to proposed cat control legislation. *Aust. Vet. J.* **2002**, *80*, 536–543. [CrossRef] [PubMed]

40. Biben, M. Predation and predatory play behaviour of domestic cats. *Anim. Behav.* **1979**, *27*, 81–94. [CrossRef]

41. Holzapfel, S.; Robertson, H.A.; McLennan, J.A.; Sporle, W.; Hackwell, K.; Impey, M. *Kiwi (Apteryx Spp.) Recovery Plan: 2008–2018*; Department of Conservation: Wellington, New Zealand, 2008.

42. Fountain, J.; Espiner, S.; Xie, X. A cultural framing of nature: Chinese tourists' motivations for, expectations of, and satisfaction with, their New Zealand tourist experience. *Tour. Rev. Int.* **2010**, *14*, 71–83. [CrossRef]

43. Hall, C.M. Tourism destination branding and its effects on national branding strategies: Brand New Zealand, clean and green but is it smart? *Eur. J. Tour. Hosp. Recreat.* **2010**, *1*, 68–98.

44. Statistics New Zealand. Tourism Satellite Account: 2015. Available online: http://www.stats.govt.nz/browse_for_stats/industry_sectors/Tourism/tourism-satellite-account-2015/Summary_results.aspx (accessed on 21 November 2016).

45. Kellert, S.R.; Berry, J.K. Attitudes, knowledge, and behaviors toward wildlife as affected by gender. *Wildl. Soc. B* **1987**, *15*, 363–371.

46. Pifer, L.; Shimizu, K.; Pifer, R. Public attitudes toward animal research: Some international comparisons. *Soc. Anim.* **1994**, *2*, 95–113. [CrossRef] [PubMed]

47. Mathews, S.; Herzog, H.A. Personality and attitudes toward the treatment of animals. *Soc. Anim.* **1997**, *5*, 169–175. [CrossRef]

48. Bjerke, T.; Ødegårdstuen, T.S.; Kaltenborn, B.P. Attitudes toward animals among Norwegian adolescents. *Anthrozoös* **1998**, *11*, 79–86. [CrossRef]

49. Phillips, C.; Izmirli, S.; Aldavood, J.; Alonso, M.; Choe, B.; Hanlon, A.; Handziska, A.; Illmann, G.; Keeling, L.; Kennedy, M. An international comparison of female and male students' attitudes to the use of animals. *Animals* **2010**, *1*, 7–26. [CrossRef] [PubMed]

50. Walker, J.K.; McGrath, N.; Nilsson, D.L.; Waran, N.K.; Phillips, C.J. The role of gender in public perception of whether animals can experience grief and other emotions. *Anthrozoös* **2014**, *27*, 251–266. [CrossRef]

51. Herzog, H.A., Jr.; Betchart, N.S.; Pittman, R.B. Gender, sex role orientation, and attitudes toward animals. *Anthrozoös* **1991**, *4*, 184–191. [CrossRef]

52. Eldridge, J.J.; Gluck, J.P. Gender differences in attitudes toward animal research. *Ethics Behav.* **1996**, *6*, 239–256. [CrossRef] [PubMed]

53. Serpell, J.A. Factors influencing human attitudes to animals and their welfare. *Anim. Welf.* **2004**, *13*, 145–151.

54. Gunaseelan, S.; Coleman, G.J.; Toukhsati, S.R. Attitudes toward responsible pet ownership behaviors in Singaporean cat owners. *Anthrozoös* **2013**, *26*, 199–211. [CrossRef]

55. Harrod, M.; Keown, A.; Farnworth, M. Use and perception of collars for companion cats in New Zealand. *N. Z. Vet. J.* **2016**, *64*, 121–124. [CrossRef] [PubMed]

56. Jay, M. The political economy of a productivist agriculture: New Zealand dairy discourses. *Food Policy* **2007**, *32*, 266–279. [CrossRef]

57. Bonnington, C.; Gaston, K.J.; Evans, K.L. Fearing the feline: Domestic cats reduce avian fecundity through trait-mediated indirect effects that increase nest predation by other species. *J. Appl. Ecol.* **2013**, *50*, 15–24. [CrossRef]

58. Farnworth, M.J.; Campbell, J.; Adams, N.J. What's in a name? Perceptions of stray and feral cat welfare and control in Aotearoa, New Zealand. *J. Appl. Anim. Welf. Sci.* **2011**, *14*, 59–74. [CrossRef] [PubMed]

59. Dabritz, H.A.; Atwill, E.R.; Gardner, I.A.; Miller, M.A.; Conrad, P.A. Outdoor fecal deposition by free-roaming cats and attitudes of cat owners and nonowners toward stray pets, wildlife, and water pollution. *J. Am. Vet. Med. Assoc.* **2006**, *229*, 74–81. [CrossRef] [PubMed]

60. Lord, L.K. Attitudes toward and perceptions of free-roaming cats among individuals living in Ohio. *J. Am. Vet. Med. Assoc.* **2008**, *232*, 1159–1167. [CrossRef] [PubMed]

61. Loyd, K.A.T.; Hernandez, S.M. Public perceptions of domestic cats and preferences for feral cat management in the Southeastern United States. *Anthrozoös* **2012**, *25*, 337–351. [CrossRef]

62. Slater, M.R. The welfare of feral cats. In *The Welfare of Cats*; Springer: Berlin, Germany, 2007; pp. 141–175.

63. Levy, J.K.; Gale, D.W.; Gale, L.A. Evaluation of the effect of a long-term trap-neuter-return and adoption program on a free-roaming cat population. *J. Am. Vet. Med. Assoc.* **2003**, *222*, 42–46. [CrossRef] [PubMed]

64. Stoskopf, M.K.; Nutter, F.B. Analyzing approaches to feral cat management—One size does not fit all. *J. Am. Vet. Med. Assoc.* **2004**, *225*, 1361–1964. [CrossRef] [PubMed]

65. Foley, P.; Foley, J.E.; Levy, J.K.; Paik, T. Analysis of the impact of trap-neuter-return programs on populations of feral cats. *J. Am. Vet. Med. Assoc.* **2005**, *227*, 1775–1781. [CrossRef] [PubMed]

66. Andersen, M.C.; Martin, B.J.; Roemer, G.W. Use of matrix population models to estimate the efficacy of euthanasia versus trap-neuter-return for management of free-roaming cats. *J. Am. Vet. Med. Assoc.* **2004**, *225*, 1871–1876. [CrossRef] [PubMed]

67. Natoli, E.; Maragliano, L.; Cariola, G.; Faini, A.; Bonanni, R.; Cafazzo, S.; Fantini, C. Management of feral domestic cats in the urban environment of Rome (Italy). *Prev. Vet. Med.* **2006**, *77*, 180–185. [CrossRef] [PubMed]

8

Direct Observation of Dog Density and Composition during Street Counts as a Resource Efficient Method of Measuring Variation in Roaming Dog Populations over Time and between Locations

Elly Hiby * (iD) and Lex Hiby

Conservation Research Ltd., 110 Hinton Way, Great Shelford, Cambridge CB22 5AL, UK; lexhiby@gmail.com

* Correspondence: ellyhiby@gmail.com

Simple Summary: Roaming dogs are a common sight in many countries; they can be undernourished and unwell and may be a risk to public health. Different ways of improving the situation are proposed and attempted in many locations. To see which work, we suggest measuring dog density by counting dogs along standard routes across locations and repeating those counts at the same time of year and day, being careful to count the same way each time. It is not necessary to estimate the total number of dogs because it is the number per km of street that determines how many dogs a resident will meet on their way to school or work, and reducing density and healthier dogs would be considered a success. Smartphone applications make it easy to stick to standard routes and record dogs of different types, so we can also track things like the percentage of females with pups and the percentage of dogs that are emaciated. We present examples of such counts demonstrating large differences in densities between countries. There are few examples of counts over several years but we present one showing a definite reduction in density in a location that has provided spay and neuter services for several years.

Abstract: Dog population management is conducted in many countries to address the public health risks from roaming dogs and threats to their welfare. To assess its effectiveness, we need to monitor indicators from both the human and dog populations that are quick and easy to collect, precise and meaningful to intervention managers, donors and local citizens. We propose that the most appropriate indicators from the roaming dog population are population density and composition, based on counting dogs along standard routes using a standard survey protocol. Smart phone apps are used to navigate and record dogs along standard routes. Density expressed as dogs seen per km predicts the number of dogs residents will encounter as they commute to work or school and is therefore more meaningful than total population size. Composition in terms of gender, age and reproductive activity is measured alongside welfare, in terms of body and skin condition. The implementation of this method in seven locations reveals significant difference in roaming dog density between locations and reduction in density within one location subject to intervention. This method provides a resource efficient and reliable measure of roaming dog density, composition and welfare for the assessment of intervention impact.

Keywords: dog; stray dog; dog population management; animal welfare; survey; population density; strip transect; monitoring; evaluation

1. Introduction

Domestic dogs have evolved alongside humans for many thousands of years, and are currently almost ubiquitous in human society. Global estimates of dog population size are over 700 million [1].

In many countries, owned dogs are allowed to roam freely outside their owner's property for at least a portion of the day. For example, 68.5% of dogs were reported by their owners to be unconfined for at least part of the day in Todos Santos, Guatemala [2]; this was 37% in Iringa, Tanzania [3]; and between 27% and 67% in different sized urban areas in the Coquimbo region of Chile [4]. In addition, those dogs that do not have an owner also roam freely in the same space, in search of resources such as shelter and food, in the form of edible garbage and handouts from sympathetic people. The presence of roaming dogs, both owned roaming and unowned dogs, on streets and public property is therefore not uncommon. The density of this roaming dog population appears to differ between locations; however, there is limited objective data exploring this variation.

Due to the public health risks that these dogs may present and the threats to their own welfare many governments, municipalities and non-governmental organisations implement interventions to manage dog populations. The goals are often to reduce the number of dogs on the street and to improve the welfare and safety of the remaining population. However, there is limited published data detailing the impact of these efforts on dog density or welfare. In a scoping review of the literature [5], 26 studies assessing the impact of dog population management (DPM) were found, including seven which attempted to measure the impact on dog population density, of which only two were in peer-review journals [6,7], the remaining four were a book, conference proceedings or unpublished reports. This paucity of data leaves those responsible for managing dog populations limited in their ability to make evidence-based decisions on which interventions to establish, or to evaluate and improve the impact of their own interventions. Further, a failure to present evidence of impact may reduce the chances of ongoing funding and the political will to sustain an intervention.

An estimate of the total roaming dog population may be requested for planning or evaluating an intervention. However, this measure of abundance is time-consuming to establish, requiring repeated surveys of naturally or artificially marked samples of roaming dogs (for example [7] and [8]); the estimates are also subject to biases that are difficult to quantify. Abundance also requires clear definition in the context of a population consisting of a mixture of unowned and unconfined owned dogs, should it for example include those owned dogs that may only venture out of their owner's property for a few minutes each morning? Or should some threshold of roaming apply, such as only those owned dogs that roam for at least 20% of the day? Such definitions rely upon the knowledge of owners, which is time-consuming to measure and will be subject to unquantifiable error. Where the budget available for research is generous, assessing well defined dog population abundance, including sub-populations of dogs with different levels of ownership and confinement, may be possible; however, this is rarely the case in those locations where roaming dog density is a significant problem. An alternative is to focus on roaming dog population density as the appropriate indicator for evaluating the impact of a DPM intervention. We can define density as the expected number of roaming dogs (regardless of ownership status which is usually unidentifiable at the time of observation), that would be encountered by trained observers moving along every street within the region of interest divided by the total surveyed street length. Again, we need additional specifications: how fast observers should move, at what time of day and year, the extent to which observers should search under cars and so on. It is however easy to comply with such specifications once defined.

Assuming that there is insufficient time to move along every street, we can estimate population density by selecting a random sample of streets, counting the roaming dogs encountered along that route and dividing by its length. To select a purely random sample, each unit of street length within the region of interest would need to have the same probability of inclusion. Although we cannot ensure that is the case, we can try to make the selected route representative of the region of interest by having the route drawn by someone naïve to the expected spatial variation in roaming dog density. Any resulting biases affect comparison of density between different regions, but by using the same route for successive surveys we avoid bias invalidating estimates of change over time on that route.

A notable benefit of this measure is that most citizens are not affected directly by the total number of roaming dogs in their city whereas roaming dog density, expressed as dogs seen per km, determines the number of dogs they will encounter as they commute to a regular destination, for example their place of work or school. Hence, a change in roaming dog density along public streets is more meaningful to the potential beneficiaries of the intervention. In addition, most urban areas are growing in size; in the developing world this rate of growth can be staggeringly high. In such an urban area, the total number of roaming dogs may increase along with expansion and development of the city. Thus, even if an intervention succeeds in reducing the density of roaming dogs on a city's streets to the benefit of the residents, it may be incorrectly deemed to have failed if the absolute population size has not reduced. Finally, if carefully conducted, measurements of population density have much higher precision than estimates of total abundance obtained using the same level of effort, and are therefore more sensitive to any changes resulting from intervention.

Observers also have the opportunity to record the type of each dog encountered and its visible body and skin condition, resulting in estimates of the composition of the roaming dog population. Interventions commonly include reproduction control to reduce unwanted puppies and breeding behaviours that are considered a nuisance. By monitoring the percentage of females that show visible signs of lactation, the extent to which the intervention is accessing the roaming dog population can be assessed. In addition, monitoring body and skin condition may provide a measure of an intervention's impact on dog welfare.

The authors hence set out to establish a method of measuring roaming dog population density and composition that would be sensitive to differences between location and changes within location over time, but also simple and cost effective to implement. It is an adaptation of index monitoring, primarily used for wildlife (for example, see [9] and [10] for discussions of ideal index monitoring methodologies and analyses in several wildlife species), to a domestic species. It assumes constant average detectability of roaming dogs by applying consistent search effort over time, achieved by observers adhering closely to the survey protocol and routes. The methodology utilises counts of roaming dogs along routes following urban and suburban streets, effectively providing strip transects along the roads, pavements and verges between buildings to measure density [11]. Utilising the physical structures of buildings to create strip transects has been used for measuring density of other species in urban areas, including bird species, e.g., [12]. The method presented here has been trialed in several locations and refined based on implementation experience and results. It builds on the method utilised by Reece and Chawla [6] in Jaipur, India, where counts of roaming dogs are conducted along streets with almost exhaustive coverage of a particular area of the city. However, the method described here utilises routes that extend across urban areas to integrate over spatial variation in roaming dog density.

2. Materials and Methods

To measure change in population density we need a standard unit of survey effort (e.g., "catch per unit effort" in fisheries). In the case of roaming dogs we selected the number of roaming dogs seen per kilometre along standard routes using a standard survey protocol. As these same routes must be maintained for all future surveying the initial selection of routes must be done with care. Routes were drawn using the "add driving route" tool in Google My Maps (www.google.co.uk/maps/about/mymaps); two approaches to designing routes were used:

● Representative routes. A "representative" route is drawn by someone naïve to the expected spatial variation in roaming dog density. The route is drawn to take in an approximately representative proportion of residential and larger roads, and areas of different housing types using the satellite view in My Maps (see Figure 1).

● "Hotspot" routes. The term "hotspot" was used because these routes were drawn to focus on areas known to have high density of roaming dogs. People local to the area with an interest in roaming dogs were asked to indicate on maps where they tended to see the most roaming dogs. The routes were then drawn to bisect as many of these areas as possible within the shortest distance.

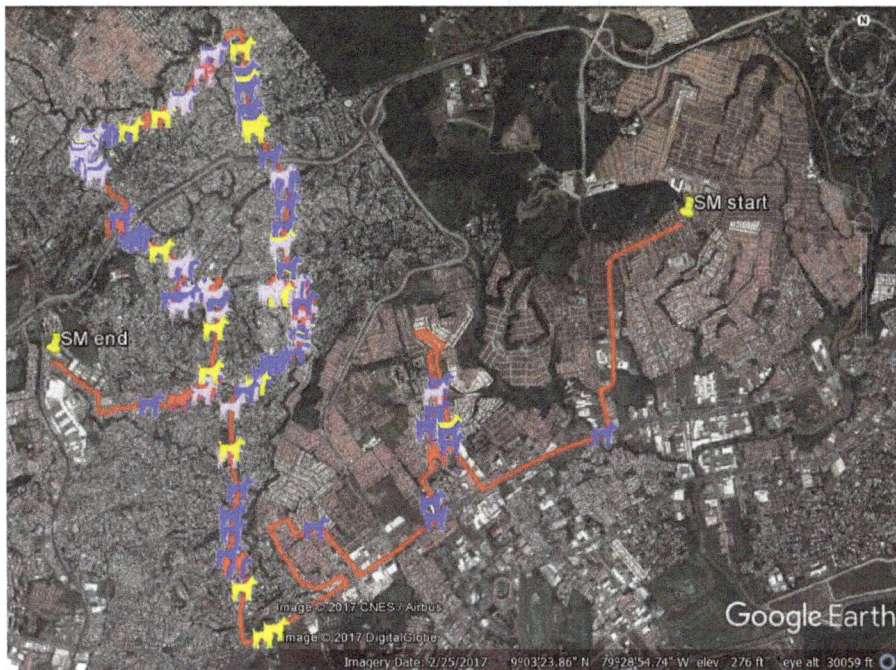

Figure 1. Google Earth image of the "San Miguelito" route in Panama City. The red line shows the route surveyed, the dog icons show the location of the observer when the roaming dog was recorded; blue dogs are male, yellow dogs are female, grey dogs are adults of unknown gender and red dogs are lactating females. Where a sterilisation programme has taken place, using visible marks of sterilisation status such as ear notches or ear tags, black and green icons are used to represent castrated males and spayed females.

Where representative routes are used, the average number of dogs per km of street can be extrapolated to make an estimate of the total number of dogs visibly roaming on public streets at the time of the survey, using the total road length for the area. Where an estimate of detectability is available, this can be used in a further stage of extrapolation to estimate the total number of roaming dogs at the outset of an intervention.

Navigation along the routes was supported by the use of mapping apps on smart phones. The routes were saved as kml files and then displayed on mapping apps, such as Google Maps, Maps.Me or Locus.

Direct observation of the dogs was done by a team of at least two observers. These observers would walk, cycle, drive or ride a motorcycle along the route. The mode of transport was chosen according to the accessibility of the roads and the preference of the surveyors. Once a mode of transport was selected this had to be maintained for future monitoring surveys.

The length of the route was dictated by the mode of transport as the aim was to create a route that took no longer than 2 h to complete, usually 20 km maximum in length when using a car or motorcycle.

Observers move as quickly as possible along the route, allowing sufficient time to assess gender and welfare, but attempting to move faster along the route than the dogs to avoid double counting. Interaction with the dogs is minimised to avoid influencing their movement; this either encourages them to come with observers or causes them to run away which increases the chances they will interact with other dogs. Interactions between dogs may lead to increased movement, therefore greater potential for double counting and risks aggressive encounters which endanger dog welfare and human safety.

A survey event required each route to be surveyed at least twice to establish a measure of day-to-day variation that could then be used to calculate the significance of any observed change in dog density over time.

Observation of dogs was recorded using the smart phone app OSMtracker with a layout designed specifically for dog surveys; the observer taps an icon on the app display to record the observed dog type (see Figure 2). This is an event recording app that notes the GPS location of the observer at the time of event logged (see Figure 1 for an example of dog type icons displayed on Google Earth using GPS information recorded at the time of observation). Each dog was scored for the following:

- Gender/age
  - ○ Male
  - ○ Female
  - ○ Lactating female
  - ○ Unknown adult
  - ○ Pup (under 4 months of age)
  - ○ Sterilised male (only in those locations where marking of sterilised dogs is used)
  - ○ Sterilised female (only in those locations where marking of sterilised dogs is used)
- Visible welfare
  - ○ Body condition score (BCS) on a 5 point scale (using visual cues only, as described in [13])
  - ○ Presence or absence of a visible skin condition

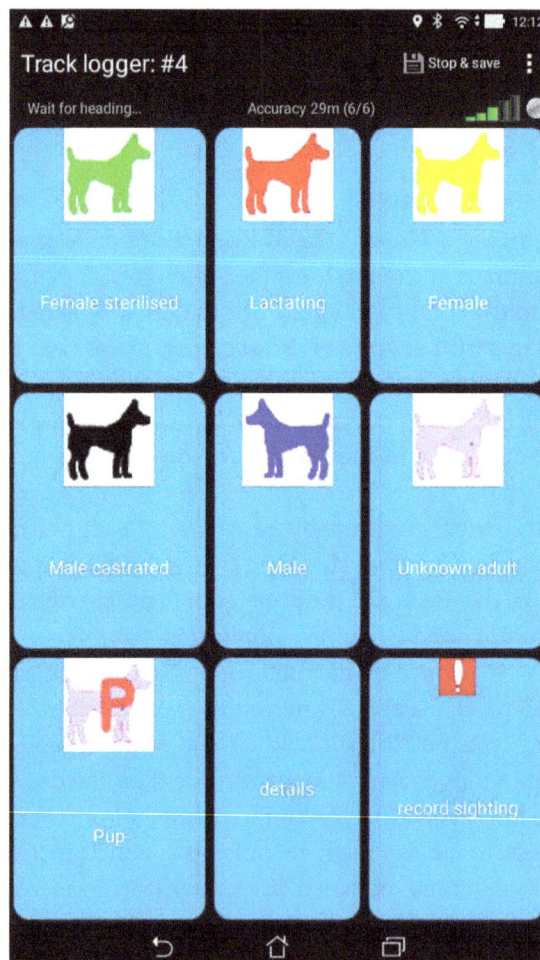

Figure 2. Image of OSMtracker app display on a mobile phone, showing an icon for each dog type recorded during surveying.

In each location, the protocol used for survey was recorded to ensure future monitoring surveys were conducted with consistent search effort. This included the start time for each route, average speed, mode of transport, acceptable weather conditions (e.g., do not survey during rain as fewer dogs will be visible), whether the observers should check under parked cars and how far down a side street off their route should they look.

Data were uploaded to an Access database and analysed. The differences between location in percentage of females lactating, the percentage of dogs with low body condition and the percentage with skin conditions were tested using a Kruskal-Wallis H-test. The difference in dogs per km between locations was tested using Analysis of Variance (ANOVA), differences in dogs per km over time and lactation over time within Panama City were tested using regression analysis.

2.1. Power to Detect Change in Density

We consider the situation where a survey following some level of intervention is to be compared to a baseline survey conducted prior to the intervention to detect any significant change in average density. Replicating the baseline surveys along each route then allows the power to detect change to be estimated simply as a minimum required observed change. The differences between the densities recorded on the replicate surveys, averaged over the routes and then divided by their standard error has a Student's t distribution based on $n-1$ degrees of freedom where n equals the number of routes. Those differences can therefore be used to calculate the minimum percentage change observed by a future survey that would be required to detect a significant change in actual population density.

For example, a roaming dog survey of Mumbai in January 2014 [14] counted dogs seen per km along 21 predesigned routes, repeating the counts on the following day. A mean of 10.54 dogs were seen per km. As expected, the average difference between the replicate counts was close to zero at 0.097, with a standard error of 0.29. To use those same routes to show a change in current roaming dog density as compared to January 2014, significant at the 95% level, would therefore require that currently observed density is less than or more than 10.54 times 0.29 times $t_{0.05,20}$, i.e., by approximately 6% or 0.63 dogs per km.

If a series of surveys are conducted, then selecting a pair that happen to show a desired change would invalidate the size of the test, which would need to be based on just the final survey or on a time series analysis and therefore a model of change over time.

2.2. Power to Detect Change in Composition

Replicate counts of roaming dogs of certain types, for example of lactating females, can also be used to estimate the power to detect change in their population density. However, the power to detect change in, for example, the percentage of females that are lactating can be estimated without replication if the number of lactating females counted can be assumed to have a binomial distribution. In that case the fraction of females that are seen to be lactating has approximately a normal distribution with standard deviation $\sqrt{\frac{1}{n}p(1-p)}$ where n equals the number of females counted and p equals the fraction that were lactating. Under a null hypothesis that the current population fraction lactating is unchanged as compared to an earlier survey, the difference between current and previous observed fractions would have zero expectation and standard deviation $\sqrt{\left(\frac{1}{n_1} + \frac{1}{n_2}\right)p(1-p)}$ where p is a combined estimate based on the n_1 and n_2 females counted in the two surveys. The observed fractions would then have to differ by 1.96 times that estimated standard deviation to reject the null hypothesis and conclude at the 95% level that a change in the fraction lactating had occurred.

Using the Mumbai survey as an example; 0.08 of the 3236 females recorded during the street counts were lactating whereas 0.11 of the females counted in "slum" areas were lactating, an increase of 0.03. However the total number of females counted in the slum areas (n_2) was less than the 463 required to make the increase in the observed fraction significant at the 95% level.

Table 1. Indicators relating to density, reproductive activity and welfare of roaming dogs for two or more routes in seven locations; resulting from application of the method of direct observation of dogs along public streets. BCS, body condition score.

Country	Route Type	Name of Route	Date Surveyed	Dogs Per km	% Lactating	% BCS 1	% BCS 1 or 2	% Visible Skin Condition
Bosnia	Hotspot	Kljuc	16 June	9.07	0.0%	0.0%	0.0%	4.2%
		Mrkonjic Grad	16 June	0.78	0.0%	0.0%	0.0%	10.7%
		Trebinje	16 September	1.49	11.1%	0.0%	17.9%	
Bogatic municipality, Serbia	Representative	Badovinci	16 May	0.855	50.0%	0.0%	4.2%	0.0%
		Bogatic		0.6	33.3%	0.0%	11.1%	0.0%
		Crna Bara		0.52	0.0%	0.0%	0.0%	0.0%
		Dublje		0.145	0.0%	0.0%	5.6%	0.0%
		Klenje		0.72	0.0%	0.0%	18.8%	0.0%
Constanta county, Romania	Hotspot	Cernavoda	16 July	4.79	6.8%	0.0%	8.3%	1.4%
	Representative	Agigea	16 September	6.52	25.9%	0.0%	44.4%	18.5%
Panama City, Panama	Representative	San Miguelito	November–December 2013	5.62	11.1%	4.0%	38.7%	28.2%
		Casco Viejo		1.07	8.0%	2.3%	15.9%	11.8%
		Juan Diaz		1.87	0.0%	5.1%	22.0%	22.8%
		Kuna Nega		5.83	4.6%	2.5%	18.6%	14.5%
Puerto Rico	Representative	Aguadilla	14 March	1.13	0.0%	0.0%	2.6%	9.4%
		Fajardo/Ceiba		1.73	4.3%	0.0%	11.3%	22.7%
		Toa Alta		1.73	0.0%	0.0%	2.0%	9.5%
San Jose, Costa Rica	Representative	San Jose	14 June	2.59	8.8%	0.0%	5.6%	6.2%
		Heredia Y Belen		1.50	0.0%	0.0%	2.0%	6.3%
		Cartago		3.09	11.1%	1.0%	9.0%	5.1%
		Alajuela		2.28	20.0%	1.1%	9.6%	6.2%
		Rancho Redondo		4.09	6.5%	1.3%	6.4%	2.0%
Kathmandu, Nepal	Representative	Zone 1	16 March	12.30	12.3%	0.0%	*	0.9%
		Zone 2		27.14	6.2%	0.1%		3.3%
		Zone 3		12.28	6.0%	0.0%		2.7%
		Zone 4		14.41	6.6%	0.1%		2.6%
		Zone 5		15.66	4.1%	0.1%		3.0%
		Zone 6		8.40	8.3%	0.0%		6.5%
		Zone 7		11.37	20.3%	0.0%		1.8%
		Zone 8		11.76	10.3%	0.0%		0.9%

* Only emaciated dogs with BCS 1 had their body condition score recorded during the survey in Kathmandu; this was due to the high number of roaming dogs to record within limited survey time.

3. Results

This method has been conducted in many locations to date. Table 1 shows the data from 7 of these locations across Europe, Latin America and Asia. The number of roaming dogs observed per km of street surveyed in these locations is also shown in Figure 3.

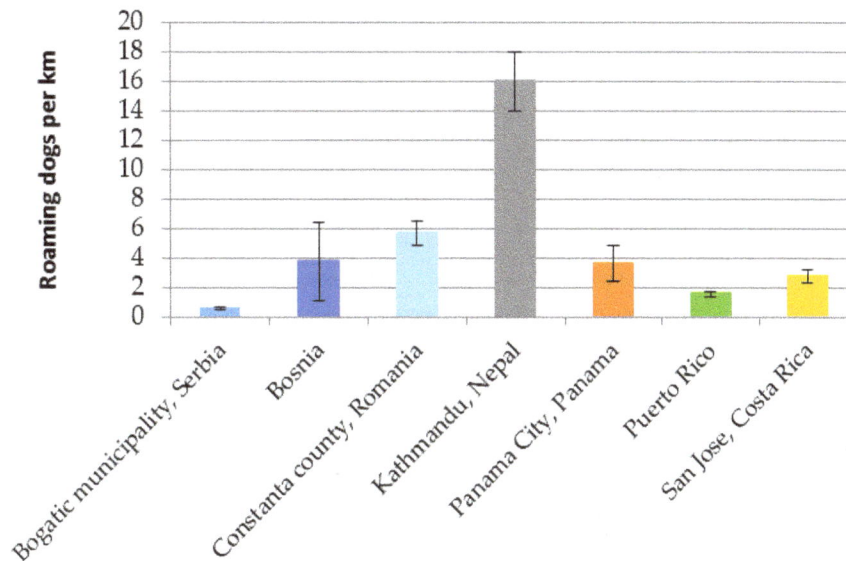

Figure 3. Bar chart showing the difference in average roaming dog density per km along both hotspot and representative routes in seven locations (it should be noted that both the design of the routes and the degree of urbanization along these routes varies between location, hence the average density along routes cannot be taken to represent national or regional roaming dog density), error bars shown are +/− one standard error.

The density of roaming dogs per km differed significantly between the locations listed in Table 1 ($F = 10.943$, $df = 6$, $p < 0.001$). Table 1 also provides three additional indicators. The percentage of females that are lactating, which did not differ significantly between country ($H = 3.450$, $df = 6$, $p = 0.751$); and two indicators of welfare state, visible skin problems and body condition score. The percentage of dogs with a visible skin problem showed a significant difference between the locations ($H = 20.621$, $df = 6$, $p < 0.01$). Body condition score was explored through both the percentage of dogs that were recorded as BCS 1 emaciated and the percentage that were either BCS 1 emaciated or BCS 2 thin. Neither of these indicators were significantly different between locations (BCS 1 $H = 10.690$, $df = 6$, $p = 0.098$; BCS 1 or 2 $H = 8.907$, $df = 5$, $p = 0.179$).

Monitoring using the same survey protocol has been carried out in some of the locations listed in Table 1. Table 2 displays the monitoring data from five locations, the number of repeat surveys that have been conducted ranging from 1 to 4.

The dogs per km of street survey in Tables 1 and 2 are averages within route, resulting from two or more replicate surveys along the same route, using the same protocol, on consecutive days. An example of these replicates over time is given in Figure 4, which displays the dogs per km of street recorded at every survey, both replicates within survey event and repeated surveys over time for the four routes in Panama City.

Table 2. Monitoring data resulting from repeat surveying along standard routes in five locations.

Country	Route Type	Name of Route	13 December	14 June	14 December	15 October	16 September
Panama City, Panama	Representative	San Miguelito	5.62	5.453	5.887	5.73	5.895
		Casco Viejo	1.07	1.03	0.95	0.79	0.44
		Juan Diaz	1.87	2.99	2.735	2.035	1.805
		Kuna Nega	5.83	4.8167	3.883	4.73	4.435
Country	Route Type	Name of Route	14 March	15 April	16 March		
Puerto Rico	Representative	Aguadilla	1.13	0.98	0.60		
		Fajardo/Ceiba	1.73	1.23	1.25		
		Toa Alta	1.73	1.20	1.04		
Country	Route Type	Name of Route	16 June	16 September			
Bosnia	Hotspot	Kljuc	9.07	7.04			
Country	Route Type	Name of Route	16 July	16 October			
Constanta county, Romania	Hotspot	Cernavoda	4.79	4.34			
Country	Route Type	Name of Route	16 March	16 November			
Kathmandu, Nepal	Representative	Zone 1	12.30	15.45			
		Zone 2	27.14	29.565			
		Zone 3	12.28	12.675			
		Zone 4	14.41	13.54			
		Zone 5	15.66	18.42			
		Zone 6	8.40	10.905			
		Zone 7	11.37	14.425			
		Zone 8	11.76	12.835			

Regression analysis of the data shown in Figure 4 reveals the Casco Viejo route has shown a statistically significant change in density over time, with a decreasing density of roaming dogs per km of street across the five survey events ($R^2 = 0.5934$, $p < 0.05$); this route covers an area of the city that has undergone intervention over a number of years, including sterilisation of male and female dogs.

Again, although not statistically significant ($R^2 = 0.1578$, $p = 0.179$), Casco Viejo shows a reduction in percentage of females lactating over time, see Figure 5; percentage lactating is expected to be the first indicator to respond to an intervention that involves spaying of female dogs that roam.

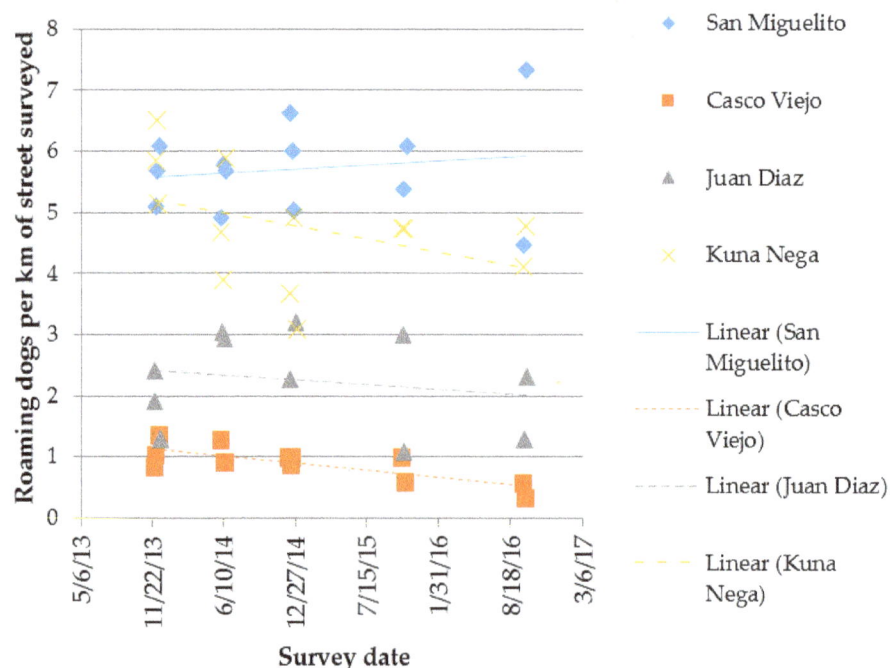

Figure 4. Roaming dogs per km of street surveyed for all four Panama City routes, showing the data for the two or three replicates at each survey event and five survey events across time.

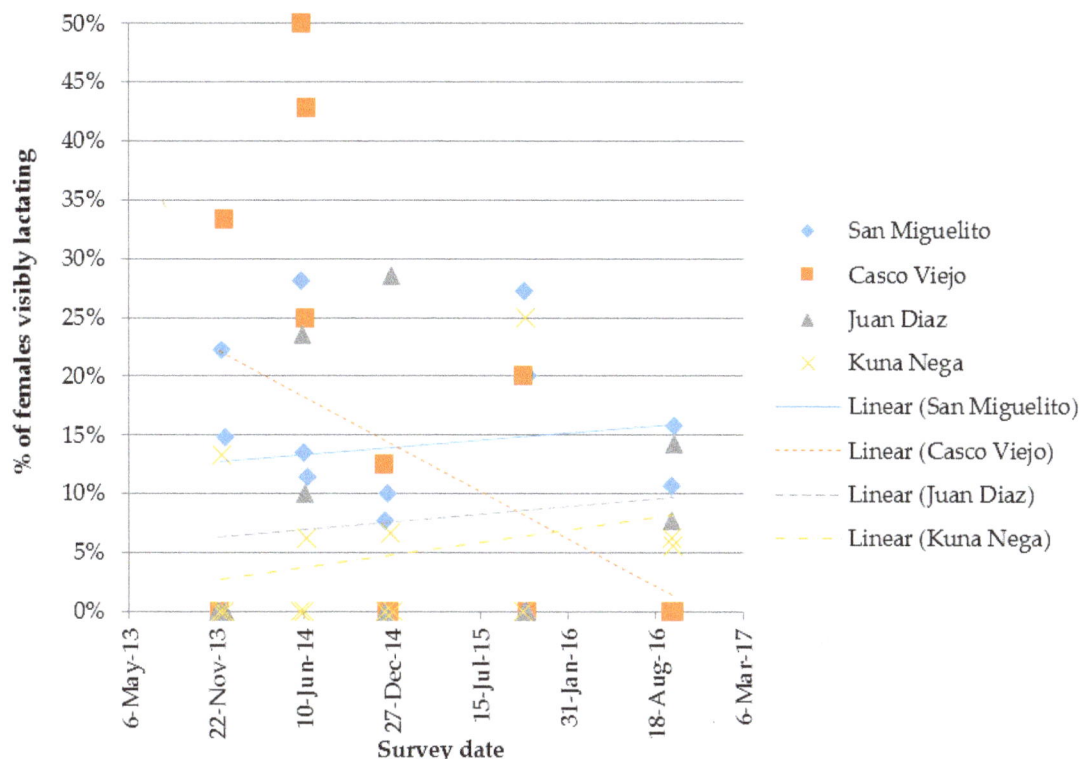

Figure 5. Percentage of females lactating at the time of observation; percentage for each of the four Panama City routes, at each survey event (comprised of two or three replicate surveys per route).

4. Discussion

The method of direct observation of roaming dogs along routes provides data for measuring a range of important indicators for roaming dog populations. Its uptake in several locations, including persistent use for monitoring over time, is evidence for its simplicity of implementation.

Where a consistent survey protocol is used to compare changes in the density of dogs observed along standard routes, this represents a novel indicator of the probability of encountering a dog along these routes and their average welfare and reproductive state. As such there is no comparable method against which to validate this method. However, where the method is extended by the use of representative routes and total street length to estimate the total number of dogs visibly roaming in an area, there is the potential to compare this against other approaches. Conducting exhaustive searches of all streets could be used to validate whether the route selected was indeed representative of the true average density across the area. Another potential comparison could be made with the estimate resulting from applying mark-recapture methods [7,8,15], however, as this method suffers from unknown error from potentially violated assumptions, this may not be true validation, but a useful comparison nonetheless.

Implementing this method requires consistent motivation and interest in the data it produces. We have found that those locations that have maintained ongoing monitoring are those that benefit from a local team of surveyors, as opposed to those that require outside personnel. In addition, these local teams require ongoing support in data analysis and interpretation to ensure they are able to use the data in meaningful ways.

A potential weakness of the method is its reliance on consistency in protocol when conducting the street survey to reduce the impact of confounding variables. Hence it is important to ensure surveyors are required to survey at the same time of day and avoid days of unusual human activity, such as national holidays or market days, when dog visibility could be affected. The track taken by the surveyors and their speed is recorded by the OSMtracker app, so that their adherence to the route can be checked and their speed indicates search effort, which needs to be kept constant. To minimise observer differences, local teams are trained by experts in the survey method and, as far as possible, the same observers are used for both the replicate and repeat surveys. Roaming dogs have been shown to display quite prominent seasonal breeding in some locations [16], leading to changes in percentage lactating and density across the year. Hence surveys should be conducted at the same time of year, and where multiple surveys are conducted within the year, comparisons of changes over time must be made between surveys at the same time of year and not across seasons.

The density of roaming dogs, as indicated by the number of roaming dogs recorded per km of street surveyed is sufficiently sensitive to expose significant difference between locations and, in one location, a significant reduction over time. We argue it is also an important and relevant indicator, as it reflects the experience citizens have of roaming dogs in their community, for example as they commute to work and school.

The percentage of females that are visibly lactating has potential as an early stage indicator of change in response to DPM interventions that use spaying of females. If one assumes that the puppies born to roaming females (both owned dogs that are roaming away from home or unowned females) are more likely to be unwanted and suffer high mortality, roaming females become a principle target for spaying. Following implementation of a project that spays female dogs, an observed reduction in lactating females indicates that the roaming dog population is less reproductively active. Reduction in density may follow as roaming dogs die and are not replaced by pups at the same rate due to reduced breeding. However, there may be little reduction in adult roaming dog density if very few pups born on the streets survive and the roaming population is actually sustained by dispersal or abandonment of owned and currently confined dogs. There may even be an initial increase in adult roaming density if female survival improves as a result of spaying.

The importance of the proportion of lactating females in the roaming dog population has also been highlighted by Reece et al. [17]; human animal-bite incidents reported by the SMS Hospital in Jaipur appear to show seasonal variation, with a peak in bites following 10 weeks after the estimated peak whelping time for street dogs in that city. It is hypothesised by the authors that maternal defensive aggression may be the motivation for at least some of these bites from dogs, as this peak occurs when there will be the highest number of puppies at 2–3 months, an age when they are visible and attractive to people, yet still under protection of their dam.

The indicators of body condition score and skin condition are basic measures of welfare state; there was a significant difference in the percentage of dogs with a visible skin problem between locations. Many DPM interventions aim to improve welfare and hence these indicators may provide valuable evidence of impact where they show a change over time. Dogs with an emaciated body condition (BCS 1) were rare in the surveys presented here, with a maximum of 5.1% recorded on one of the routes in Panama City; most routes did not record any emaciated dogs at all, possibly because a dog in an emaciated state is unlikely to survive for long. Nevertheless, the percentage of emaciated dogs is a valuable indicator as this body condition suggests a serious welfare problem that an intervention may be aiming to address. However, where this percentage is very low, the combined percentage of dogs that are emaciated or thin (BCS 2) can also be monitored. Although a thin dog may not necessarily be suffering a serious welfare problem, a high percentage of dogs that are thin or emaciated suggests the population is challenged in terms of health or access to resources. In some locations, such as Kathmandu, where observers are recording high numbers of dogs during the survey, the team may elect to only record the presence of emaciated dogs, because of the time required to assess and record dogs with BCS 2–5.

A limitation of this method is that it does not address the issue of the composition of the roaming dog population with regards to ownership status. As described in the introduction, it is known that a proportion of owned dogs will roam on public streets without owner supervision; this proportion varies considerably between locations and will depend on attitudes of both owners towards confinement and neighbours towards roaming dogs, as well as the structure of homes and fencing which will have cultural and economic drivers. Estimating the ratio of owned to ownerless dogs within a roaming dog population is hypothetically possible by utilising methods of mark-resight combined with a questionnaire of owners; where a known number of the owned dog population that is reportedly allowed to roam is marked, followed by street surveying where observers count roaming dogs and record whether they are marked or unmarked. However, this method is subject to several assumptions and requires intensive effort to implement a questionnaire, mark dogs and survey streets; hence it was considered beyond the scope of a resource efficient method for measuring change over time. Arguably, changes in indicators of dog density, composition and welfare measured through street surveying alone, following the course of an intervention, will provide signs of dog ownership. For example, an intervention that focuses on sterilisation of owned dogs may observe a steep decline in the percentage of roaming females that are lactating, suggesting that the majority of the roaming dogs are indeed owned dogs allowed to roam unsupervised.

5. Conclusions

By increasing the use of direct observation of dog density and composition during street counts, the authors hope to contribute to the use of objective data in evaluating and managing DPM interventions. Although the data gathered through this method can be used to compare locations, its real strength is in monitoring changes over time. Since the method is simple and efficient, the surveys can be repeated consistently and relatively frequently along the same routes. Such monitoring has been conducted in several locations; the example of Panama City is provided. However, in most locations only monitoring baselines have been established, because the interventions are in early stages and changes in the roaming dog population are not yet expected.

This method alone will not be sufficient for reliable evaluation or predictions of how a roaming dog population will respond to an intervention; dogs exist within a close relationship with people, those that own, care or dislike them, all impact on their survival, reproduction and welfare. Therefore, additional methods that attempt to measure the attitudes and behaviours of people and how they change in response to intervention will be required for more meaningful evaluation of the mechanisms behind any changes in dog density.

Acknowledgments: Preparation of the manuscript was unfunded. Implementation of the method was funded by different sources according to location: Bogatic municipality, Serbia was implemented with Organisation for Respect and Care of Animals (ORCA) and co-funded by the Bogatic Municipality and ORCA; Bosnia was funded by the International Fund for Animal Welfare (IFAW); Constanta country, Romania was implemented with Save The Dogs and Other Animals and co-funded by the International Companion Animal Management (ICAM) Coalition and World Animal Protection; Kathmandu, Nepal was implemented with Humane Society International (HSI) and co-funded by ICAM Coalition and HSI; Panama City was implemented with Spay Panama and funded by HSI; Puerto Rico and San Jose, Costa Rica were funded by HSI.

Author Contributions: Elly Hiby and Lex Hiby contributed equally to design, performance, analysis and writing.

Conflicts of Interest: The authors declare no conflict of interest. The funders of individual locations had no role in the design of the study, analyses, or interpretation of data; in the writing of the manuscript, or in the decision to publish the results.

References

1. Hughes, J.; Macdonald, D.W. A review of the interactions between free-roaming domestic dogs and wildlife. *Biol. Conserv.* **2013**, *157*, 341–351. [CrossRef]

2. Pulczer, A.S.; Jones-Bitton, A.; Waltner-Toews, D.; Dewey, C.E. Owned dog demography in Todos Santos Cuchumatán, Guatemala. *Prev. Vet. Med.* **2013**, *108*, 209–217. [CrossRef] [PubMed]

3. Gsell, A.S.; Knobel, D.L.; Kazwala, R.R.; Vounatsou, P.; Zinsstag, J. Domestic dog demographic structure and dynamics relevant to rabies control planning in urban areas in Africa: The case of Iringa, Tanzania. *BMC Vet. Res.* **2012**, *8*, 236. [CrossRef] [PubMed]

4. Acosta-Jamett, G.; Cleaveland, S.; Cunningham, A.A.; Bronsvoort, B.M.D. Demography of domestic dogs in rural and urban areas of the Coquimbo region of Chile and implications for disease transmission. *Prev. Vet. Med.* **2010**, *94*, 272–281. [CrossRef] [PubMed]

5. Hiby, E.; Atema, K.N.; Brimley, R.; Hammond-Seaman, A.; Jones, M.; Rowan, A.; Fogelberg, E.; Kennedy, M.; Balaram, D.; Nel, L.; et al. Scoping review of indicators and methods of measurement used to evaluate the impact of dog population management interventions. *BMC Vet. Res.* **2017**, *13*, 1–20. [CrossRef] [PubMed]

6. Reece, J.F.; Chawla, S.K. Control of rabies in Jaipur, India, by the sterilisation and vaccination of neighbourhood dogs. *Vet. Rec.* **2006**, *159*, 379–383. [CrossRef] [PubMed]

7. Totton, S.C.; Wandeler, A.I.; Zinsstag, J.; Bauch, C.T.; Ribble, C.S.; Rosatte, R.C.; McEwen, S.A. Stray dog population demographics in Jodhpur, India following a population control/rabies vaccination program. *Prev. Vet. Med.* **2010**, *97*, 51–57. [CrossRef] [PubMed]

8. Punjabi, G.A.; Athreya, V.; Linnell, J.D.C. Using natural marks to estimate free-ranging dog Canis familiaris abundance in a MARK-RESIGHT framework in suburban Mumbai, India. *Trop. Conserv. Sci.* **2012**, *5*, 510–520. [CrossRef]

9. Pollock, K.H.; Nichols, J.D.; Simons, T.R.; Farnsworth, G.L.; Bailey, L.L.; Sauer, J.R. Large scale wildlife monitoring studies: Statistical methods for design and analysis. *Environmetrics* **2002**, *13*, 105–119. [CrossRef]

10. Ficetola, G.F.; Romano, A. Optimizing monitoring schemes to detect trends in abundance over broad scales. *Anim. Conserv.* **2017**. [CrossRef]

11. Hayne, D.W. An Examination of the Strip Census Method for Estimating Animal Populations. *J. Wildl. Manag.* **1949**, *13*, 145–157. [CrossRef]

12. Munyenyembe, F.; Harris, J.; Hone, J. Determinants of bird populations in an urban area. *Aust. J. Ecol.* **1989**, *14*, 549–557. [CrossRef]

13. ICAM Coalition. *Are We Making a Difference? A Guide to Monitoring and Evaluating Dog Population Management Interventions*; ICAM Coalition: Yarmouth Port, MA, USA, 2015.

14. Hiby, L.; (Conservation Research Ltd., Cambridge, UK). Roaming dog population survey of Greater Mumbai conducted with HSI-Asia. Unpublished data, 2014.

15. Hiby, L.R.; Reece, J.F.; Wright, R.; Jaisinghani, R.; Singh, B.; Hiby, E.F. A mark-resight survey method to estimate the roaming dog population in three cities in Rajasthan, India. *BMC Vet. Res.* **2011**, *7*, 46. [CrossRef] [PubMed]

16. Reece, J.F.; Chawla, S.K.; Hiby, E.F.; Hiby, L.R. Fecundity and longevity of roaming dogs in Jaipur, India. *BMC Vet. Res.* **2008**, *4*, 6. [CrossRef] [PubMed]

17. Reece, J.F.; Chawla, S.K.; Hiby, A.R. Decline in human dog-bite cases during a street dog sterilisation programme in Jaipur, India. *Vet. Rec.* **2013**, *172*, 473. [CrossRef] [PubMed]

9

American Citizens' Views of an Ideal Pig Farm

Patrycia Sato [1], **Maria J. Hötzel** [2] **and Marina A.G. von Keyserlingk** [1,*]

[1] Animal Welfare Program, 2357 Main Mall, Faculty of Land and Food Systems,
University of British Columbia, Vancouver, BC V6T 1Z4, Canada; sato.patrycia@gmail.com

[2] Laboratório de Etologia Aplicada e Bem-Estar Animal,
Departamento de Zootecnia e Desenvolvimento Rural, Universidade Federal de Santa Catarina,
Florianópolis 88034-001, Brazil; maria.j.hotzel@ufsc.br

[*] Correspondence: marina.vonkeyserlingk@ubc.ca

Simple Summary: The public, who also make up the largest proportion of consumers of animal products, often criticize farm animal industries in regards to their care and handling of farm animals. The U.S. swine industry has not been exempt from such criticisms. The aim of this study was to explore the views of the people not affiliated with the swine industry on what they perceived to be the ideal pig/pork farm, and their associated reasons. Through an online survey, participants were invited to respond to the following open-ended question: "What do you consider to be an ideal pig/pork farm and why are these characteristics important to you?". Respondents considered animal care, profitability, farm size, compliance with sanitary, environmental rules and regulations, farm cleanliness and sanitary standards, and workers' rights and welfare important, but also raised concerns relating to pigs' quality of life including space to move, feeding, contact with outdoors or nature, absence of pain, suffering and mistreatment. Perspectives were also raised regarding the ideal farm as a profitable business operation, clean, and with optimal sanitary conditions. Respondents also emphasized naturalness, frequently stating that pigs should have access to the outdoors, and rejected the use of hormones, antibiotics, and other chemicals for the purposes of increasing production.

Abstract: Food animal production practices are often cited as having negative animal welfare consequences. The U.S. swine industry has not been exempt from such criticisms. Little is known, however, about how lay citizens who are not actively engaged in agricultural discussions, think about swine production. Thus, the aim of this study was to explore the views of people not affiliated with the swine industry on what they perceived to be the ideal pig/pork farm, and their associated reasons. Through an online survey, participants were invited to respond to the following open-ended question: "What do you consider to be an ideal pig/pork farm and why are these characteristics important to you?". Generally respondents considered animal welfare (e.g., space, freedom to move, and humane treatment), respondents considered the business operation role important for pork production (e.g., profitability, compliance with sanitary, environmental rules and regulations, and workers' rights), and naturalness (e.g., natural feeding, behaviours and life) important for pork production. Concerns relating to pigs' quality of life included space to move, feeding, contact with outdoors or nature, absence of pain, suffering and mistreatment. Perspectives were also raised regarding the ideal farm as a profitable business operation, clean, and with optimal sanitary conditions. Respondents also emphasized naturalness, frequently stating that pigs should have access to the outdoors, and rejected the use of hormones, antibiotics, and other chemicals for the purposes of increasing production. In summary, the findings of this study suggest that the U.S. swine industry should strive to adopt animal management practices that resonate with societal values, such as ensuring humane treatment, and the failure to do so could risk the sustainability of the swine industry.

Keywords: animal welfare; attitude; business operation; consumer; ethics; naturalness

1. Introduction

As the United States (U.S.) came out of the Great Depression food shortages were addressed by improving efficiencies of food animal production, resulting in dramatic changes in the way farm animals were housed [1]. Confinement indoor housing methods became the norm, particularly after the Second World War, for poultry, pigs, veal calves, and laying hens [2]. Over the last century much of the global pork industry has transitioned from small, outdoor herds, to large, intensive indoor systems [3]. Currently, the U.S. is the world's third-largest producer and consumer of pork products, representing an important activity in the agricultural economy, with exports averaging approximately 20% of commercial production [4].

However, intensive pork production has come under scrutiny from stakeholders external to the industry; these concerns are focused primarily on the quality of life afforded to pigs [5,6], and have resulted in dramatic changes in how pigs are housed and cared for in the European Union [7]. However, despite these changes, producer-led changes in other parts of the world have been slow, with many farmers defending their current practices, often arguing that urban citizens are ignorant of farm practices, and therefore should not be consulted [5]. More recently, retailers and processors have become globally active participants in the discussion of how farm animals should be cared for on farms (see review [8]); these initiatives have no doubt increased public awareness and ensuing concerns for farm animal welfare in the U.S. [9].

Given the continued pressure placed on U.S. animal agriculture by stakeholders external to the pig industry (e.g., retailers and animal advocates), it is important to understand what lay individuals believe are ideal characteristics that result in a good life for pigs on U.S. farms. Although there is vast literature on public perceptions regarding pig welfare in European countries (see review by [10]), less is known regarding citizens of other countries [11], including the U.S. [12–14]. Thus, the aim of this study was to explore the views of U.S. citizens with little experience with the U.S. pork industry on what they perceived to be the ideal pig farm and their associated reasons. In a survey conducted in Denmark, Lassen et al. [15] found that, when talking about pork, the interviewees characteristically limited their remarks to price and what can be described as the material quality of pork. Thus, an additional objective of this study was to assess whether there would be differences in response patterns by adopting the expression "pig farming" or "pork farming", considering that maybe the latter could dispel aspects related to the animals as sentient beings [16].

2. Materials and Methods

This survey was completely anonymous and approved by the University of British Columbia Behavioural Research Ethics Board (H13-01466). Data were collected via the online platform Fluid Surveys (Fluid Surveys, http://fluidsurveys.com/), and participants were recruited via Amazon's Mechanical Turk (MTurk, Provo, UT). Several studies have assessed MTurk and shown that this approach results in high-quality and reliable data (e.g., [17–19]). This survey is a convenience sample, and thus is not meant to be representative of the entire US population. Upon completion the participants were paid (U.S. $0.50). The survey was launched on 10 April 2015. The cohort consisted of 200 U.S. residents, who were recruited within 48 h of launching the survey. The goal of this type of qualitative work is not to focus on frequencies and relative importance of the arising themes per se, but eliciting all possible views. This can be done by increasing the number of participants sampled until such time no new views arise, normally referred to as data saturation. The work that arises from these types of studies can then be used to inform future work that is then based on representative sampling, which can then be used to make strong inferences of the views of a population.

Upon entering the on line platform, participants were given the following information before taking the survey, which was adapted from [20]: "Take a short survey asking your opinion of pig farms. We want to know what characteristics you think make the 'ideal' pig farm". Due to the possibility of these different interpretations, we used both terms "pig farm" and "pork farm", and thus randomized these two treatments given to participants. Participants were then asked to give written informed consent and then provided access to a single open-ended question: *"What do you consider to be an ideal (pig, pork) farm and why are these characteristics important to you?"*. They were free to express any aspects they felt were important. Participants were then asked 11 multiple-choice demographic questions after answering the study question (see Supplementary Material).

Survey Analysis

Open-ended responses (on average 65 words) were analyzed based on methods described initially by Huberman and Miles [21]: *Data reduction* (information is coded to find themes), *data display* (organization of the information permitting to reach conclusions), and *conclusion drawing and verification* (noting of patterns and themes and using confirmatory tactics such as consistency between coders).

Applied thematic analysis was the analytical framework used in this study. Three trained evaluators blind to demographic information, initially independently examined a subset of the responses, that included inductive, data-driven coding that was used to develop themes that answered our research question—What is an ideal pig/pork farm? Then the first author did the analyses, which included initial line-by-line coding, a process of defining and labeling segments of data with words or short phrases [22]. Inter-coder agreement, a process whereby another researcher analyzes the same data and compares and discusses the results [22] was undertaken, and any discrepancies were discussed among the three authors.

Three readers compared results and reconciled any discrepancies before the final analysis was undertaken. The thematic analysis of the responses identified six primary themes (Table 1). The main themes arose from the responses rather than being determined *a priori*. The quotes were selected to represent examples of excerpts within responses that had been classified under a given code within each theme; preference was given to statements that contained a concept shared by many responses, or those that better expressed a given concept.

Table 1. Emergent themes in response to the question, "What do you consider to be an ideal pig/pork farm and why are these characteristics important to you?".

Theme	Pork Farm $n = 105$	Pig Farm $n = 94$	Total $n = 199$
	%	%	%
Animal welfare	72	77	74
Business operation	44	43	44
Naturalness	25	30	27
Ethical considerations	25	24	25
Use of antibiotics, hormones, and "chemical residues"	22	15	19
Environment	10	16	13

3. Results

Demographic data are presented on Table 2. Of the two hundred responses, 94 were related to an ideal pig farm, and 105 to an ideal pork farm. Respondents were from 30 U.S. States (no responses were obtained from Alaska, Arkansas, Delaware, Idaho, Indiana, Iowa, Kansas, Kentucky, Maine, Maryland, Minnesota, Mississippi, Montana, New Mexico, North Dakota, Rhode Island, South Dakota, Utah, West Virginia, and Wyoming). Overall our participants were largely from the millennial generation, ranging in age from 25–34, with the majority holding at least a Bachelor's degree. The participants declared themselves largely unfamiliar with pork production; 86.2% of respondents from the pig cohort (C1), and 85.7% of respondents from the pork cohort (C2) self reported as not being involved with pig farming. We noted no clear differences in the responses between both cohorts; respondents of both cohorts understood a pig or pork farm as a commercial unit that produced pork for human consumption, resulting in similar concerns raised by both cohorts (Table 1). We therefore report the results together, but when providing a quote we clarify whether it was a respondent from the C1 (pig) or C2 (pork) cohort.

Table 2. Participant demographics of the cohorts that participated in an online survey where they were asked to respond to the question, "What do you consider to be an ideal pig/pork farm and why are these characteristics important to you?".

Demographics	Variable	Pig Farm (%)	Pork Farm (%)
		n = 94	*n* = 105
Sex	Male	57.4	65.7
	Female	42.6	34.3
Age	18–24	25.5	18.1
	25–34	39.4	47.6
	35–44	19.2	18.1
	>45	16.0	16.2
Level of education	Some high school	1.1	0.0
	High school graduate or equivalent	5.3	13.3
	Trade or vocational degree	0.0	1.0
	Some college	22.3	26.7
	Associate degree	12.8	10.5
	Bachelor's degree	50.0	37.1
	Graduate or professional degree	8.5	11.4
Area of residence	Urban	31.9	23.8
	Rural	25.5	27.6
	Suburban	42.6	48.6
Time with household pet	Never	10.6	9.5
	<1 year	3.2	2.9
	1–5 years	16.0	15.2
	>5 years	70.2	72.4
Familiarity with Pig/Pork Farming	Very familiar	1.1	4.8
	Somewhat familiar	45.7	42.9
	Not familiar	53.2	52.4
Involvement with Pig/Pork farming	Farmer	1.1	2.9
	Veterinarian	0.0	1.0
	Agronomist or Animal Scientist	0.0	1.0
	Agricultural Science	1.1	1.9
	Pig/Pork Industry Professional	0.0	1.0
	Animal Advocate	9.6	7.6
	Not Involved	86.2	85.7
	Other	3.2	4.8
Vegetarian or vegan	Yes	7.4	7.6
	No	92.6	92.4

Results of the qualitative responses are described per main themes, which are described per order of prevalence.

3.1. Animal Welfare

Animal welfare was the most mentioned theme: 74% of the respondents addressed it when describing or justifying the features they considered important or essential in an ideal farm. The majority of respondents focused their responses in terms of concerns relating to animal welfare, including space to move, feeding, contact with outdoors or nature, absence of pain, suffering, and mistreatment; a number of references in relation to animal sentience were also made, with participants using positive terms such as "happiness" and "intelligence". The ethical background underpinning animal welfare concerns was clearly present in a large proportion of the respondents in that they used words such as "respect", "decency", "dignity", and most notably, "humane" to refer to animal treatment.

3.1.1. Space and Animal Freedom

The most frequently noted characteristic of the *ideal pig farm* was space, mentioned by 44% of the respondents—reflecting concerns about the animals' housing. For example, respondents stated that in an ideal pig farm: *"The pigs have room to roam and aren't trapped in pens until they are fat enough to slaughter."* (Resp. C1 1); *"It would be a farm where the pigs are kept in a sanitary environment, and not overcrowded."* (Resp. C1 199); *"Where animals are given space to roam and not piled on top of one another."* (Resp. C2 146).

In the context of space, some respondents (9%) criticized the confined system: *"The use of cages should not be permitted"* (Resp. C2 125); *"Plenty of room for the pigs! Those I've seen are normally too small and too cramped with far too many pigs in such a tiny pen."* (Resp. C1 81); *"I think an ideal pork farm should be spacious. I read a lot about the horrid conditions that pigs are kept in such as severe overcrowding. I would want the pigs to have plenty of room to move around."* (Resp. C2 156). A few respondents (4%) seemed to consider confined housing acceptable, as long it provides sufficient space: *"They should be able to walk around on grass in penned areas and be able to move freely in their pens"* (Resp. C1 56). *"There should be plenty of space for them in their pen, for when they breed and needed for the piglets to grow."* (Resp. C1 87).

Another frequently mentioned feature (by 20% of the respondents) was the need for an outdoor area for pigs where they could move around, interact with each other and perform natural behaviors: *"The pigs will have access to the outdoors, to grass, to vegetation"* (Resp. C1 8); *"I think the pigs should have enough room to move about and socialize with other pigs while they are there. They should have access to outdoors as well as shelter. Mud is mandatory"* (Resp. C2 147); *"The ideal pork farm to me would be a large designated area where the pigs are free to roam and forage for food as they would normally and naturally."* (Resp. C2 156). Interestingly 12 people (6%) mentioned the term "free range".

Some people also acknowledged pigs as intelligent animals, emphasizing the importance of the facilities for a happy life. For example, one participant described that at the ideal pig farm animals *"Are given plenty of space and clean living conditions. Pigs are intelligent animals and deserve a good life"* (Resp. C1 92); *"The ideal pig farm would probably be relatively cruelty free as pigs are relatively intelligent animals and I see no point in them suffering unduly before they are killed and butchered"* (Resp. C1 69).

Some respondents related offering more space and free-range housing to meat quality: *"I think proper living space for the pigs is the most important characteristic, since pigs that are able to roam and graze are happier, and provide better tasting pork"* (Resp. C1 17); *"An ideal pig farm is a farm that has wide open space for pigs to roam and feed. This is important as I feel keeping pigs cramped, enclosed space will help spread disease and infections. The pigs will also produce better meat as they are healthier and less stressed"* (Resp. C1 19). However, it was clear that many associated more space with other farm features that they believed to improve meat quality: *"The ideal pork farm is one that is small enough to have all the pork be free-range and slop fed. The pork farm has nice handlers, and kills the pigs humanely. It's important that the meat I eat be happy, and happy pigs come from being treated well."* (Resp. C2 191); *"The pigs would have humane lives before slaughter, plenty of room to roam and be fed organic, sustainable foods in order to grow. This makes for a better meat product, and something that is healthier for the general public."* (Resp. C2 186).

Respondents also referred to the need for veterinary care to be provided to the animals, such as: *"They should have adequate veterinary care"* (Resp. C1 56). Animal health was also frequently associated with meat quality; such as *"the pigs need to be raised in a healthy manner to produce the best pork to eat"* (Resp. C2 156).

3.1.2. Salient Terms and Features Used in Reference to Pigs' Welfare

Some terms used by a high proportion of the respondents were:

(1)   "Humane" (41%; e.g., *"The one of utmost importance is humane treatment of the animals"*, (Resp. C2 154); *"A farm that is productive, but humane to the animals"*, (Resp. C2 139)).

(2)   For 36% of the respondents, pigs should be "well fed" (including appropriate type and amount of feed, grass-fed or natural, free of chemical residues, or organic feed): *All pigs should be well fed, appropriate medical care, and lead a relatively enjoyable life until it's time for them to become food.* (Resp. C2 147). Similarly, one participant stated *"an ideal farm should have the animals roaming relatively freely and feeding on natural foods like grass."* (Resp. C2 189).

(3)   Specific objection to "animal mistreatment", and calls for good animal treatment were mentioned by 21% of the participants. The quality of treatment of animals was raised regarding slaughter

("*The pigs would be treated humanely and would be slaughtered in a honest and safe manner*", (Resp. C1 66), general animal care ("*A farm where all the pigs are well cared for and treated humanely*", (Resp. C1 43), human handling ("*The pig should be treated in an ethical manner as well, they should not be beaten or treated in a manner that is inhumane*", (Resp. C2 194), and animal health ("*This (good care) is important because diseases and sickness can spread more easily where the pigs are forced to group together too tightly.*", (Resp. C2 158).

(4)   "Free" or "freedom" (16%; e.g., "*Somewhere where the pigs are allowed outside to live freely and roam and play.*" (Resp. C1 36); "*An ideal pig farm would be one where pigs have a lot of space to move around and plenty of food. These are important because we should give pigs freedom for their lives and not limit things for them*", (Resp. C1 91)).

(5)   Overall, the "absence of pain and suffering" was mentioned by 12% of the respondents: "*It is important to know that the animals did not suffer*" (Resp. C2 104); "*Well I'd like the pigs to lead lives of minimal pain.*" (Resp. C2 109); "*I would also want the farm to slaughter them in the most humane method possible to avoid as much pain as possible*" (Resp. C1 61); "*They would get some toys or something to enjoy life. Mother pigs would be able to rear their piglets. Piglets wouldn't be castrated or teeth clipped without some form of pain killer*" (Resp. C1 21).

(6)   "Happy pig" (10%; e.g., "*My ideal pig farm has happy pigs. They are able to roam and exercise and eat healthy foods. They live a long, full life before being butchered and are treated with the utmost respect*" (Resp. C1 34).

3.2. Business Operation

The second most mentioned theme was the business operation (43%), which included a variety of opinions concerning cleanliness and optimal sanitary conditions (21%), and production efficiency/profitability (11%).

Many respondents pointed out cleanliness of the pigs' environment as an important feature associated with animal health conditions and, consequently, with human health: "*The facility is well maintained and clean*" (Resp. C1 64); "*It is important that the farm is clean so the pigs don't become ill and become contaminated when they are slaughtered*" (Resp. C2 102). Some of the respondents also extended their responses to include good sanitary conditions "*the ideal farm has safe practices that lead to food being produced that is safe for human consumption*" (Resp. C2 116); "*An ideal pork farm would have a healthy environment for the livestock and wouldn't use unnecessary antibiotics, etc.*" (Resp. C2 130).

For some, profitability production efficiency and low cost production were essential for the business, for example: "*The main objective of farm plan is to obtain maximum returns*" (Resp. C2 176); "*Another aspect of a perfect pig farm is the use of technology and automation. This will make the farm more efficient and more likely to keep the farm profitable*" (Resp. C1 19); "*The ideal pork farm will have a cost efficient operation. It will have a good HR department that paints a picture of happy hogs, but in reality the bottom dollar is important*" (Resp. C2 160).

Other aspects that respondents (5%) mentioned in relation to the business operation were that a pig farm should follow rules and regulations: "*An ideal pig farm would be a sanitary livestock facility that was constructed, maintained and utilized in a state and federally approved manner, where the workers are credentialed and properly trained in the proper, humane treatment of livestock. The equipment would pass all safety inspections and follow all approved operational regulations. The pigs would be feed to proper nutrients as outlined by the respective governmental agency. The farm would be regularly inspected and all inspection results posted in a public manner*" (Resp. C1 22); "*One that complies with all humane animal treatment regulations*", (Resp. C1 15). Additionally, the facility will train, respect and value its workers (4%), produce at low cost (3%), be located away from urban areas (2%, e.g., "*The ideal pig farm would probably be remote so others don't suffer from the smell, laid out well for maximum efficiency*", (Resp. C1 69)), produce locally (1%), and make good use of technology (1%, e.g., "*Another aspect of a perfect pig farm is the use of technology and automation. This will make the farm more efficient and more likely to keep the farm profitable*", (Resp. C1 19)).

A few mentioned farm size, some stating that the farm should be small or "not too big" (3%) while others, stated that it should be big (3%). A few said an ideal pig farm should be family run (3%), e.g., "*A family run farm. They will put more into keeping the animals well since it means more to them money wise as well as personally instead of only bottom line for a big company*" (Resp. C2 98).

For a few respondents production related aspects were the only concern, for example: "*Organization, efficiency, and cleanliness is pretty much the main goals in my mind.*" (Resp. C2 164); "*The ideal one would have a giant air filtration system around so the stink doesn't get out. Those things smell horrible when you drive by them. I don't really care about the "quality of life for a pig", it's food to me.*" (Resp. C2 192).

3.3. Naturalness

Respondents (27%) mentioned naturalness, referring to natural feeding, natural behaviors, natural lives, natural farming, and nature. Many people expressed the wish that these animals were fed only with natural products: "*They would consume natural foods, and as a result of a mostly natural lifestyle they would be healthier*" (Resp. C2 123); *Pigs with enough space to run around freely, fed on a vegetarian diet and not injected with hormones or antibiotics. I think these are all important to ensure quality product that won't harm people eating it.* (Resp. C2 131); *A farm where pigs can roam free and not be confined, where they are allowed to be outside or inside at any time, and where they can eat a variety of food that it's natural for them to eat.*" (Resp. C1 7).

Others referred to the life of animals ("*One where the pigs are living a more natural life*", (Resp. C1 15)), or more specifically to the ability of pigs to express their natural behaviors: "*Pigs would have mud to rest and play in*". (Resp. C2 108); "*The females would be allowed to care for her offspring until such a time that separation would be natural*" (Resp. C2 120). Some expressed these preferences in terms of "natural farming": "*An ideal pig farm should have a large amount of land/space for the pigs to roam, and a proper place for them to stay in the barns. They should be given a healthy diet, and shouldn't be fed hormones for growth. All natural is important to me because I try to encourage the use of all natural farming methods.*" (Resp. C1 52); "*The ideal pig farm would be based on principles of sustainability and harmony with nature*". (Resp. C1 39).

3.4. Ethical Considerations and Recognition of Trade-Offs

When conveying their opinions approximately 25% of the respondents provided their views from an ethical perspective, for example: "*I believe that the ideal pork farm is clean and that the animals are treated humanely. This is important to me because it is in line with my ideals and morals*" (Resp. C2 155). Some (10%) used terms like "decent" or "decency", "respect", and "dignity": "*These characteristics are important to me because I believe that if they are going to be slaughtered for human benefit, we owe it to them to give them a decent life*". (Resp. C1 32); "*I like bacon, and I feel better about eating bacon from places where the animals were treated at least decently before being killed for bacon consumption.*" (Resp. C2 199); "*First and foremost would be humane treatment—pigs that can go outside, sows that aren't cooped up in those god awful (sic) farrowing crates, adequate space per animal, animals treated with kindness and dignity and provided with medical care when necessary and adequate and nutritious feed, no overbreeding*" (Resp. C2 106).

Some respondents stated that they eat pork and support pork production before emphasizing that they expect ethical treatment of the animals, for example: "*I believe that pigs, although it is acceptable to eat them, should be treated with respect while they are alive.*" (Resp. C2 119); "*An ideal pork farm is where pigs are treated properly and are not abused in any way. They are fed properly with good feed and their living conditions are good. This means a healthy environment for them to live, play, and roam. These characteristics are important to me because I think animals deserve to be treated properly. They are living and breathing so despite the fact that many end up as food, they don't deserve any less while they're alive.*" (Resp. C2 114).

Some identified a need for a balance between good practices, profitability, and meat quality, but also highlighted the importance of meeting government standards: "*An ideal pork farm is one that maximizes yield without causing the animals undue harm or compromises food safety*" (Resp. C2 165); "*The ideal pig farm should balance the animals' welfare with the need to keep the meat sanitary*". (Resp. C1 57);

"The entire process must comply with all state, local, and federal laws. The business must be as transparent as possible, to demonstrate to the public that they are doing everything that their industry considers to be important . . . the process must be efficient. Just because the company should care for the welfare of the animals doesn't mean that they should be wasteful in spending or create a product that is incredibly expensive. They should streamline their operations and follow a business plan in order to keep costs low for the consumers" (Resp. C2 151).

Others argued that keeping production costs low should be secondary to food safety, animal welfare, or environmental sustainability:

"I would consider a pork farm to have enough room to allow the pigs to maintain a healthy lifestyle. This will also ensure that the pigs would have a less of a chance to pass on sicknesses to each other. I understand that this would raise the cost of manufacturing, but this price increase would be valuable to both the pig farm, and to the people who consume the product."

(Resp. C2 190)

"I'd rather pay a little more money for pork knowing these animals were treated well and fed well."

(Resp. C2 146)

"An ideal pig farm goes above and beyond by making sure that the pigs are raised in as good environment. It is important that they are well fed and have space to move around. The pig farm would not place such a high priority in maximizing profits. These characteristics are important because it is the decent thing to do."

(Resp. C1 13)

"Humane treatment of the animals. They should be treated to a normal, natural life and not overcrowded and confined in their own waste until they are ready to be slaughtered. Less production would be a fair price to pay for humane treatment."

(Resp. C1 12)

"A non-polluting, environmentally friendly farm where the animals are treated as kindly as possible and are dispatched as painlessly as possible. I don't think profitability can justify cruelty. No business has a right to contaminate the community or its common resources."

(Resp. C1 24)

However, a few statements dismissed any farm goals pertaining to animal welfare, instead favoring productivity, for example: *"As cruel as it might be I'd consider the best pig farm to be one that can stuff as many pigs into as small a space as possible while maintaining decent cleanliness. The higher the efficiency, the lower the cost for me"* (Resp. C1 70); *"Whatever gets the pork to me fastest and cheapest"* (Resp. C2 148).

3.5. Overuse of Antibiotics, Hormones, and "Chemical Residues"

Some people (19%) described the ideal farm from the perspective that the farmers should engage in the rational use of chemicals: *"An ideal pork farm would have humanely treated pigs who are fed organically. It's important that my meat sources are as humane as possible with as few chemicals as possible"* (Resp. C2 183); *"Antibiotics should be used only when needed"* (Resp. C2 196); but others were less tolerant regarding the use of these substances: *"The animals should not be getting antibiotics or hormones"* (Resp. C2 189); *"I consider an ideal pork farm to be organic. Meaning, the pigs are not injected with steroids, hormones, or antibiotics, and the feed they are given is not just slop, but rather decent non-pesticide soaked leftovers and feed"* (Resp. C2 141); *"It would practice sustainable and GMO free farming practices free of hormones"* (Resp. C2 187).

3.6. Impact on the Environment

A relatively small proportion of respondents discussed environmental impacts of pig production systems, suggesting that at least for these survey respondents this was likely not a primary concern. Some participants raised the issue of pollution generated by livestock and argued that manure management, in addition to the rational use of resources, such as water, should be addressed. In total, 13% mentioned some feature related to this theme, with 6% using the term "environmentally friendly": *"It would have good drainage and be low in pollution. The owner would be mindful of best environmental practices for both air and water quality"* (Resp. C2 184); *"and a way to properly treat waste from the farm"* (Resp. C1 60); *"Acceptably low environmental impact is important because there is little sense in spoiling aquifers and other groundwater solely for the production of pig products; maintaining a potable water supply is far more important than maintaining a pork supply in the long run. As such, the pig farm must balance the need for pork against the weightier need for water"* (Resp. C1 53); *"I would say that the ideal pig farm is very sustainable meaning that the water use of the entire farm is kept to an absolute minimum"* (Resp. C1 18).

4. Discussion

Overall respondents described a pig or pork farm as an animal production unit that produces the pork that they eat, and from this perspective they discussed what conditions they considered important for pork production, such as animal care, profitability, farm size, compliancy with sanitary, environmental rules and regulations, farm cleanliness and sanitary standards, and workers' rights and welfare. As our main objective was to identify important concerns regarding pig farming by individuals living in the U.S., we did not expect participants to rank the importance they attribute to each feature they mentioned. So, although more participants expressed concerns about pig welfare than any other issue, this does not mean that this is their first priority, or even that this influences their purchasing habits.

Space, largely associated with animals' freedom to move and the ability to perform innate natural behaviors, was the main theme addressed by the respondents. Many described their desire for housing systems that are not overcrowded and that do not limit restriction of movement. Restriction of space has been shown to be a main pig welfare concern for European [23] and U.S. [12] citizens. Other studies have also reported that space, especially in relation to freedom of movement, is a major concern in current pig production systems (e.g., Germany [24], China [25], Brazil [26]). For the U.S. citizens who responded to our survey, it is possible that the salience of this concern reflects, at least in part, the effect of campaigns related to ballot initiatives in several U.S. states in recent years [27,28]. Alternatively, it may be argued that the animal protection organizations that led these initiatives recognized space and freedom as primary social values associated with livestock welfare, giving priority to this issue in their campaigns, which may have influenced some of the participants.

Providing pigs with access to the outdoors is highly valued, and inherently associated with higher animal welfare standards by European citizens [15,29,30]. In the current survey, providing pigs access to the outdoors or free-range housing was mentioned as a desired characteristic by fewer than 40% of the participants; but when it was raised it was almost always in response to concerns about the space provided to the animals, suggesting that lack of space and overcrowding represents a greater concern for our participants than a confined housing system per se. We see provision of more space as a possible opportunity for the swine industry, given that attempts to improve confined systems to comply with society's expectations should lead to possible increased acceptance. For instance, Vanhonacker et al. [23] also concluded that the animal welfare image among the public in the case of confined pigs may benefit from providing farm animals with more space.

Other animal welfare related topics mentioned by respondents included the absence of pain and suffering, naturalness, and especially humane treatment. Accordingly, in a systematic review of the literature, Clark et al. [31] concluded that naturalness and humane treatment are the two top consumer concerns associated with farm animal welfare. In our study, slaughter was mentioned by 18% of the respondents, many demanding that it be humane, while others were more specific referring to wanting assurance that it occurs in the absence of pain and suffering. Two explanations suggested by McKendree et al. [12] for this elevated concern about slaughter in their survey with U.S. citizens (exposure to videos in the media showing mistreatment of animals at slaughterhouses and an inherent discomfort with killing animals for food consumption) were confirmed by statements made by respondents in our survey. Other important issues shown to reduce the welfare of pigs, including transportation [32] and tail docking [33] were not raised by our participants—and castration [34] was mentioned only by one participant. This could be an indication of a lack of awareness and may also reflect the focus on slaughter and restriction of movement (housing) by animal advocacy groups (and in turn the media) [12].

To our surprise, in contrast with other studies that discuss farm size as being a major concern identified by lay citizens, very few respondents raised this issue in our study. For example, large-scale industrial production has been heavily criticized in Europe [30,35]. In contrast to the Europeans, Chinese urban citizens seem to prefer industrial farms [36,37], a response that was echoed by some Brazilian consumers [38,39]. The preference for large industrial farms in some countries, particularly in emerging economies, by pork consumers may be associated with the perception that sanitary conditions and food safety standards are higher on these types of farms [36,37,40]. In the current survey, cleanliness and sanitary aspects were also highly valued as desired features of an ideal pig farm. Interestingly, consumer attitude surveys in general indicate that, even though consumers from different countries value animal welfare, food safety is the highest-ranking attribute mentioned by survey participants [13,41–43]. However, despite interview based surveys reporting that food safety and animal welfare concerns are highly valued, others have reported that these values are not reflected in consumer-purchasing behavior, as point-of-sale price remains a high priority [10,35,44].

Some participants considered it important to abolish the use of chemicals in pigs' feed, e.g., antibiotics, hormones, and pesticides, a position likely reflecting concerns regarding a perceived overuse of antibiotics, hormones, and other chemicals for animal production purposes, in both developed [24,45] and developing countries [25,46,47]. This finding was also in agreement in studies covering other livestock species [20,48,49], where, collectively, respondents raised concerns about animals receiving natural, healthy, or organic feed, indicating a growing concern about this topic. In the same context, experimental work has focused on the intensive housing systems (and the associated conditions for pigs) and the overuse of antibiotics, hormones, and other similar products and their associated effects on food safety and meat quality [10,24,25,30].

Intensification of livestock production has been associated with negative effects on the environment, rural populations, biodiversity, and farm animal welfare [2,50], resulting in intense criticisms from social, animal, and environmental protection movements. Some participants in our study stated that farms should be located far from cities to avoid pollution, and mentioned the issue of smell coming from pig operations, echoing other research from the U.S. [14]. However, only a few participants discussed environmental impacts of pig farming or agriculture sustainability in a broader context, suggesting that the U.S. public has been largely absent from agriculture policy discussions [51–53]. One argument frequently used to defend the intensification of livestock production are the tremendous efficacies that can be realized in these types of systems, thus allowing for increases in the amount of food animal products needed to meet the perceived demand for food for the projected 9 billion global population by 2050 [54]. However, some have argued that large intensive animal production systems will be less well accepted despite being associated with practices that are viewed to be more sustainable, including reduced consumption of animal products and use of technologies [55–57]. However, others have shown that people do not seem willing to eat less meat or accept meat substitutes such as artificial meat [58–60]. It has also been suggested that equity, access, and distribution should be greater priorities than increased production [61]. However, in some countries policy discussions of this nature have only recently included animal welfare trade-offs [56,62]. Our study provides evidence that, at least for the respondents in our study, farm animal welfare and food safety are primary concerns and thus both should be given due consideration. We suggest greater efforts by U.S. policy makers to include the lay public's views and expectations in these types of discussions. Failure to address this gap between farm practices, policy discussion, and societal expectations (see also von Keyserlingk, et al. [63]), could potentially threaten the long term sustainability of the U.S. pig industry.

Respondents highlighted linkages between different features that they considered necessary for an ideal pig/pork farm. For example, they linked animal welfare with economics and meat quality, meat quality with human health or nutrition, naturalness with animal welfare, and production systems with environmental sustainability. Several respondents also stated that reducing cost of production did not justify what they considered animal "abuse". In some cases respondents stated their position by relaying perceived trade-offs between their preferences and other potentially competing factors. However, they never went beyond two-way relations, in other words they appeared to be largely unaware of the complexity associated with agriculture sustainability [64,65]. This may explain, at least in part, the disconnect between different stakeholders regarding animal agriculture, including the conception of animal welfare [5,66,67]. Farmers have argued that the lay public lacks information and familiarity with pig farming issues, and therefore have unrealistic opinions (e.g., [5]). However it has been argued that simply increasing people's information may not change this scenario [68,69], given that increased knowledge of animal agriculture in general [24], specific practices [46,70], or having visited a farm [14] appears to increase, rather than decrease, concerns regarding the welfare of agricultural animals.

This study utilized the online survey tool Amazon's Mechanical Turk (MTurk), which enabled quick access to participants who are at least as diverse and more representative of non-college populations previously used in typical Internet and traditional sampling regimes [17]. These authors also provided evidence that despite the financial compensation, payment does not appear to affect data quality. We also recognize that our results may have been influenced to some extent by respondents' social desirability bias (i.e., respondents appearing more sensitive to issues than they are in reality), however, it has been shown that online self-administered surveys minimize this effect (e.g., [71]).

One objective of this study was to assess whether there would be differences in response patterns by adopting the expression "pig farming" or "pork farming", considering that maybe the latter could dispel concerns, related to the animals as sentient beings. In a survey conducted in Denmark, Lassen et al. [15] found that, when talking about pork, the interviewees characteristically limited their remarks to price and what can be described as the material quality of pork. However, in our study we noted no clear differences in the responses between both cohorts; respondents of both cohorts understood a pig or pork farm as a commercial unit that produced pork for human consumption, resulting in similar concerns raised by both cohorts. Also of interest, 14% of our participants indicated that they had some involvement with the pork industry; however, they raised similar issues such as space, humane care, access to the outdoors, and animal welfare as those with no involvement in pork production. However, equally interesting was that those with no involvement in pork production also raised issues normally viewed to be of concern by those working in the industry, such as production and economics.

Lastly, this study, based on a relatively small, convenience sample of participants living in 30 of the 50 U.S. states, and as such does not represent the views of the American society. When compared with a representative sample of Americans, our sample contained primarily respondents who are 18–35 years of age, referred to by many as the millennial generation. The technology used for sampling itself may have resulted in a skewed population response, favoring younger or more technologically savvy respondents, a point, which should be raised and discussed. However, this generation arguably represents the up incoming group of Americans who will be the primary purchasers of food, and that arguably will be influential in determining policies associated with food animal agriculture.

This study made use of a single open-ended question, which allows us to use well established social science methods to analyse the qualitative responses and to identify the connection of themes at an individual participant level. This type of qualitative research can provide important insights into which factors about pig/pork farms are the most important to the general public, as well as to identify potential areas of concern. Two logical follow up studies from this one would be firstly, to do in-depth interviews to further understand the beliefs and values of citizens, and secondly, to identify the proportions of individuals who have similar attitudes—this type of question would be better suited to a quantitative approach that uses a larger, representative sample. Our results can be useful and arguably important to consider when developing a quantitative survey targeting a representative sample, with full stratification across states, ages, and income groups, etc.

5. Conclusions

Participants expressed concerns about animal welfare that were both moral and ethical in nature, but also appeared supportive of swine production systems and practices that promote high sanitary and food safety standards. In general, they also desired rearing conditions for pigs that are associated with high meat quality, findings that are similar from studies done in many other countries. In summary, we encourage the U.S. swine industry to continually reflect on the types of practices they use, particularly in relation to the restriction of movement, when caring for their animals as practices that fail to resonate with societal values could risk the long terms sustainability of their industry.

Acknowledgments: We thank Jesse Robbins (UBC Animal Welfare Program) for his help at the outset of this project and Katelyn Mills (UBC Animal Welfare Program) for her comments on an earlier draft of the manuscript.

Author Contributions: Marina A.G. von Keyserlingk and Patrycia Sato conceived, designed and performed the experiments; Marina A.G. von Keyserlingk, Patrycia Sato and Maria J. Hötzel analysed the data and wrote the paper.

Conflicts of Interest: The authors declare no conflict of interest.

References

1. Mench, J.A.; James, H.; Pajor, E.A.; Thompson, P.B. *The Welfare of Animals in Concentrated Animal Feeding Operations*; Pew Commission: Washington, DC, USA, 2008.
2. Fraser, D. Animal welfare and the intensification of animal production. In *Ethics of Intensification: Agricultural Development and Cultural Change*; Thompson, P.B., Ed.; FAO: Rome, Italy, 2008; Volume 16, pp. 167–189.
3. Kittawornrat, A.; Zimmerman, J.J. Toward a better understanding of pig behavior and pig welfare. *Anim. Health Res. Rev.* **2011**, *12*, 25–32. [CrossRef] [PubMed]
4. United States Department of Agriculture (USDA). *Hogs & Pork—Overview*; United States Department of Agriculture: Washington, DC, USA, 2016; p. 29.
5. Benard, M.; de Cock Buning, T. Exploring the potential of dutch pig farmers and urban-citizens to learn through frame reflection. *J. Agric. Environ. Ethics* **2013**, *26*, 1015–1036. [CrossRef]
6. Dockès, A.C.; Kling-Eveillard, F. Farmers' and advisers' representations of animals and animal welfare. *Livest. Sci.* **2006**, *103*, 243–249. [CrossRef]
7. Broom, D.M. *Animal Welfare in the European Union*; European Parliament: Brussels, Belgium, 2017; p. 75.
8. Von Keyserlingk, M.A.G.; Hötzel, M.J. The ticking clock: Addressing farm animal welfare in emerging countries. *J. Agric. Environ. Ethics* **2015**, *28*, 179–195. [CrossRef]
9. Richards, T.; Allender, W.; Fang, D. Media advertising and ballot initiatives: The case of animal welfare regulation. *Contemp. Econ. Policy* **2013**, *31*, 145–162. [CrossRef]
10. Thorslund, C.A.H.; Sandøe, P.; Aaslyng, M.D.; Lassen, J. A good taste in the meat, a good taste in the mouth—Animal welfare as an aspect of pork quality in three european countries. *Livest. Sci.* **2017**, *125*, 37–45. [CrossRef]
11. Ryan, E.B.; Fraser, D.; Weary, D.M. Public attitudes to housing systems for pregnant pigs. *PLoS ONE* **2015**, *10*, e0141878. [CrossRef] [PubMed]
12. McKendree, M.G.S.; Croney, C.C.; Widmar, N.J.O. Effects of demographic factors and information sources on united states consumer perceptions of animal welfare. *J. Anim. Sci.* **2014**, *92*, 3161–3173. [CrossRef] [PubMed]

13. Cummins, A.M.; Widmar, N.J.O.; Croney, C.C.; Fulton, J.R. Understanding consumer pork attribute preferences. *J. Econ. Lett.* **2016**, *6*, 166–177. [CrossRef]
14. Cummins, A.M.; Widmar, N.J.O.; Croney, C.C.; Fulton, J.R. Exploring agritourism experience and perceptions of pork production. *Agric. Sci.* **2016**, *7*, 239–249. [CrossRef]
15. Lassen, J.; Sandøe, P.; Forkman, B. Happy pigs are dirty! Conflicting perspectives on animal welfare. *Livest. Sci.* **2006**, *103*, 221–230. [CrossRef]
16. Croney, C.C.; Reynnells, R.D. The ethics of semantics: Do we clarify or obfuscate reality to influence perceptions of farm animal production? *Poult. Sci.* **2008**, *87*, 387–391. [CrossRef] [PubMed]
17. Buhrmester, M.; Kwang, T.; Gosling, S.D. Amazon's mechanical turk: A new source of inexpensive, yet high-quality, data? *Perspect. Psychol. Sci.* **2011**, *6*, 3–5. [CrossRef] [PubMed]
18. Saunders, D.R.; Bex, P.J.; Woods, R.L. Crowdsourcing a normative natural language dataset: A comparison of amazon mechanical turk and in-lab data collection. *J. Med. Internet Res.* **2013**, *15*, e100. [CrossRef] [PubMed]
19. Rouse, S.V. A reliability analysis of mechanical turk data. *Comp. Hum. Behav.* **2015**, *43*, 304–307. [CrossRef]
20. Cardoso, C.S.; Hötzel, M.J.; Weary, D.M.; Robbins, J.A.; von Keyserlingk, M.A.G. Imagining the ideal dairy farm. *J. Dairy Sci.* **2016**, *99*, 1663–1671. [CrossRef] [PubMed]
21. Huberman, A.M.; Miles, M.B. Data management and analysis methods. In *Handbook of Qualitative Research*; Denzin, N.K., Lincoln, Y.S., Eds.; SAGE: Thousand Oaks, CA, USA, 1994; p. 643.
22. Guest, G.; MacQueen, K.; Namey, E. *Applied Thematic Analysis*; SAGE: Thousand Oaks, CA, USA, 2012; p. 253.
23. Vanhonacker, F.; Verbeke, W.; van Poucke, E.; Buijs, S.; Tuyttens, F.A.M. Societal concern related to stocking density, pen size and group size in farm animal production. *Livest. Sci.* **2009**, *123*, 16–22. [CrossRef]
24. Weible, D.; Christoph-Schulz, I.; Salamon, P.; Zander, K. Citizens' perception of modern pig production in germany: A mixed-method research approach. *Br. Food J.* **2016**, *118*, 2014–2032. [CrossRef]
25. You, X.; Li, Y.; Zhang, M.; Yan, H.; Zhao, R. A survey of chinese citizens' perceptions on farm animal welfare. *PLoS ONE* **2014**, *9*, e109177. [CrossRef] [PubMed]
26. Yunes, M.C.; Cardoso, C.S.; Roslindo, A.; von Keyserlingk, M.A.G.; Hötzel, M.J. Farm animal production systems in brazil: Citizens' opinions and preferences. In Proceedings of the XXIV Congreso de la Asociación Latinoamericana de Producción Animal, Puerto Varas, Chile, 9–13 November 2015; Volume 24.
27. Centner, T.J. Limitations on the confinement of food animals in the united states. *J. Agric. Environ. Ethics* **2010**, *23*, 469–486. [CrossRef]
28. Tonsor, G.T.; Wolf, C.A. Drivers of resident support for animal care oriented ballot initiatives. *J. Agric. Appl. Econ.* **2010**, *42*, 419–428. [CrossRef]
29. Carlsson, F.; Frykblom, P.; Lagerkvist, C.J. Consumer preferences for food product quality attributes from swedish agriculture. *AMBIO* **2005**, *34*, 366–370. [CrossRef] [PubMed]
30. Miele, M. *Report Concerning Consumer Perceptions and Attitudes Towards Farm Animal Welfare*; Official Experts Report Eawp (Task 1.3); Uppsala University: Uppsala, Sweden, 2010.
31. Clark, B.; Stewart, G.B.; Panzone, L.A.; Kyriazakis, I.; Frewer, L.J. A systematic review of public attitudes, perceptions and behaviours towards production diseases associated with farm animal welfare. *J. Agric. Environ. Ethics* **2016**, *29*, 455–478. [CrossRef]
32. Velarde, A.; Fàbrega, E.; Blanco-Penedo, I.; Dalmau, A. Animal welfare towards sustainability in pork meat production. *Meat Sci.* **2015**, *109*, 13–17. [CrossRef] [PubMed]
33. Sutherland, M.A.; Tucker, C.B. The long and short of it: A review of tail docking in farm animals. *Appl. Anim. Behav. Sci.* **2011**, *135*, 179–191. [CrossRef]
34. Rault, J.-L.; Lay, D.C., Jr.; Marchant-Forde, J.N. Castration induced pain in pigs and other livestock. *Appl. Anim. Behav. Sci.* **2011**, *135*, 214–225. [CrossRef]
35. Krystallis, A.; de Barcellos, M.D.; Kuegler, J.O.; Verbeke, W.; Grunert, K.G. Attitudes of european citizens towards pig production systems. *Livest. Sci.* **2009**, *126*, 46–56. [CrossRef]
36. De Barcellos, M.D.; Grunert, K.G.; Zhou, Y.; Verbeke, W.; Perez-Cueto, F.J.A.; Krystallis, A. Consumer attitudes to different pig production systems: A study from mainland china. *Agric Hum. Values* **2013**, *30*, 443–455. [CrossRef]
37. Cicia, G.; Caracciolo, F.; Cembalo, L.; Del Giudice, T.; Grunert, K.G.; Krystallis, A.; Lombardi, P.; Zhou, Y. Food safety concerns in urban china: Consumer preferences for pig process attributes. *Food Control* **2016**, *60*, 166–173. [CrossRef]

38. De Barcellos, M.D.; Perin, M.G.; Perez-Cueto, F.; Saab, M.; Grunert, K.G. Consumers' values and attitudes and their relation to the consumption of pork products: A study from q-porkchains in brazil. *J. Chain Netw. Sci.* **2012**, *12*, 41–54. [CrossRef]

39. De Barcellos, M.D.; Krystallis, A.; de Melo Saab, M.S.; Kuegler, J.O.; Grunert, K.G. Investigating the gap between citizens' sustainability attitudes and food purchasing behaviour: Empirical evidence from brazilian pork consumers. *Int. J. Consum. Stud.* **2011**, *35*, 391–402. [CrossRef]

40. Dhein Dill, M.; Palma Revillion, J.P.; Jardim Barcellos, J.O.; Antunes Dias, E.; Zara Mércio, T.; Esteves de Oliveira, T. Procedural priorities of the pork loin supply chain. *J. Technol. Manag. Innov.* **2014**, *9*, 84–92. [CrossRef]

41. Vanhonacker, F.; Van Poucke, E.; Tuyttens, F.; Verbeke, W. Citizens' views on farm animal welfare and related information provision: Exploratory insights from flanders, belgium. *J. Agric. Environ. Ethics* **2010**, *23*, 551–569. [CrossRef]

42. Ingenbleek, P.; Immink, V. Consumer decision-making for animal-friendly products: Synthesis and implications. *Anim. Welf.* **2011**, *20*, 11–19.

43. Miranda-de la Lama, G.C.; Estévez-Moreno, L.X.; Sepúlveda, W.S.; Estrada-Chavero, M.C.; Rayas-Amor, A.A.; Villarroel, M.; María, G.A. Mexican consumers' perceptions and attitudes towards farm animal welfare and willingness to pay for welfare friendly meat products. *Meat Sci.* **2017**, *125*, 106–113. [CrossRef] [PubMed]

44. Harvey, D.; Hubbard, C. Reconsidering the political economy of farm animal welfare: An anatomy of market failure. *Food Policy* **2013**, *38*, 105–114. [CrossRef]

45. Wolf, C.A.; Tonsor, G.T.; McKendree, M.G.S.; Thomson, D.U.; Swanson, J.C. Public and farmer perceptions of dairy cattle welfare in the united states. *J. Dairy Sci.* **2016**, *99*, 5892–5903. [CrossRef] [PubMed]

46. Hötzel, M.J.; Roslindo, A.; Cardoso, C.S.; von Keyserlingk, M.A.G. Citizens' views on the practices of zero-grazing and cow-calf separation in the dairy industry: Does providing information increase acceptability? *J. Dairy Sci.* **2017**, *100*, 4150–4160. [CrossRef] [PubMed]

47. Yunes, M.C.; von Keyserlingk, M.A.G.; Hötzel, M.J. Brazilian citizens' opinions and attitudes about farm animal production systems. *PLoS ONE*, submitted.

48. Hall, C.; Sandilands, V. Public attitudes to the welfare of broiler chickens. *Anim. Welf.* **2007**, *16*, 499–512.

49. Ellis, K.A.; Billington, K.; McNeil, B.; McKeegan, D.E.F. Public opinion on uk milk marketing and dairy cow welfare. *Anim. Welf.* **2009**, *18*, 267–282.

50. Croney, C.C.; Anthony, R. Invited review: Ruminating conscientiously: Scientific and socio-ethical challenges for us dairy production. *J. Dairy Sci.* **2011**, *94*, 539–546. [CrossRef] [PubMed]

51. Steinfeld, H.; Gerber, P.; Wassenaar, P.; Castle, V.; Rosales, M.; De Haan, D. *Livestock's Long Shadow: Environmental Issues and Options*; Food and Agriculture Organization of the United Nations: Rome, Italy, 2006; p. 407.

52. Foley, J.A.; Ramankutty, N.; Brauman, K.A.; Cassidy, E.S.; Gerber, J.S.; Johnston, M.; Mueller, N.D.; O'Connell, C.; Ray, D.K.; West, P.C.; et al. Solutions for a cultivated planet. *Nature* **2011**, *478*, 337–342. [CrossRef] [PubMed]

53. Tilman, D.; Balzer, C.; Hill, J.; Befort, B.L. Global food demand and the sustainable intensification of agriculture. *Proc. Natl. Acad. Sci. USA* **2011**, *108*, 20260–20264. [CrossRef] [PubMed]

54. Godfray, H.C.J.; Beddington, J.R.; Crute, I.R.; Haddad, L.; Lawrence, D.; Muir, J.F.; Pretty, J.; Robinson, S.; Thomas, S.M.; Toulmin, C. Food security: The challenge of feeding 9 billion people. *Science* **2010**, *327*, 812–818. [CrossRef] [PubMed]

55. Steinfeld, H.; Gerber, P. Livestock production and the global environment: Consume less or produce better? *Proc. Natl. Acad. Sci. USA* **2010**, *107*, 18237–18238. [CrossRef] [PubMed]

56. Garnett, T.; Appleby, M.C.; Balmford, A.; Bateman, I.J.; Benton, T.G.; Bloomer, P.; Burlingame, B.; Dawkins, M.; Dolan, L.; Fraser, D.; et al. Sustainable intensification in agriculture: Premises and policies. *Science* **2013**, *341*, 33–34. [CrossRef] [PubMed]

57. Hötzel, M.J. Improving farm animal welfare: Is evolution or revolution needed in production systems? In *Dilemmas in Animal Welfare*; Appleby, M.C., Weary, D.M., Sandoe, P., Eds.; CABI: Oxfordshire, UK, 2014; pp. 67–84.

58. Macdiarmid, J.I.; Douglas, F.; Campbell, J. Eating like there's no tomorrow: Public awareness of the environmental impact of food and reluctance to eat less meat as part of a sustainable diet. *Appetite* **2016**, *96*, 487–493. [CrossRef] [PubMed]

59. Hartmann, C.; Siegrist, M. Consumer perception and behaviour regarding sustainable protein consumption: A systematic review. *Trends Food Sci. Technol.* **2017**, *61*, 11–25. [CrossRef]

60. Hocquette, A.; Lambert, C.; Sinquin, C.; Peterolff, L.; Wagner, Z.; Bonny, S.P.F.; Lebert, A.; Hocquette, J.-F. Educated consumers don't believe artificial meat is the solution to the problems with the meat industry. *J. Integr. Agric.* **2015**, *14*, 273–284. [CrossRef]

61. Loos, J.; Abson, D.J.; Chappell, M.J.; Hanspach, J.; Mikulcak, F.; Tichit, M.; Fischer, J. Putting meaning back into "sustainable intensification". *Front. Ecol. Environ.* **2014**, *12*, 356–361. [CrossRef]

62. Röös, E.; Bajželj, B.; Smith, P.; Patel, M.; Little, D.; Garnett, T. Protein futures for western europe: Potential land use and climate impacts in 2050. *Reg. Environ. Chang.* **2017**, *17*, 367–377. [CrossRef]

63. Von Keyserlingk, M.A.G.; Martin, N.P.; Kebreab, E.; Knowlton, K.F.; Grant, R.J.; Stephenson, M., II; Sniffen, C.J.; Harner, J.R., III; Wright, A.D.; Smith, S.I. Invited review: Sustainability of the us dairy industry. *J. Dairy Sci.* **2013**, *96*, 5405–5425. [CrossRef] [PubMed]

64. Gomiero, T.; Pimentel, D.; Paoletti, M.G. Is there a need for a more sustainable agriculture? *Crit. Rev. Plant Sci.* **2011**, *30*, 6–23. [CrossRef]

65. Croney, C.C.; Apley, M.; Capper, J.L.; Mench, J.A.; Priest, S. Bioethics symposium: The ethical food movement: What does it mean for the role of science and scientists in current debates about animal agriculture? *J. Anim. Sci.* **2012**, *90*, 1570–1582. [CrossRef] [PubMed]

66. Te Velde, H.; Aarts, N.; Van Woerkum, C. Dealing with ambivalence: Farmers' and consumers' perceptions of animal welfare in livestock breeding. *J. Agric. Environ. Ethics* **2002**, *15*, 203–219. [CrossRef]

67. Vanhonacker, F.; Verbeke, W.; Van Poucke, E.; Tuyttens, F.A.M. Do citizens and farmers interpret the concept of farm animal welfare differently? *Livest. Sci.* **2008**, *116*, 126–136. [CrossRef]

68. Hötzel, M.J. Letter to the editor: Engaging (but not "educating") the public in technology developments may contribute to a socially sustainable dairy industry. *J. Dairy Sci.* **2016**, *99*, 6853–6854. [CrossRef] [PubMed]

69. Weary, D.M.; von Keyserlingk, M.A.G. Public concerns about dairy cow welfare: How should the industry respond? *Anim. Prod. Sci.* **2017**, *57*, 1201–1209. [CrossRef]

70. Ventura, B.A.; von Keyserlingk, M.A.G.; Wittman, H.; Weary, D.M. What difference does a visit make? Changes in animal welfare perceptions after interested citizens tour a dairy farm. *PLoS ONE* **2016**, *11*, e0154733. [CrossRef] [PubMed]

71. Heerwegh, D. Mode differences between face-to-face and web surveys: An experimental investigation of data quality and social desirability effects. *Int. J. Public Opin. Res.* **2009**, *21*, 111–121. [CrossRef]

10

The Effect of *Lupinus albus* on Growth Performance, Body Composition and Satiety Hormones of Male Pigs Immunized against Gonadotrophin Releasing Factor

Karen Moore [1,2,*], Bruce Mullan [2], Jae Cheol Kim [2,†] and Frank Dunshea [1]

[1] Faculty of Veterinary and Agricultural Sciences, The University of Melbourne, Parkville, Victoria 3010, Australia; fdunshea@unimelb.edu.au
[2] Grains and Livestock Industries, Department of Agriculture and Food Western Australia, South Perth, Western Australia 6151, Australia; bruce.mullan@agric.wa.gov.au (B.M.); jae.kim@abvista.com (J.C.K.)
* Correspondence: karen@klmconsulting.com.au
† Current Address: AB Vista Asia, 329682 Singapore, Singapore.

Academic Editor: Clive J. C. Phillips

Simple Summary: Pigs immunized against gonadotrophin releasing factor (immunocastrates; IC males) have an increased feed intake, growth rate, back fat and fat deposition compared to entire males. A previous experiment found that *Lupinus albus* L. (albus lupins) has the potential to reduce feed intake and fat deposition in IC males. The current experiment aimed to develop a dietary management strategy using albus lupins for either 14 or 28 days pre-slaughter to reduce the increase in feed intake and subsequent increase in carcass fatness in IC males.

Abstract: Two hundred and ninety four pigs were used with the aim to develop a dietary management strategy using *Lupinus albus* L. (albus lupins) to reduce the increase in feed intake and subsequent increase in carcass fatness in pigs immunized against gonadotrophin releasing factor (immunocastrates; IC males) and entire male pigs in the late finishing stage. From day (d) 0 to 28, IC males fed the control diet grew faster ($p = 0.009$) than entire males fed the control diet but there was no difference in growth rate between sexes for pigs fed albus lupins for 14 days pre-slaughter (Albus 14) or pigs fed albus lupins for 28 days pre-slaughter (Albus 28). From d 15 to 28, IC males receiving the Albus 14 diet grew more slowly ($p < 0.001$) than entire males receiving the Albus 14 diet. From d 15 to 28 ($p < 0.001$), IC males fed the control diet ate more feed than entire males fed the control diet, although there was no difference between sexes in feed intake of the Albus 14 and Albus 28 diet. Immunocastrates had a lower backfat when fed either Albus 14 or Albus 28 compared to the control diet, although there was no difference between diets for entire males. There was also a trend for pigs on the Albus 14 and Albus 28 diets to have a higher lean deposition ($p = 0.055$) and a lower fat deposition ($p = 0.056$) compared to the pigs on the control diet. Pigs fed the Albus 28 diet had a lower plasma ghrelin concentration compared to pigs fed the Albus 14 or the control diet ($p = 0.002$). Pigs fed the Albus 28 diet had a higher peptide YY concentration than those fed the control or albus 14 diet ($p = 0.004$). The inclusion of albus lupins at 20% in the diets of IC male pigs for either 14 or 28 days pre-slaughter was successful in reducing feed intake, body fat and backfat to similar levels of entire males. However, the growth rate of the IC male pigs was impacted more than would be desirable.

Keywords: albus lupins; body composition; growth performance; immunocastrated male pigs; satiety hormones

1. Introduction

Lupinus albus L. (albus lupins) have been reported to reduce feed intake in several pig experiments [1–3]. The most likely mechanism by which albus lupins reduce feed intake is by delayed transit in the stomach and small intestine. This delayed transit then feedbacks on satiety signals [1].

Moore et al. [3] investigated albus lupins inclusion in the diet of pigs immunized against gonadotrophin releasing factor (GnRF) in an attempt to reduce feed intake and fat deposition associated with the production of these pigs. However, the initial inclusion of albus lupins in Moore et al. [3] resulted in a greater reduction in feed intake than what was anticipated and so the concentration was reduced after the first week. For the final two-week period before slaughter, the feed intake and growth performance of immunocastrated (IC) male pigs on the albus lupin diet was similar to the entire males who received the control diet. The inclusion of albus lupins at 20% in the diet also appeared to have had some success in decreasing fat deposition in both entire males and IC males. For example, at a similar carcass weight, the back fat of IC males receiving the albus lupin diet was less than the back fat of entire males receiving the control diet (8.7 vs. 9.3 cm) [3]. Given the positive results, it is proposed to determine the effect of using albus lupins at a constant concentration on feed intake and fat deposition over a four-week period after the second immunization against GnRF.

The increase in fat deposition and feed intake of IC males occurs to a greater extent in the second two-week period after the second immunization against GnRF [3,4]. Therefore, it is proposed to investigate albus lupins inclusion in the final two-week period to minimize the increase in feed intake and fat deposition.

The aim of this project was to develop a dietary management strategy using albus lupins to reduce the increase in feed intake and subsequent increase in carcass fatness in IC male pigs. The hypotheses were (1) pigs immunized against GnRF which are fed a diet containing albus lupins for either 14 or 28 days prior to slaughter will have a reduced feed intake and growth rate compared to pigs immunized against GnRF receiving a standard finisher diet; (2) pigs fed albus lupins will have less fat compared to pigs receiving a standard finisher diet; (3) pigs immunized against GnRF and fed a diet containing albus lupins for either 14 or 28 days prior to slaughter will have a similar backfat compared to entire males receiving a standard finisher diet and; (4) pigs immunized against GnRF and fed albus lupins for 28 days prior to slaughter will have a lower overall daily feed intake but a similar fat composition compared to pigs immunized against GnRF and fed albus lupins for 14 days prior to slaughter.

2. Materials and Methods

The experimental protocol was approved by the Department of Agriculture and Food Western Australia's Animal Research Committee and by the Animal Ethics Committee (Activity number 15-5-17). The animals were handled according to the Australian Code of Practice for the Care and Use of Animals for Scientific Purposes [5]. A total of 294 Large White × Landrace × Duroc entire male and immunocastrated male pigs were used in this experiment. The experiment was a 2 × 3 factorial with the main treatments being: (i) sex and lysine concentration [sex; entire males fed a diet with 0.64 g standardized ileal digestible (SID) lysine/MJ DE (mega joule digestible energy) for 28 days prior to slaughter (entire males) or IC males fed a diet with 0.64 g SID lysine/MJ DE for 14 days after second immunization against GnRF followed by 0.50 g SID lysine/MJ DE for 14 days prior to slaughter (IC male)]; and (ii) feeding strategy [control; 200 g/kg albus lupins for 28 days prior to slaughter (Albus 28); or control diet for 14 days after second immunization against GnRF followed by 200 g/kg albus lupins for the last 14 days prior to slaughter (Albus 14)].

2.1. Allocation and Housing

Two hundred and ninety four entire male pigs were sourced from a high health status commercial herd at 39.4 ± 2.79 kg liveweight (LW). Upon arrival, the pigs were individually identified with ear tags, weighed and stratified on their LW. The pigs allocated to being immunocastrated received a priming dose of an anti-gonadotrophin releasing factor immunological product (Improvac®, Zoetis Australia, Rhodes, Australia) on day (d) −28 (where d 0 is when all pigs received the second dose of the anti-gonadotrophin releasing factor vaccine). The entire males did not receive a placebo injection. The pigs were group housed (n = 7) in a naturally ventilated grower/finisher shed and they had ad libitum access to water and a commercial feed via a single-spaced feeder.

2.2. Diets and Feeding Regime

On d 0, all pigs received the experimental diet and pigs who had received the priming dose of the anti-gonadotrophin releasing factor vaccine were given their second dose. The experimental diets were formulated to the same nutrient specifications (13.5 MJ DE and 0.64 g standardized ileal digestible lysine (SID)/MJ DE (high) or 0.50 g SID/MJ DE (low)). The diets were formulated so that the IC male pigs were fed as entire males for 2 weeks (from d 0; high) and then the lysine concentration in the diet was reduced for the remaining 2 weeks (low; based on a previous lysine requirement study for IC males of this particular genetics; Moore et al. [6]). The entire male pigs continued to receive the diet adequate for an entire male pig (high). The composition of the experimental diets is given in Table 1. The diets were also analyzed for quantitative AA composition (Australian Proteome Analysis Facility, Sydney, NSW, Australia) and the results are presented in Table 2. The diets fed for each sex and feeding strategy for d 0 to 14 and d 15 to 28 are described in Table 3.

Table 1. Composition of the experimental diets.

Ingredients g/kg, as-Fed	Control Low [1]	Control High [2]	Albus Low [1]	Albus High [2]
Barley	400	400	400	579
Wheat	384	257	260	101
Mill run	50	85	91	10
Lupins, angustifolius	100	100	0	0
Lupins, albus	0	0	200	200
Canola meal	20	100	10	49
Soybean meal	10	10	10	14.5
Bloodmeal	1.28	15.2	2	20
Tallow	15.3	15.7	10	10
Limestone	11.1	11.1	11.5	11.0
DiCal Phosphorus	1.31	0	0	0
Salt	2	2	2.48	2
L-Lysine HCL	2.43	2.29	0.61	0.83
Methionine	0.51	0.56	0	0.70
Phytase [3]	0.20	0.20	0.20	0.20
Choline chloride, 60%	1.02	0.32	1.76	1.53
Vitamins and minerals [4]	1.0	1.0	1.0	1.0
Nutrient Composition [5]				
DE, MJ/kg	13.5	13.5	13.5	13.5
CP, g/kg	144	176	172	190
Ca, g/kg	8.00	8.00	8.00	8.00
Total P, g/kg	6.35	6.85	6.53	6.25
Available P, g/kg	4.50	4.50	4.49	4.50
NDF, g/kg	175	196	188	182
ADF, g/kg	53.3	49.5	59.2	64.8
g SID Lys/MJ DE [6]	0.50	0.64	0.50	0.64

[1] Low—lysine concentration was 0.50 g standardized ileal digestible lysine/MJ DE, fed to immunocastrated males for 14 days prior to slaughter; [2] High—Lysine concentration was 0.64 g standardized ileal digestible lysine/MJ DE, fed to entire males for entire 28 days prior to slaughter and to immunocastrated males for 14 days after the second immunization against GnRF; [3] Phytase from Phyzyme, Danisco Australia Pty Ltd. (Banksmeadow, Australia); [4] Provided per kg of final diet: 7000 IU Vitamin A, 1400 IU Vitamin D3, 20 g Vitamin E, 1 g Vitamin K, 1 g Vitamin B1, 3 g Vitamin B2, 1.5 g Vitamin B6, 15 mg Vitamin B12 12 g niacin, 10 mg pantothentic acid, 0.19 g folic acid, 30 mg biotin, 10.6 g Calcium pantothenatic, 60 g iron, 100 g zinc, 40 g manganese, 10 g copper, 0.2 g cobalt, 0.5 g iodine, 0.3 g selenium, and 20 g antioxidant.; [5] Calculated composition.; [6] SID: standardized ileal digestible lysine/MJ digestible energy.

Table 2. Quantitative amino acid analysis of the diets.

Amino Acid g/kg, as-Fed	Control Low [1]	Control High [2]	Albus Low [1]	Albus High [2]
Histidine	3.6	4.7	3.7	4.9
Isoleucine	5.6	6.4	6.2	6.9
Leucine	10.1	12.7	11.1	14.2
Lysine	7.4	9.2	7.2	9.6
Methionine	1.8	2.4	1.6	1.9
Phenylalanine	6.7	8.2	7.0	9.1
Threonine	5.1	6.5	5.7	7.1
Valine	7.0	9.3	7.6	10.2
Alanine	5.5	7.7	5.9	8.1
Arginine	9.5	10.8	11.9	12.3
Aspartic acid	10.5	12.5	12.4	14.8
Glycine	6.3	8.8	6.8	8.4
Glutamic acid	34.0	37.4	35.1	38.1
Proline	11.1	13.6	10.7	14.0
Serine	6.8	8.0	7.6	8.7
Tyrosine	2.8	3.5	3.7	4.0

[1] Low—lysine concentration was 0.50 g standardized ileal digestible lysine/MJ DE; [2] High—Lysine concentration was 0.64 g standardized ileal digestible lysine/MJ DE.

Table 3. Diets fed to each sex and feeding strategy for the periods day 0 to 14 and day 15 to 28.

Sex Feeding Strategy	Day 0 [1] to 14	Day 15 to 28	Number of Pens/Treatment [2]
Entire males			
Control	Control high [3]	Control high	7
Albus 14	Control high	Albus high	7
Albus 28	Albus high	Albus high	7
Immunocastrated males			
Control	Control high	Control low [4]	7
Albus 14	Control high	Albus low	7
Albus 28	Albus high	Albus low	7

[1] Day 0 = second immunization against GnRF given to immunocastrated males; [2] 7 pigs/pen; [3] High—lysine concentration was 0.64 g standardized ileal digestible lysine/MJ DE; [4] Low—lysine concentration was 0.50 g standardized ileal digestible lysine/MJ DE.

2.3. Growth Performance

Pigs were weighed weekly and feed intake was determined on day 0, 7, 14, 21 and 28 to measure average daily gain and voluntary feed intake. The feed conversion ratio was calculated on a weekly basis from when the feeding of the experimental diets commenced.

2.4. Dual X-Ray Absorptiometry

Twelve pigs per treatment (three pigs/pen randomly selected from four replicate pens, so 72 in total (12 pigs × 6 treatments)) were scanned on day 27 using dual-energy x-ray absorptiometry (DXA) to determine the percentage of bone mass composition, lean and fat. The pigs were removed from feed and fasted for approximately 16 h before scanning. Immediately before scanning, the pigs were weighed and then transferred to the DXA facility. They were injected intramuscularly with Stresnil® (azaperone 40 mg/mL, Stresnil Neuroleptic Injection for Pigs, Ausrichter Pty Ltd., Newtown, NSW, Australia) at 2 mL/10 kg LW. When sufficiently sedated, the pigs were transferred to the DXA machine (Norland XR46 Densitometer Machine, Norland Products Inc., Cranbury, NJ, USA) [7]. The pigs were scanned in ventral-recumbency, with hind legs extended and forelegs positioned caudally. Whole body mode was used to scan and the scan was subsequently analyzed using whole body analysis. Measurements made by DXA included lean tissue mass, fat tissue mass and bone mineral content. After scanning, the pigs were placed in a recovery room until they were able to stand and were then returned to their pens. The pigs were given their respective diets on return to their pens.

2.5. Slaughter Procedure

Four weeks after the diets were introduced, the pigs were individually tattooed, removed from feed overnight and transported to a commercial abattoir (approximately 90 min transport time). The pigs were stunned using a carbon dioxide, dip-lift stunner set at 85% CO_2 for 1.8 min (Butina, Denmark). Exsanguination, scalding, dehairing and evisceration were performed using standard commercial procedures. Hot carcass weight (HCW, AUSMEAT Trim 13; head off, fore trotters off, hind trotters on; AUS-MEAT Ltd, South Brisbane, Qld, Australia) and P2 backfat depth, 65 mm from the dorsal midline at the point of the last rib (PorkScan Pty Ltd., Canberra, Australia) were measured approximately 35 min after exsanguination, prior to chiller entry (2 °C, airspeed 4 m/s).

2.6. Satiety Hormones

Blood samples (20 mL in lithium heparin tubes) were collected on d 14 and 28 from the same pigs that were selected for DXA scanning. The blood samples were centrifuged at 2000× g for 15 min to recover plasma and were stored at −20 °C until analyzed. Plasma insulin, peptide tyrosine tyrosine (peptide YY), cholecystokinin (CKK), glucagon-like peptide 1 (GLP-1) and ghrelin were quantified using commercial kits (Mercodia Porcine Insulin ELISA 10-1200-01, Sapphire BioSciences Pty Ltd. (Redfern, Australia); Pig Peptide tyrosine tyrosine, PYY ELISA Kit MyBioSource MBS903317, Resolving Images Pty Ltd. (Melbourne, Australia); Porcine Cholecystokinin (CKK) ELISA kit MyBioSource MBS264395, Resolving Images Pty Ltd.; Pig glucagon-like peptide 1, GLP1 ELISA kit, MyBioSource MBS943508, Resolving Images Pty Ltd. and; Porcine Ghrelin (GHRL) ELISA kit MyBioSource MBS2019385, Resolving Images Pty Ltd.; respectively).

2.7. Statistical Analysis

General analysis of variance was performed with the GENSTAT 18 program (VSN International Ltd., Hemel Hempstead, UK) to analyze the main effects of sex and lysine concentration and diet on growth performance, carcass quality, body composition and satiety hormones. For growth performance and carcass data, the pen was the experimental unit. For the DXA and satiety hormone measures, pig was the experimental unit. Repeated measures analysis of variance was used to analyze the satiety hormones. A level of probability of < 0.05 was used to determine statistical difference between the means. A level of probability of < 0.1 but > 0.05 was determined to be a trend. Fisher's-protected least significant differences were used to determine differences among treatments.

3. Results

3.1. Growth and Carcass Performance

Immunocastrated males grew faster ($p = 0.005$), ate more feed ($p = 0.046$) and had a better feed conversion ($p = 0.032$) compared to entire males between d 0 and 14. Pigs fed Albus 28 had a lower daily gain ($p < 0.001$), lower feed intake ($p < 0.001$) and tended to have a poorer feed conversion ratio ($p = 0.077$) compared to pigs fed Control or Albus 14 from d 0 to 14. From d 0 to 28, there was trend for pigs fed Albus 14 to have a poorer feed conversion ($p = 0.091$) than those fed either the Control diet or Albus 28 (Table 4).

Table 4. Growth and carcass performance for entire male and immunocastrated male pigs fed three different feeding strategies from 72.3 to 101.1 kg liveweight (n = 7).

	Entire Male			Immunocastrated Male			SED [d]	p-Value		
	Control [a]	Albus 14 [b]	Albus 28 [c]	Control	Albus 14	Albus 28		Sex	Feeding Strategy	Sex × Feeding Strategy
Daily gain (kg/day)										
d 0–14	1.11	1.04	0.861	1.18	1.14	0.950	0.050	0.005	<0.001	0.93
d 15–28	1.12 [j]	0.929 [i]	1.09 [j]	1.28 [k]	0.726 [h]	0.929 [i]	0.060	0.062	<0.001	<0.001
d 0–28	1.11 [i]	0.985 [h]	0.974 [h]	1.23 [j]	0.933 [h]	0.940 [h]	0.040	0.67	<0.001	0.009
Feed intake (kg/day)										
d 0–14	2.72	2.64	2.29	2.78	2.83	2.34	0.084	0.046	<0.001	0.42
d 15–28	3.05 [i]	2.49 [h]	2.72 [h]	3.86 [j]	2.49 [h]	2.74 [h]	0.134	0.001	<0.001	<0.001
d 0–28	2.88 [i]	2.57 [h]	2.51 [h]	3.32 [j]	2.67 [h]	2.54 [h]	0.094	0.001	<0.001	0.009
Feed conversion ratio										
d 0–14	2.47	2.55	2.69	2.37	2.49	2.47	0.097	0.032	0.077	0.49
d 15–28	2.73 [h,i,j]	2.68 [h,i]	2.52 [h]	3.01 [j]	3.51 [k]	2.97 [i,j]	0.148	<0.001	0.006	0.034
d 0–28	2.59	2.61	2.58	2.70	2.87	2.70	0.067	<0.001	0.091	0.25
CW [e] (kg)	67.7 [j,k]	65.3 [h,i,j]	65.9 [i,j]	69.8 [k]	64.4 [h,i]	62.8 [h]	1.28	0.42	<0.001	0.027
DP [f] (%)	65.4 [i]	65.6 [i]	65.6 [i]	65.7 [i]	65.2 [i]	64.2 [h]	0.421	0.059	0.11	0.028
P2 backfat (mm) [g]	9.28 [h,i]	9.07 [h,i]	8.90 [h]	11.1 [j]	9.49 [h,i]	9.66 [i]	0.391	<0.001	0.047	0.042

[a] Control: Control diet; [b] Albus 14: fed diet containing 20% albus lupins for 14 days pre-slaughter; [c] Albus 28: fed diet containing 20% albus lupins for 28 days pre-slaughter; [d] SED for Sex × Feeding strategy; [e] CW: carcass weight; [f] DP: dressing percentage; [g] Carcass weight used as a covariate; [h–k] different superscripts within the same row are significantly different.

From d 15 to 28, IC males receiving either Albus 14 or Albus 28 grew slower ($p < 0.001$) than entire males receiving Albus 14 or Albus 28, however IC males on the control diet grew faster than entire males on the Control diet. From d 0 to 28 ($p = 0.009$), there was a sex by feeding strategy interaction in that IC males fed the Control diet grew faster than entire males fed the Control diet but there was no difference in growth rate between sexes for either Albus 14 or Albus 28. There was a sex by feeding strategy interaction for feed intake for d 15 to 28 ($p < 0.001$) and d 0 to 28 ($p = 0.009$) where IC males fed the Control diet ate more feed than entire males fed the Control diet, however, there was no difference between sexes in feed intake of the Albus 14 and Albus 28 diet. There was a sex by feeding strategy interaction for the feed conversion ratio from d 15 to 28 ($p = 0.034$) where IC males fed Albus 14 had a worse feed conversion ratio compared to those fed either Albus 28 or the Control diet. There was no difference between feeding strategies for the entire males.

There was a sex by feeding strategy interaction ($p = 0.027$) for carcass weight where IC males fed either Albus 14 or Albus 28 had a lower carcass weight compared to those on the Control diet, however, there was no difference between feeding strategies for entire males. There was also a sex by feeding strategy interaction ($p = 0.028$) for dressing percentage where IC males fed Albus 28 had a lower dressing percentage compared to the other feeding strategies, however, there was no difference between diets for entire males. There was a sex by feeding strategy interaction ($p = 0.042$) for backfat where IC males had a lower backfat when fed either Albus 14 or Albus 28 compared to the Control diet, however, there was no difference between feeding strategies for entire males.

3.2. Body Composition

There was a sex by feeding strategy interaction ($p = 0.001$) for percentage bone mineral content (BMC) in that IC males on the Control diet had a lower BMC than those fed Albus 28, however entire males on the Control diet had a higher BMC than those fed Albus 28. Immunocastrated males had a lower percentage lean mass ($p < 0.001$) and a higher percentage fat deposition ($p < 0.001$) compared to entire males. There was a trend for pigs fed Albus 14 and Albus 28 to have a higher lean deposition ($p = 0.055$) and a lower fat deposition ($p = 0.056$) compared to the pigs on the Control diet. There were no interactions for lean deposition or fat deposition (Table 5).

Table 5. Body composition for entire male and immunocastrated male pigs fed three different feeding strategies from 72.3 to 101.1 kg LW ($n = 12$).

	Entire Male			Immunocastrated Male				p-Value		
	Control [a]	Albus 14 [b]	Albus 28 [c]	Control	Albus 14	Albus 28	SED [e]	Sex	Feeding Strategy	Sex × Feeding Strategy
% BMC [e]	1.88 [h]	1.82 [g,h]	1.75 [f,g]	1.70 [f]	1.79 [f,g,h]	1.86 [h]	0.053	0.28	0.91	0.001
% Lean	82.5	82.9	83.7	79.1	81.7	81.4	1.071	<0.001	0.055	0.33
% Fat	15.6	15.3	14.6	19.2	16.5	16.8	1.083	<0.001	0.056	0.29

[a] Control: Control diet; [b] Albus 14: fed diet containing 20% albus lupins for 14 days pre-slaughter; [c] Albus 28: fed diet containing 20% albus lupins for 28 days pre-slaughter; [d] SED for Sex × Feeding strategy; [e] BMC—bone mineral content; [d-f] different superscripts within the same row are significantly different.

3.3. Satiety Hormones

There was no main effect of sex or feeding strategy on plasma CKK concentration ($p > 0.05$; Figure 1). There was a time × feeding strategy interaction where plasma CKK concentration increased from d 14 to d 28 for pigs fed the Control, however there was no change from d 14 to d 18 for pigs on Albus 14 or Albus 28 ($p = 0.002$).

The majority of pigs (95%) had GLP-1 concentrations below the level of detection. There was no effect of sex, feeding strategy, time or any interactions for plasma glucagon-like peptide 1 ($p > 0.05$, data not shown).

There was no effect of sex or feeding strategy or any interactions on plasma insulin concentration ($p > 0.05$). Plasma insulin concentration increased from d 14 to d 28 ($p = 0.037$; Figure 2).

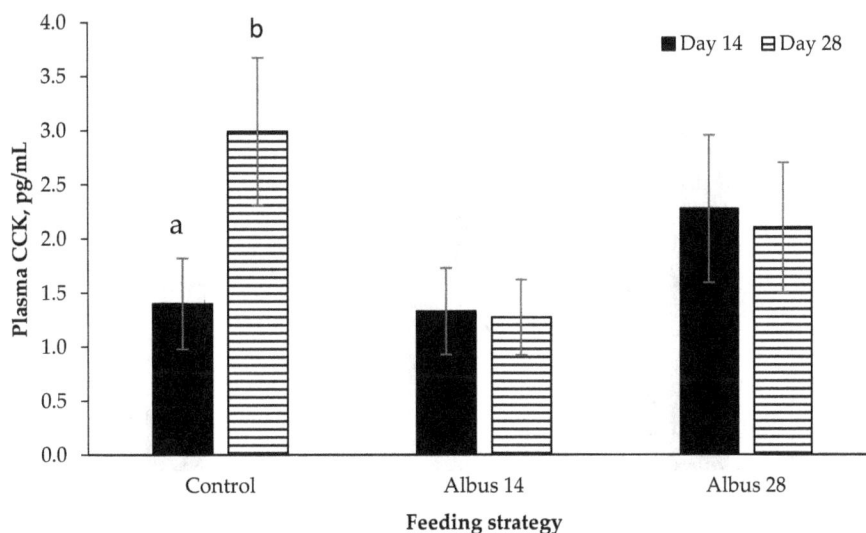

Figure 1. Plasma cholecystokinin (CYY) concentration on day 14 and day 28 after the implementation of the feeding strategy (mean $\pm$ SE; $n = 24$). There was a time $\times$ diet interaction ($p = 0.002$). Data for entire males and IC males have been pooled as there was no effect of sex or any interactions ($p > 0.05$). [a,b] Different superscripts within diets are significantly different.

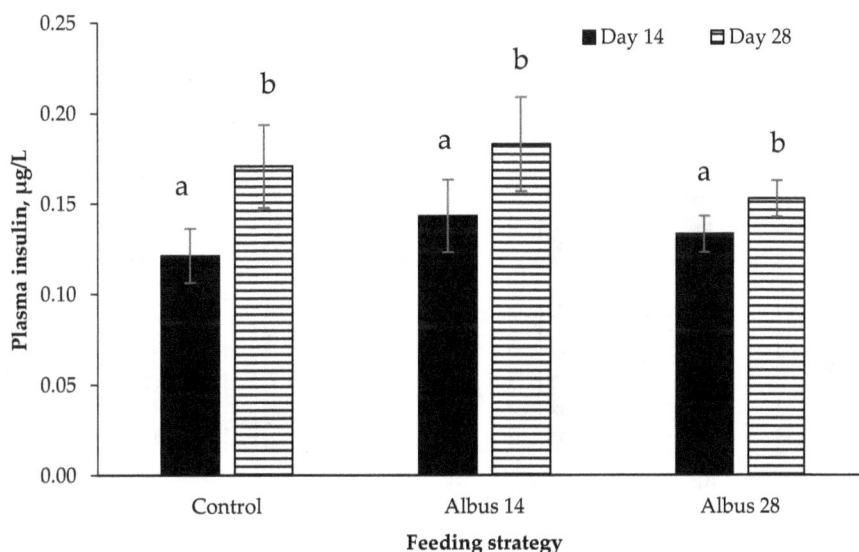

Figure 2. Plasma insulin concentration on day 14 and day 28 after the after the implementation of the experimental diets (mean $\pm$ SE; $n = 24$). Plasma insulin increased with time ($p = 0.037$). Data for entire males and IC males have been pooled as there was no effect of sex or any interactions ($p > 0.05$). [a,b] Different superscripts within diets are significantly different.

There was no effect of sex or time or any interactions on plasma ghrelin concentration ($p > 0.05$; Figure 3). Pigs fed Albus 28 had a lower plasma ghrelin concentration compared to pigs fed the Control or Albus 14 ($p = 0.002$).

Immunocastrated male pigs had a higher plasma PYY concentrations than entire male pigs ($p < 0.001$, Figure 4). Pigs fed Albus 28 had a higher PYY concentration than those fed the Control diet or Albus 14 ($p = 0.004$). Peptide YY concentration increased from d 14 to d 28 ($p < 0.001$). There was a time $\times$ sex interaction where there was no difference in PYY concentration for entire males from d 14 to d 28, however, the PYY of IC males increased from d 14 to d 28 ($p = 0.002$). There were no other interactions ($p > 0.05$).

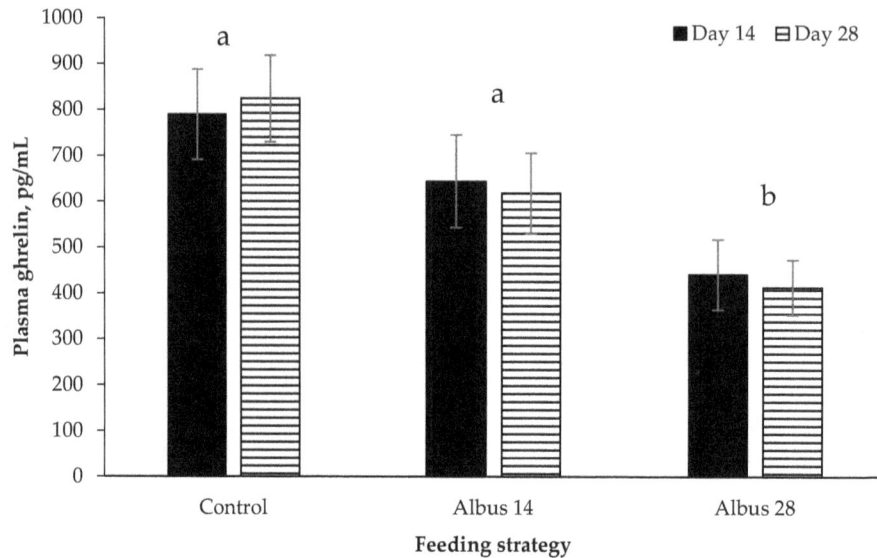

Figure 3. Plasma ghrelin concentration on day 14 and day 28 after the implementation of the experimental diets (mean $\pm$ SE; $n = 24$). There was a significant effect of diet ($p = 0.002$). Data for entire males and IC males have been pooled as there was no effect of sex or any interactions ($p > 0.05$). [a,b] Different superscripts between diets are significantly different.

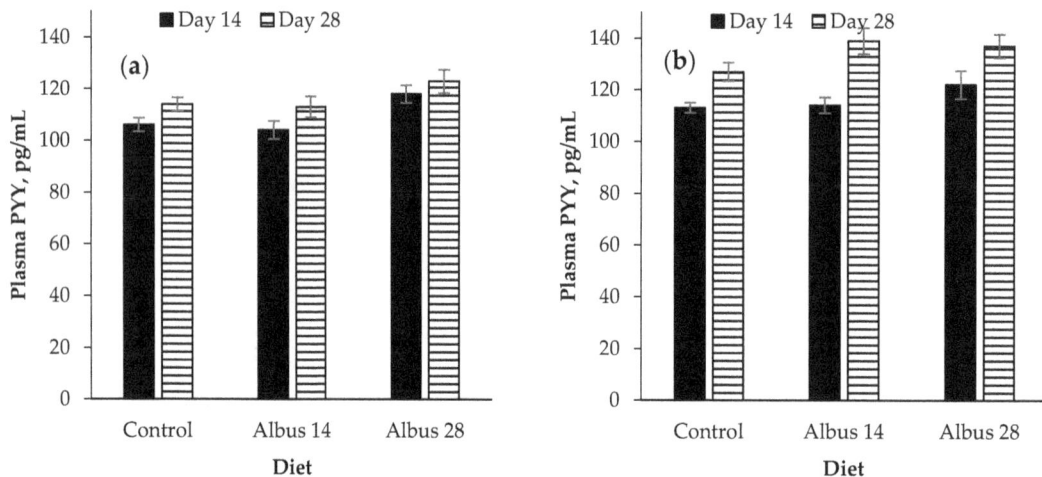

Figure 4. Plasma peptide YY (PYY) concentration on day 14 and day 28 after the implementation of the experimental diets for (**a**) entire male pigs and (**b**) immunocastrated male pigs (mean $\pm$ SE; $n = 12$). The p-values for sex, diet, time and time by sex were $p < 0.001$, $p = 0.004$, $p < 0.001$ and $p = 0.002$, respectively. There were no other significant interactions ($p > 0.05$).

4. Discussion

The hypothesis that pigs immunized against GnRF which are fed a diet containing albus lupins for either 14 or 28 days prior to slaughter will have a reduced feed intake and growth rate compared to pigs immunized against GnRF fed a standard finisher diet was supported. The feed intake of IC males was 23% less for pigs on the Albus 28 diet and 20% less for the Albus 14 diet compared to the IC males receiving the control diet. The growth rate was 23% less for IC males on the Albus 28 diet and 24% less for those fed the Albus 14 diet compared to control. The reduction in feed intake and growth rate of pigs fed albus lupins concurs with Moore et al. [3]. Albus lupins are thought to decrease feed intake by delayed transit through the stomach and small intestine. This may then feedback through satiety signals [1].

Although there was a reduction in feed intake as expected when the IC male pigs were fed albus lupins, the reduction was greater than anticipated (approximately 25% compared to the predicted 15%). The analyzed standardised ileal digestible lysine levels of the diets were as estimated and the IC males that received the control diet with the low lysine concentration consumed the feed and grew as expected. It appears that the largest decrease in feed intake was associated with the albus low lysine diet (diet received from d 15 to 28 for the IC males). It is suggested that perhaps there was increased acceptability issues with the albus low diet (associated with the albus lupins rather than the lysine concentration) in older or heavier pigs which was not expected and it is unknown why this may have been the case. Perhaps this is related to the large increase in feed intake that is generally observed in IC males around 2 weeks after secondary immunization that could not be exhibited in pigs that had only just been introduced to the albus diet.

The increased reduction in feed intake affected the daily gain of IC males to a greater extent than entire males. This was probably because the entire males have faster and leaner growth than IC males at a similar level of energy intake as they have a greater capacity for lean tissue growth [8].

The desired outcome was for the feed intake and backfat of IC males to be similar to that of entire males whilst maintaining a slight improvement in growth rate of the IC males. However, from d 15 to 28, the daily gain, feed intake and feed conversion of the IC males on the albus diets were lower than the entire males on the control diet. In contrast, Moore et al. [3] found that the IC males fed a 20% albus lupin diet had a similar daily gain, feed intake and feed conversion ratio compared to entire males fed the control diet from d 15 to 28. The differences between the two experiments may be due to acceptability issues of the albus low diet in the current experiment. Due to the inconsistent results, it is suggested that further work on including albus lupins in the diet be conducted. This should include titrating the inclusion level of albus lupins to ensure they are included at the appropriate rate to maximize growth performance whilst reducing feed intake of the IC males.

The performance of pigs in this research facility is often superior to that observed in commercial production systems due to its very high health status and so the impact of the albus lupin diets on growth rate and feed intake are discussed further in relation to previous experiments conducted in this facility using IC male pigs of the same genotype and similar liveweights. The average daily gain and feed intake of IC male pigs fed the equivalent of a control diet ad libitum in this research facility for the second two-week period after the second immunization against GnRF are 1.18 kg/d and 3.54 kg/d, respectively [3,4,6]. In the current experiment, IC male pigs fed either the Albus 14 or Albus 28 diet from d 15 to 28 had a 38% and 15% lower daily gain and 30% and 23% lower feed intake, respectively, compared to the standard growth rates and feed intakes of IC males fed a control diet in this research facility. No measures of welfare, pig behavior and hunger were incorporated in the current experiment, so definitive conclusions on the possible impact of the reduction in feed intake beyond the reduction in growth rate on welfare cannot be drawn.

The reduction in the feed intake of IC male pigs fed Albus 14 from d 15 to 28 was equivalent to a restriction of approximately 2.5 times maintenance (calculated using the equation MEm (kJ/d) = 444 kJ $\times$ BW$^{0.75}$, where MEm = metabolic energy maintenance and BW = liveweight [9]). Moore et al. [4] restricted individually housed IC males to 2.5 times maintenance by restricting the amount of feed fed to the pigs. At similar liveweights and hence feed intakes, the growth rate was similar to that of the IC males fed Albus 14 from d 15 to 28 in the current experiment (0.80 vs. 0.73 kg/d, respectively).

This experiment used a similar strategy as qualitative restriction to restrict feed intake in an attempt to reduce backfat and increase carcass leanness. Qualitative restriction refers to offering feed ad libitum but reducing feed quality (for example by including bulky ingredients containing dietary fibre or with non-fibrous nutrients known to suppress appetite) [10,11]. Less energy is consumed from low-quality food by ad libitum fed pigs so intake is restricted [12,13]. An alternative strategy is to restrict feed intake by restricting the amount of feed (quantitative restriction). Restrictively fed IC male pigs have been found to have a reduced backfat [14] and increased carcass leanness [15]. However, in group-housed pigs, restricting the feed intake by restricting the amount of feed has welfare issues in terms of increased aggression [15]. Other researchers have also noted that quantitative restriction is also associated with signs of hunger (review by Tolkamp and D'Eath [16]).

D'Eath et al. [17] and Tolkamp and D'Eath [16] reviewed the two methods of restricted feeding and conclude that there is controversy on the welfare benefits of qualitative versus quantitative restriction. Some researchers have concluded that qualitative feed restriction has welfare advantages over quantitative feed restriction because it promotes satiety and more normal feeding behavior [16]. In contrast, other researchers conclude that there are no welfare improvements in quantitative versus qualitative restriction because the pigs are still experiencing 'metabolic hunger'. Tolkamp and D'Eath [16] and D'Eath et al. [17] conclude that the differences between researchers can be attributed to (i) the methodologies used to measure animal hunger and their perceived value; (ii) assumptions about what controls food intake and feeding behavior and (iii) how 'naturalness' of behavior is weighted as a determinant of animal welfare. In the present experiment, measures of animal welfare were not incorporated and it is suggested that further research using albus lupins to reduce feed intake incorporate some measures of welfare and animal hunger. However, as noted by Tolkamp and D'Eath [16], better methodologies to measure animal hunger and a greater understanding of what is controlling feed intake may be required for this to be effective.

The hypothesis that pigs fed albus lupins will have less fat compared to pigs receiving a standard finisher diet was supported. Pigs on both of the albus lupin diets had approximately 2.5% less body fat and 0.9 mm lower backfat compared to pigs fed the control diet. This concurs with findings from Quiniou et al. [14] who when restricting feed intake to 2.5 or 2.75 kg/d, which equated to 15% and 22% lower feed intake than ad libitum, found that backfat thickness was reduced by between 0.6 and 1.0 mm in the restricted fed pigs compared to the ad libitum fed pigs. Van Nevel et al. [2] and Moore et al. [3] also found that backfat was reduced when albus lupins were included in diets. The reduced backfat and an increase in lean in van Nevel et al. [2] was attributed to the slower growth rate of the pigs fed albus lupins.

The reduction in body fat percentage and backfat for pigs fed the albus lupin diets was greater for IC males compared to entire males. This is likely because of the increased fat deposition associated with IC males two weeks after the second immunization against GnRF, as demonstrated by Moore et al. [3] and Moore et al. [4].

The hypothesis that pigs immunized against GnRF and fed a diet containing albus lupins for either 14 or 28 days prior to slaughter will have a similar backfat compared to entire males receiving a standard finisher diet was supported in principle as the p-value was 0.042 which can be considered equivocal. When combined with the lower body fat percentage and decreased feed intake, this provides further support in principle for albus lupins to be included in the diet of IC males in markets where producers are penalized for excessive back fats provided the large decrease in growth rate can be overcome. Moore et al. [3] found that IC male pigs fed albus lupins for 28 days had a similar backfat to entire males fed the control diet for 28 days. Further work may be required to confirm if the reduction in backfat of IC males fed diets containing albus lupins for either 14 or 28 days prior to slaughter to similar levels as entire males fed a standard finisher diet is a real effect.

The hypothesis that pigs immunized against GnRF and fed albus lupins for 28 days prior to slaughter will have a lower overall daily feed intake but a similar fat composition compared to pigs immunized against GnRF and fed albus lupins for 14 days prior to slaughter was also supported. Immunocastrated male pigs fed albus lupins for 28 days ate 5% less feed overall than IC males fed albus lupins for 14 days pre-slaughter, while their percentage fat composition was similar. However, when the feed intake was compared over the period between d 15 and 28 only, IC males that were fed albus lupins for this period only (Albus 14) had a 9% lower feed intake than those that had received albus lupins for the entire 28 days (Albus 28). Therefore, the albus lupin diet would only need to be fed for the final two-week period before slaughter to minimize fat deposition and the increase in backfat provided, as mentioned already, decrease in growth rate can be alleviated. This could possibly be achieved with a lower inclusion rate of albus lupins.

Pigs on the albus feeding strategies tended to have a higher percentage lean mass compared to those on the Control. This is supported by van Nevel et al. [2] who found that when albus lupins were included at 30%, there was a tendency for the percentage of lean content to increase. The trend for an increase in lean content and a decrease in fat content is most likely associated with the decrease in feed intake of the pigs fed albus lupins resulting in a decreased growth rate. In contrast, when Quiniou et al. [14] restrictively fed pigs by reducing the amount of feed, there was no difference in lean meat when using an X-ray computed tomography scanner to measure the volumetric lean content in half carcasses. The growth rate was also decreased when feed intake was reduced by approximately 22% [14].

There was no effect of albus lupins on dressing percentage in this experiment. In contrast, other researchers have found a decrease in dressing percentage when pigs were fed diets containing varying concentrations of albus lupins [1,2,18]. The decrease in dressing percentage supports the theory of the delayed transit of the albus lupins through the stomach and small intestine [1].

Several satiety hormones were also investigated to try to determine how the albus lupins were reducing feed intake. Gut hormones such as CCK and GLP-1 and stomach distension are short-term signals which have a direct effect on gastric emptying and meal termination. Signals that work in the long term determine the sensitivity to these short-term signals. This includes hormones such as leptin, insulin, PYY and ghrelin. These hormones have longer-lasting postprandial effects on meal initiation and satiety [19]. The consistent results in satiety hormones across a wide range of mammals suggest that outcomes from human studies are relevant to feed consumption in agricultural animals and gastrointestinal hormone functions [20] and therefore some of the results are discussed in relation to this.

There was a time by feeding strategy interaction where plasma CCK concentration increased from d 14 to d 28 for pigs fed the control diet, however there was no change from d 14 to d 28 for pigs on Albus 14 or Albus 28. Pigs fed the diets containing albus lupins had a lower feed intake than those on the control diet for the period d 15 to 28 after the second immunization against GnRF. Given that CCK is a short-term signal that determines meal termination [19], perhaps the higher concentrations of CCK observed in the control diet occur to curb food consumption. In comparison, the feed intake of those pigs fed the albus diets had already decreased and therefore a longer acting hormone is contributing to the decrease in food intake. Cholecystokinin is released into the blood when carbohydrates, fats and protein are present in the duodenum [21–23]. It is one determinant of meal termination, with a necessary condition for the appetite-suppressing effect of CCK being a full stomach [19]. Cholecystokinin is thought to have a peripheral effect on the induction of satiety, with one means being the inhibition of gastric emptying [24]. However, other work has suggested that this is unlikely to be the main mechanism by which CCK affects satiety [25].

In the current experiment, there was no diet or sex effect on GLP-1 or insulin. Glucagon-like peptide-1 is produced by endocrine L-cells which are mostly found in the distal ileum and colon [26,27]. Therefore, it is suggested that the effect the albus lupins are having on decreasing food intake was independent to the GLP-1 signaling system. Glucagon-like peptide-1 is also thought to stimulate insulin secretion [1,28] and as there was no effect of GLP-1, it is not unexpected that there was also no difference in insulin levels between diets.

Plasma ghrelin was decreased in pigs fed Albus 28 compared to the Control and Albus 14. Ghrelin is secreted in the stomach and stimulates eating with concentrations decreasing following meals [20]. Although ghrelin is secreted in the stomach, the stomach does not appear to contain the sensing mechanisms that suppress ghrelin secretion after meals [20]. The signals which suppress ghrelin appear to originate further in the small intestine [29]. The decrease in ghrelin in pigs receiving Albus 28 concurs with the suggestion by Dunshea et al. [1] that albus lupins possibly feedback on satiety signals by delayed transit in the stomach and small intestine. However, it does not explain why there was no difference in ghrelin concentration between d 14 and d 28 in pigs fed Albus 14 as up until d 14 these pigs had received the control diet.

There was a time × sex interaction for peptide YY where there was no difference in PYY concentration for entire males from d 14 to d 28, however, the PYY of IC males increased from d 14 to d 28. This is opposite to what would be expected as an increase in peptide-YY would traditionally be associated with a decrease in food intake, but in this experiment the IC males had a higher feed intake compared to the entire males. It is proposed that perhaps the increase in concentration was not enough of an increase as it has been found that significant reductions in food intake were only associated with PYY concentrations which were higher than a high-calorie meal [20].

Pigs fed Albus 28 had a higher plasma PYY concentration than those fed the control or Albus 14. The feed intake of pigs fed both Albus 28 and Albus 14 was reduced on d 28 compared to the control diet. It would be expected that the PYY concentration of pigs fed Albus 14 would also be higher on d 28 but this was not observed and may suggest that other satiety hormones are playing a larger role in decreasing the feed intake of pigs fed albus lupins.

Peptide YY is produced and secreted in the distal ileum and colon from the endocrine L-cells which also express GLP-1 [20]. Although peptide-YY and GLP-1 are secreted from the same cells, their plasma concentrations can be a different pattern to their bioactive forms because dipeptidyl peptidade-IV, which is found circulating in plasma, activates PYY but inactivates GLP-1 [20]. This may partly explain why there was a difference in PYY concentrations but not GLP-1 concentrations in this experiment. Peptide YY is one of the hormones which play a role in the ileal brake mechanism [20]. The ileal brake refers to the feedback mechanism which ensures nutrient digestion and absorption is optimized by controlling the transit of a meal through the gastrointestinal tract [30].

Further study is required to clarify how albus lupins are depressing feed intake. The delayed passage of the albus lupins through the digestive tract, as observed by Dunshea et al. [1], is resulting in a long-term depression of feed intake due to the action of hormones such as peptide YY and ghrelin which are released by the digestive tract [31]. However, there may also be a combination of other factors in play such as excessive volatile fatty acid production in the hindgut and the presence of saponins which have bitter and astringent characteristics which may inhibit feed intake and/or increase retention time [1].

5. Conclusions

The inclusion of albus lupins at 20% in the diets of IC male pigs was successful at reducing feed intake, body fat and backfat to similar levels of entire males. However, the growth rate of the IC male pigs was impacted more than would be desirable. In comparison, in Moore et al. [3] where albus lupins were included at 20% for the last 14 days pre-slaughter, the feed intake, growth rate and backfat of IC males were similar to that of entire males. Due to the inconsistent results on the growth rate of IC males, further investigation on the effect of albus lupins in the diets of immunocastrated male pigs is warranted. It is suggested that the effect of albus lupins on growth performance and backfat be further investigated using titrated levels of albus lupins, for example, from 10% to 20% to determine an appropriate level to include in order to maximize the decrease in feed intake and fat deposition whilst minimizing the effect on growth rate. If possible, measures of welfare and hunger should also be included to determine the effect that the qualitative feed restriction is having.

Acknowledgments: The authors wish to acknowledge funding provided by Australian Pork Limited (2014/445). This research has been facilitated by access to the Australian Proteome Analysis Facility which is funded by an initiative of the Australian Government as part of the National Collaborative Research Infrastructure Strategy.

Author Contributions: Karen Moore designed and conducted the experiment, analyzed the results and wrote the research paper. Frank Dunshea and Bruce Mullan designed and supervised the experiment. Jae Kim formulated the diets, provided advice on the experiment and research paper and assisted with the experiment.

Conflicts of Interest: The authors declare no conflict of interest.

References

1. Dunshea, F.R.; Gannon, N.J.; van Barneveld, R.J.; Mullan, B.P.; Campbell, R.G.; King, R.H. Dietary lupins (*Lupinus angustifolius* and *Lupinus albus*) can increase digesta retention in the gastrointestinal tract of pigs. *Aust. J. Agric. Res.* **2001**, *52*, 593–602. [CrossRef]

2. Van Nevel, C.; Seynaeve, M.; Van De Voorde, G.; De Smet, S.; Van Driessche, E.; de Wilde, R. Effects of increasing amounts of *Lupinus albus* seeds without or with whole egg powder in the diet of growing pigs on performance. *Anim. Feed Sci. Technol.* **2000**, *83*, 89–101. [CrossRef]

3. Moore, K.L.; Mullan, B.P.; Kim, J.C.; Dunshea, F.R. The effect of *Lupinus albus* and calcium chloride on growth performance, body composition, plasma biochemistry and meat quality of male pigs immunized against gonadotrophin releasing factor. *Animals* **2016**, *6*, 78. [CrossRef] [PubMed]

4. Moore, K.L.; Mullan, B.P.; Kim, J.C.; Payne, H.G.; Dunshea, F.R. Effect of feed restriction and initial body weight on growth performance, body composition and hormones in male pigs immunized against gonadotrophin releasing factor. *J. Anim. Sci.* **2016**, *94*, 3966–3977. [CrossRef] [PubMed]

5. National Health Medical and Research Council. *Australian Code for the Care and Use of Animals for Scientific Purposes*, 8th ed.; National Health and Medical Research Council: Canberra, Australia, 2013.

6. Moore, K.L.; Mullan, B.P.; Kim, J.C.; Dunshea, F.R. Standardized ileal digestible lysine requirements of male pigs immunized against gonadotrophin releasing factor. *J. Anim. Sci.* **2016**, *94*, 1982–1992. [CrossRef] [PubMed]

7. Suster, D.; Leury, B.J.; Kerton, D.J.; Borg, M.R.; Butler, K.L.; Dunshea, F.R. Longitudinal DXA measurements demonstrate lifetime differences in lean and fat tissue deposition between boars and barrows under individual and group-penned systems. *Aust. J. Agric. Res.* **2006**, *57*, 1009–1015. [CrossRef]

8. Campbell, R.G.; Taverner, M.R. Effect of strain and sex on protein and energy metabolism in growing pigs. In *Energy Metabolism of Farm Animals*; Moe, R.W., Tyrell, H.F., Reynolds, P.J., Eds.; European Association for Animal Production Publication No. 32; Rowman and Littlefield: New York, NY, USA, 1987; pp. 78–81.

9. National Research Council. *Nutrient Requirements of Swine*, 10th ed.; National Academy Press: Washington DC, USA, 1998.

10. Sandilands, V.; Tolkamp, B.J.; Savory, C.J.; Kyriazakis, I. Behaviour and welfare of broiler breeders fed qualitatively restrictive diets during rearing: Are there viable alternatives to quantitative restriction? *Appl. Anim. Behav. Sci.* **2006**, *96*, 53–67. [CrossRef]

11. Yen, J.T.; Pond, W.G.; Prior, R.L. Calcium chloride as a regulator of feed intake and weight gain in pigs. *J. Anim. Sci.* **1981**, *52*, 778–782. [CrossRef]

12. Brouns, F.; Edwards, S.A.; English, P.R. Influence of fibrous feed ingredients on voluntary food intake of dry sows. *Anim. Feed Sci. Technol.* **1995**, *54*, 301–313. [CrossRef]

13. Whittemore, E.C.; Kyriazakis, I.; Tolkamp, B.J.; Emmans, G.C. The short-term feeding behaviour of growing pigs fed foods differing in bulk content. *Physiol. Behav.* **2002**, *76*, 131–141. [CrossRef]

14. Quiniou, N.; Monziols, M.; Colin, F.; Goues, T.; Courboulay, V. Effect of feed restriction on the performance and behaviour of pigs immunologically castrated with Improvac®. *Animal* **2012**, *6*, 1420–1426. [CrossRef] [PubMed]

15. Batoek, N.; Skrlep, M.; Prunier, A.; Louveau, I.; Noblet, J.; Bonneau, M.; Candek-Potokar, M. Effect of feed restriction of hormones, performance, carcass traits, and meat quality in immunocastrated pigs. *J. Anim. Sci.* **2012**, *90*, 4593–4603. [CrossRef] [PubMed]

16. Tolkamp, B.J.; D'Eath, R.B. Hunger associated with restricted feeding systems. In *Nutrition and Welfare of Farm Animals*; Phillips, C.J.C., Ed.; Animal Welfare 16; Springer International Publishing: Cham, Switzerland, 2016; pp. 11–27.

17. D'Eath, R.B.; Tolkamp, B.J.; Kyriazakis, I.; Lawrence, R.B. 'Freedom from hunger' and preventing obesity: The animal welfare implications of reducing food quantity or quality. *Anim. Behav.* **2009**, *77*, 275–288. [CrossRef]

18. King, R.H. Lupin-seed meal (*Lupinus albus* cv. Hamburg) as a source of protein for growing pigs. *Anim. Feed Sci. Technol.* **1981**, *6*, 285–296. [CrossRef]

19. De Graaf, C.; Blom, W.A.M.; Smeets, P.A.M.; Stafleau, A.; Hendriks, H.F.J. Biomarkers of satiation and satiety. *Am. J. Clin. Nutr.* **2004**, *79*, 946–961. [PubMed]

20. Steinert, R.E.; Feinle-Bisset, C.; Geary, N.; Beglinger, C. Digestive physiology of the pig symposium: Secretion of gastrointestinal hormones and eating control. *J. Anim. Sci.* **2013**, *91*, 1963–1973. [CrossRef] [PubMed]

21. Degen, L.; Matzinger, D.; Drew, J.; Beglinger, C. The effect of cholecystokinin in controlling appetite and food intake in humans. *Peptides* **2001**, *22*, 1265–1269. [CrossRef]

22. Houpt, T.R. Controls of feeding in pigs. *J. Anim. Sci.* **1984**, *59*, 1345–1353. [CrossRef] [PubMed]

23. Roche, J.R.; Blache, D.; Kay, J.K.; Miller, D.R.; Sheahan, A.J.; Miller, D.W. Neuroendocrine and physiological regulation of intake with particular reference to domesticated ruminant animals. *Nutr. Res. Rev.* **2008**, *21*, 207–234. [CrossRef] [PubMed]

24. Moran, T.H.; McHugh, P.R. Cholecystokinin suppresses food intake by inhibiting gastric emptying. *Am. J. Physiol.* **1982**, *275*, R1308–R1319.

25. Gregory, P.C. Role of the intestine in regulation of food intake in growing pigs. In *Biology of the Intestine in Growing Animals*; Zabielski, R., Gregory, P.C., Westrom, B., Eds.; Elsevier Science, B.V.: Amsterdam, The Netherlands, 2002; pp. 428–474.

26. Holst, J.J. The physiology of glucagon-like peptide 1. *Physiol. Rev.* **2007**, *87*, 1409–1439. [CrossRef] [PubMed]

27. Goodman, M.H. Hormones of the gastrointestinal tract. In *Basic Medical Endocrinology*, 4th ed.; Academic Press: London, UK, 2009; pp. 101–127.

28. Holst, J.J.; Ørskov, C.; Nielsen, O.V.; Schwarz, T.W. Truncated glucagon-like peptide 1, an insulin-releasing hormone from the distal gut. *FEBS Lett.* **1987**, *211*, 169–174. [CrossRef]

29. Feinle-Bisset, C.; Patterson, M.; Ghatei, M.A.; Bloom, S.R.; Horowitz, M. Fat digestion is required for suppression of ghrelin and stimulation of peptide YY and pancreatic polypeptide secretion by intraduodenal lipid. *Am. J. Physiol. Endocrinol. Metab.* **2005**, *298*, E948–E953. [CrossRef] [PubMed]

30. Van Citters, G.W.; Lin, H.C. The Ileal Brake: A Fifteen-year Progress Report. *Curr. Gastroenterol. Rep.* **1999**, *1*, 404–409. [CrossRef] [PubMed]

31. Li, Q.; Patience, J.F. Factors involved in the regulation of feed and energy intake in pigs. *Anim. Feed Sci. Technol.* **2016**. [CrossRef]

11

Impact of Feed Delivery Pattern on Aerial Particulate Matter and Behavior of Feedlot Cattle [†]

Frank M. Mitloehner [1,*,‡], **Jeff W. Dailey** [2], **Julie L. Morrow** [2,§] **and John J. McGlone** [1]

[1] Department of Animal and Food Sciences, Texas Tech University, Lubbock, TX 79409, USA; john.mcglone@ttu.edu

[2] Livestock Issues Research Unit, USDA-ARS, Lubbock, TX 79409, USA; jefftadailey@gmail.com (J.W.D.); fmmitloehner@ucdavis.edu (J.L.M.)

* Correspondence: fmmitloehner@ucdavis.edu

† The use of trade, firm, or corporation names in this publication is for the information and convenience of the reader. Such use does not constitute an official endorsement or approval by the United States Department of Agriculture or the Agricultural Research Service of any product or service to the exclusion of others that may be suitable.

‡ Current address: Department of Animal Science, University of California, Davis, One Shields Avenue, Davis, CA 95616, USA.

§ Julie Morrow passed away; however, she has played a critical role in the completion of this work.

Academic Editor: Clive J. C. Phillips

Simple Summary: Fine particulate matter (with less than 2.5 microns diameter; aka $PM_{2.5}$) are a human and animal health concern because they can carry microbes and chemicals into the lungs. Particulate matter (PM) in general emitted from cattle feedlots can reach high concentrations. When feedlot cattle were given an altered feeding schedule (ALT) that more closely reflected their biological feeding times compared with conventional morning feeding (CON), $PM_{2.5}$ generation at peak times was substantially lowered. Average daily generation of $PM_{2.5}$ was decreased by 37% when cattle behavior was redirected away from PM-generating behaviors and toward evening feeding behaviors. Behavioral problems such as agonistic (i.e., aggressive) and bulling (i.e., mounting each other) behaviors also were reduced several fold among ALT compared with CON cattle. Intake of feed was less and daily body weight gain tended to be less with the altered feeding schedule while efficiency of feed utilization was not affected. Although ALT may pose a challenge in feed delivery and labor scheduling, cattle had fewer behavioral problems and reduced $PM_{2.5}$ generation when feed delivery times matched with the natural drive to eat in a crepuscular pattern.

Abstract: Fine particulate matter with less than 2.5 microns diameter ($PM_{2.5}$) generated by cattle in feedlots is an environmental pollutant and a potential human and animal health issue. The objective of this study was to determine if a feeding schedule affects cattle behaviors that promote $PM_{2.5}$ in a commercial feedlot. The study used 2813 crossbred steers housed in 14 adjacent pens at a large-scale commercial West Texas feedlot. Treatments were conventional feeding at 0700, 1000, and 1200 (CON) or feeding at 0700, 1000, and 1830 (ALT), the latter feeding time coincided with dusk. A mobile behavior lab was used to quantify behaviors of steers that were associated with generation of $PM_{2.5}$ (e.g., fighting, mounting of peers, and increased locomotion). $PM_{2.5}$ samplers measured respirable particles with a mass median diameter ≤ 2.5 μm ($PM_{2.5}$) every 15 min over a period of 7 d in April and May. Simultaneously, the ambient temperature, humidity, wind speed and direction, precipitation, air pressure, and solar radiation were measured with a weather station. Elevated downwind $PM_{2.5}$ concentrations were measured at dusk, when cattle that were fed according to the ALT vs. the CON feeding schedule, demonstrated less $PM_{2.5}$-generating behaviors ($p < 0.05$). At dusk, steers on ALT vs. CON feeding schedules ate or were waiting to eat (standing in second row behind feeding cattle) at much greater rates ($p < 0.05$). Upwind $PM_{2.5}$ concentrations were similar between the treatments. Downwind $PM_{2.5}$ concentrations averaged over 24 h were lower from ALT compared with CON pens (0.072 vs. 0.115 mg/m^3, $p < 0.01$). However, dry matter intake (DMI) was less ($p < 0.05$), and average daily gain (ADG) tended to be less ($p < 0.1$) in cattle that were fed according to the ALT vs. the CON feeding schedules, whereas feed efficiency (aka gain to feed, G:F) was not affected. Although ALT feeding may pose a challenge in feed delivery and labor scheduling, cattle exhibited fewer $PM_{2.5}$-generating behaviors and reduced generation of $PM_{2.5}$ when feed delivery times matched the natural desires of cattle to eat in a crepuscular pattern.

Keywords: behavior; feeding management; feedlot cattle; particulate matter

1. Introduction

A small portion of the particulate matter (PM) released under commercial feedlot conditions is considered fine. However, particulate matter smaller than 2.5 μm in diameter ($PM_{2.5}$) is considered a health hazard to humans and animals because it can pass through the respiratory tract to the lung alveoli [1–3] and therefore of major interest. These fine particles can carry gases and microbes into the lung [4].

Exposure to fine PM causes increased respiratory and cardiovascular health issues [5–7] and the biological response of the respiratory system varies based on particle size [8]. Fine particulate matter such as $PM_{2.5}$, more likely enters the lungs and studies have shown that components of PM, such as endotoxin or pathogens, can lead to cellular inflammation [9].

Particulate matter generation around cattle feedlots is greater in the evening compared with the morning because of increased cattle activity and is usually correlated with dry weather events [10]. Behavioral patterns of feedlot cattle differ from those displayed on pastures. Cattle kept in a pasture setting show a crepuscular pattern of activity [11,12], expressing feeding behaviors that peak (i.e., show increase in feeding behavior) at dusk and dawn. They also express less feeding behavior mid-day. In commercial feedlots, cattle are often fed during the first half of the daylight hours to maximize labor utilization and lower production costs. However, this method of feeding does not follow the natural behavior that cattle show in the pasture setting. Feed may not be available at dusk when pastured cattle naturally graze [12].

We hypothesized that by changing the feeding times of feedlot cattle from morning feeding to a more crepuscular feeding rhythm (i.e., feeding at dusk and dawn), $PM_{2.5}$-generating behaviors could be redirected into feeding and thereby decrease aerial particulate matter concentrations. The objectives of this study were to (1) determine cattle behaviors associated with $PM_{2.5}$ generation; and (2) determine if feeding in the evening can alter cattle behaviors during periods of $PM_{2.5}$ generation and lower generated particulate matter.

2. Materials and Methods

2.1. General

An experiment was conducted in a large-scale (>60,000 cattle) commercial feedlot in west Texas in order to examine the effect of altering feeding patterns on cattle behavior and resulting particulate matter generation. The experiment was conducted from April through May 2000, and was approved by the Texas Tech University Animal Care and Use Committee (IACUC#2000-02).

This experiment compared 2 feeding regimens: normal-scheduled feeding (CON) at 0700, 1000, and 1200 and alternative-scheduled feeding (ALT) at 0700, 1000 and 1830. Alternative-scheduled feeding was developed to mimic crepuscular feeding times that are normally found in grazing cattle. For CON, daily ration was fed in 3 equal portions at each scheduled time. For ALT, 30%, 20%, and 50% of the daily ration was fed at 0700, 1000, and 1830, respectively. Drinking water was provided for *ad libitum* intake.

The cattle in both treatments were fed using a clean bunk management system. In this system, the goal was to have no feed remaining in the feed bunk for a few hours before the first feeding in the morning. To ensure that cattle are eating at approximately *ad libitum* rates, feed deliveries were typically held constant for a 3-day period, after which the cattle were "challenged" to consume more feed by increasing the feed delivery by approximately 0.1 kg/animal daily (as-fed basis). If the feed bunk was empty at the desired time before the morning feeding for a period of 3 days after the "challenge," the challenge was repeated; if not, the intake was decreased to the level before the challenge.

2.2. Pens and Cattle

Figure 1 shows a schematic of 14 experimental pens (7 CON, 7 ALT, separated by one unoccupied buffer pen) with east-west orientation located at the south end of the feedlot (adjacent to a crop field). Because south winds predominated, this orientation minimized cross contamination of $PM_{2.5}$ between experimental corrals and the other corrals in the feedlot that were not part of the study. It was a practical necessity to apply the treatments in groups of pens (7 ALT and 7 CON) because animal behaviors are affected by cattle in adjacent pens. Feeding schedule (i.e., delivery times) had be grouped in spatially adjacent pens because otherwise, behavior of cattle in CON pens would have been affected by the cattle feeding activity in the ALT cattle and vice versa.

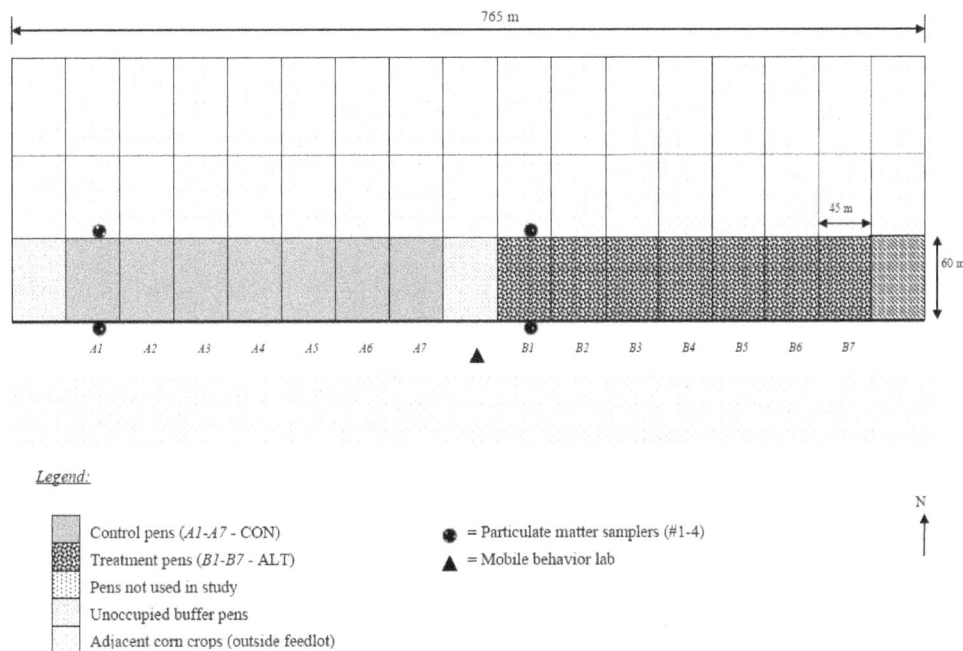

Figure 1. Schematic of experimental setup for particulate matter ($PM_{2.5}$) and behavior sampling. A total of 4 $PM_{2.5}$ samplers were used to measure $PM_{2.5}$ concentrations upwind (south side) and downwind (north side) in the south and southwest pens of the feedlot, in 1 pen per treatment per day. The 4 $PM_{2.5}$ samplers were moved daily from 1 of the 7 pens (per treatment) to the next. For example, on d 1, upwind and downwind locations were sampled in pens A1 and B1 as shown above. On day 2, upwind and downwind locations were sampled for $PM_{2.5}$ in pens A2 and B2 etc. Behavioral measures were recorded in 15 min scan sampling mode by live observation using a camera that was mounted to a 10-m high rotating tripod on top of a mobile behavior lab from 1600 and 2100 on the same days when $PM_{2.5}$ was measured. The mobile behavior lab remained at the depicted location throughout the duration of the study. Prevailing wind direction was from the South.

One pen on each side of the ALT and CON corrals was left unoccupied to avoid cross-contamination of $PM_{2.5}$ and to limit the above mentioned possible crossover effects of feeding times on behavior.

Pen surfaces (dirt lot) were not shaded and manure was removed from all 14 experimental pens before the trial began.

A total of 2813 crossbred steers, housed in 14 corral pens, were included in the study. The average number of steers per pen was 176 (15.2 m^2/steer) and with 24 cm of bunk space per steer. Before trial initiation, cattle were implanted with Synovex-S (Fort Dodge Animal Health, Overland Park, KS, USA) or Ralgro (Shering Plough, Kenilworth, NJ, USA). After receiving, cattle were weighed, blocked by arrival time, and randomly assignment to pens within blocks (paired pens) (see Figure 1).

Cattle were weighed at the onset and the conclusion of the experiment to assess BW changes. Average initial BW of steers in ALT vs. CON pens were similar (354.4 vs. 355.2 kg, SE = 8.4 kg). Both delivered and refused feed were recorded and DM assessed to allow for determination of DMI.

Steers in both treatments were adjusted to a finishing diet (Table 1) after approximately 14 days using four adaptation diets (i.e., stepped up in concentrate feed until reaching finishing feedlot ration. Measurements began 1 month after the cattle arrived at the feedlot to allow for adaptation to the environment and feeding schedules.

Table 1. Diet fed to cattle in a West Texas feedlot.

Feed Ingredients	% DM in Diet
Flaked milo	44.14
Corn silage	15.74
Supplement premix	3.33
Fat	2.59
Liquid premix	1.43
Water	0.48
Milo screen	0.34
Nutrients, %	
DM	68.04
CP	13.80
Fat	8.00
CF	4.73
Ca	0.70
P	0.30
K	0.70
Mg	0.22
Salt	0.30
S	0.24
NEm	220.76
NEg	144.32

Notes: The feed additives Tylan (7.4 mg/kg) and Rumensin (20.9 mg/kg) were added to the diet (Elanco Animal Health, Indianapolis, IN, USA) and fed throughout the trial.

2.3. Equipment

Automated DustTrak PM$_{2.5}$ samplers (Particulate Matter DustTrak, Model 8520, TSI, St. Paul, MN, USA) were used to measure PM$_{2.5}$ concentration. DustTrak samplers are not considered compliant with the Federal Reference Method for measuring PM$_{2.5}$, thus, the results may not accurately present absolute values usable for e.g., regulatory purposes, but rather data are useful to discover relative differences between treatments.

Before use, PM$_{2.5}$ samplers were factory calibrated and cleaned following the manufacturer's recommended schedule. Additionally, prior to sampling in the field, PM$_{2.5}$ samplers were compared site-by-site to rule out instrument differences as well as any kind of malfunctioning.

$PM_{2.5}$ samplers were automated and based on light scattering technology, which remotely measure PM concentration every minute and log at 15 min intervals. $PM_{2.5}$ samplers measured respirable particles with a mass median diameter ≤ 2.5 μm ($PM_{2.5}$) every 15 min over a period of 7 days in April and May. In short, the sampler draws air into a sensing chamber, which then is illuminated by a laser beam. The particles scatter light in all directions and a lens concentrates that light on a photodetector, which converts it into voltage. The scattered light is proportional to the voltage and the mass concentration of the aerosol.

A total of 4 samplers were used to measure $PM_{2.5}$ concentrations upwind and downwind in the south and southwest pens of the feedlot, in 1 pen per treatment per day. The 4 $PM_{2.5}$ samplers were moved daily from 1 of the 7 pens (per treatment) to the next. The measured particulate matter size was ≤ 2.5 μm. $PM_{2.5}$ data were collected on days when the wind was entirely from the south, southeast, or southwest wind direction to prevent cross contamination between treatments.

In addition, there was an unoccupied pen between the seven treatment and seven control pens. The instruments were housed in factory provided weatherproof environmental enclosures, which were placed inside steel cages to protect them from weather and the animals. Cages were attached to the middle of the upwind and downwind corral fence line. $PM_{2.5}$-sampler inlets were placed about 1.50 m above the ground (approximate height of steer heads when standing).

A weather station (Metos, Weiz, Austria) co-located by the mobile behavior lab, measured weather parameters (precipitation, temperature, humidity, wind speed/-direction, air pressure and light intensity) in 10 min periods over the entire study period. All weather sensors were operated at a 2 m height.

2.4. Behavior

Behaviors were measured during the periods in which $PM_{2.5}$ was generated (from 1600 until 2100) using a mobile behavior lab. Behavioral measures were recorded by live observation using a camera that was mounted to a 10 m high rotating tripod on top of a mobile behavior lab from 1600 until 2100 over 7 days. After 2100 h, during darkness, observers could not accurately record cattle behaviors. Behavioral data were measured using a 15-min scan sampling technique, in which the total number of cattle (per pen) performing a given behavior, was directly entered into a computer spreadsheet [13]. Data were expressed as a percentage of time of total observations during the period of particulate matter generation. Thus, behavioral measures are not indicative of an average of 24 h/day, but of the targeted period of $PM_{2.5}$ generation (in the evening). Percentage data were analyzed as Least Squares Means (LSM), Standard Error Means (SEM), and p-values determined by arcsine square root transforming percent data (to achieve normalized distribution).

The measured behaviors were: (a) $PM_{2.5}$-generating behaviors including locomotion (walk/run), agonistic and bulling behavior; and (b) behaviors with little effect on $PM_{2.5}$ like feeding, waiting for feed, lying and standing behavior. Behaviors were defined as described earlier [13], but in short: Locomotion was any change of body location within the pen. Agonistic behaviors were those indicative of social conflict such as threat, attack, fight, or escape. Bulling behavior was defined as mounting of a steer by its peer(s). Feeding was defined to be head over or in the bunk. Waiting for feed was an upright body posture near the bunk without actually having access to feed. Steers waiting for feed were normally waiting in the second or third row until their feeding peers were finished. Drinking was defined as the head over or in the water trough. Lying was defined as body contact with the ground and standing was considered to be an inactive upright posture (no locomotion).

2.5. Experimental Design and Analysis

Behavioral measures were collected during the period of $PM_{2.5}$ generation (1600 to 2100 h) and represent the percentage of time cattle were engaged in these behaviors during that period. Particulate matter measures were collected over 24 h and averaged for each hour of the day. The pen was the experimental unit (cattle had been randomly assigned to experimental units). Treatment pens selected were determined by location in the feedlot.

The experimental design for behavioral and $PM_{2.5}$ measures was a randomized complete block with paired pens on a given arrival date as the blocks (the assignment to treatments within blocks was random). As mentioned earlier, a total of 14 pens were used (7 pens/treatment). For measures of performance and behavior, the statistical model included treatment, block, and treatment by block interaction effects. The treatment by block effect was the error term. The effects of behaviors on the variation in $PM_{2.5}$ were analyzed with the stepwise multiple regression procedure and correlations of behaviors with $PM_{2.5}$ calculated using SAS (SAS Inst, Inc., Cary, NC, USA) in an attempt to predict aerial dust based on behavior. For $PM_{2.5}$ measures, a repeated measures analysis was employed with 24 time periods per day. The $PM_{2.5}$ model was the same as above, but also included effects of time, and treatment by time, and residual error. Performance data were analyzed as a completely randomized design with 2 treatment groups and 7 pen replications per treatment. Because treatments were determined by physical location of the pens and the predominant wind direction, pens could not be randomly assigned treatments (see earlier discussion). However, cattle were randomly assigned to pen experimental units. Means separation using the predicted difference test was governed by protected levels of significance at the alpha level reported. All analysis was conducted using PROC MIXED in SAS (SAS Inst, Inc., Cary, NC, USA).

Finally, correlation coefficients were calculated to examine relationships between cattle behaviors and the variation in aerial $PM_{2.5}$ using SAS.

3. Results

Effects of Feeding Management on Particulate Matter and Behavior

During the afternoon and early evening period, cattle experiencing the ALT treatment showed differences in most behaviors compared to those in CON (Table 2). Time spent feeding was not affected ($p = 0.40$) by treatment. Whereas CON cattle fed throughout the afternoon, the feed bunks in the corrals of ALT cattle contained no feed in the afternoon hours. Feeding behavior of cattle in the ALT treatment was concentrated after feed was delivered for a period of about 90 min (1830 to 2000). "Waiting for feed" behavior was different between cattle in CON vs. ALT treatments ($p < 0.001$).

Table 2. Behaviors of cattle (% of time) under 2 different feeding-time regimens (ALT = fed at 0700, 1000, 1830 h vs. CON = fed at 0700, 1000 and 1200 h) measured for 7 d from 1600 until 2100.

Behavior	Alternative Feeding	Control Feeding	SEM [a]	p-Value
Number of Replicates	7	7		
Number of Animals	1228	1585		
Feeding	11.0	6.5	0.80	0.40
Waiting for feed	19.3	4.6	1.57	0.001
Drinking	2.2	2.4	0.07	0.028
Standing	31.0	54.3	2.43	0.001
Lying	34.5	26.9	2.61.	0.20
Walking	1.6	2.8	0.21	0.004
Agonistic behavior	0.8	2.4	0.20	0.002
Bulling	0.003	0.013	0.003	0.050

[a] SEM = Standard error means.

Cattle fed according to ALT schedule started lining up at the feed bunks approximately 30 min before feed was delivered. Cattle fed according to CON vs. ALT treatments spent more time drinking ($p < 0.028$). Cattle experiencing CON vs. ALT treatments showed more standing behavior ($p < 0.01$). Lying behavior was not different between treatments. The locomotive behaviors walking and running were performed less among cattle experiencing the ALT than the CON treatments ($p < 0.004$).

Agonistic behavior was performed three times less among ALT versus CON treated cattle ($p < 0.002$) and bulling behavior was lower among ALT versus CON treated cattle ($p < 0.05$).

Table 3 shows correlations between behaviors and PM2.5 net concentrations for both treatments. Correlation coefficients were homogenous within treatments which indicates that PM2.5 generation, even if different in mean value in different treatments have similar causal behaviors. In ALT, net PM2.5 and the different behaviors showed significant correlations with standing ($r = 0.45$, $p < 0.01$), lying ($r = -0.43$, $p < 0.01$), and agonistic behaviors ($r = 0.35$, $p < 0.05$). The stepwise multiple regression showed that agonistic behavior predicted 17% of the variation in dust (partial $R^2 = 0.17$).

Table 3. Correlations of behaviors of cattle (% of time over 24 h) with $PM_{2.5}$ net concentration under two feeding-time regimens (ALT = fed at 0700, 1000, 1830 h vs. CON = fed at 0700, 1000 and 1200 h) measured for 7 days from 1600 until 2100.

Behavior	PM-2.5 Net Concentration	
	Alternative Feeding	Control Feeding
Feeding	0.22	−0.10
Waiting for feed	0.17	0.11
Drinking	−0.13	−0.29
Standing	0.45 *	0.34 *
Lying	−0.43 *	−0.34 *
Locomotion	0.24	0.32 †
Agonistic	0.44 **	0.35 *
Bulling	0.16	0.26

* $p < 0.05$. ** $p < 0.01$. † $p < 0.06$.

Over the 24 h period (Table 4), upwind $PM_{2.5}$ concentrations were similar between treatments. $PM_{2.5}$ concentrations measured at downwind locations were 37% lower among pens housing ALT compared to CON treated cattle ($p < 0.01$). Net $PM_{2.5}$ concentration was different between treatments; pens housing ALT vs. CON cattle had 55% lower $PM_{2.5}$ particulate matter concentrations ($p < 0.05$).

Table 4. Average particulate matter concentrations (particle size < 2.5 μm, $PM_{2.5}$) in a West Texas feedlot under 2 different feeding time regimes (ALT = 0700, 1000, 1830 h vs. CON = 0700, 1000, and 1200 h) measured during 24 h periods over 7 days.

PM Variable	ALT Experimental Feeding	CON Control Feeding	SEM [a]	p-Value
Downwind $PM_{2.5}$ concentration, mg/m^3	0.072	0.115	0.007	0.004
Upwind $PM_{2.5}$ concentration, mg/m^3	0.035	0.036	0.006	0.87
Net $PM_{2.5}$ concentration [b], mg/m^3	0.036	0.080	0.013	0.042

[a] SEM = Standard error means. [b] Net $PM_{2.5}$ concentration downwind-upwind $PM_{2.5}$ concentration, in mg/m^3.

In Figure 2a, hourly averages of upwind $PM_{2.5}$ concentrations are presented over 24 h. The two treatments had similar upwind $PM_{2.5}$ concentrations. Figure 2b shows the average hourly downwind $PM_{2.5}$ concentrations of the two treatments over 24 h. Between 2000 and 2200, pens housing CON vs. ALT treated cattle had approximately four times higher $PM_{2.5}$ concentrations ($p < 0.05$).

Initial body weights were similar between treatments. The DMI of steers in ALT was 3.6% less ($p < 0.01$) than in CON, which led to a tendency ($p = 0.095$) for a lower ADG. A post-hoc, secondary analysis was performed to determine if DMI was held constant by use of a covariate, if ADG differed between treatments. When DMI was held constant by use of a covariate, then ADG was similar ($p = 0.88$) for cattle in CON and ALT treatments (Table 5).

a)

b)

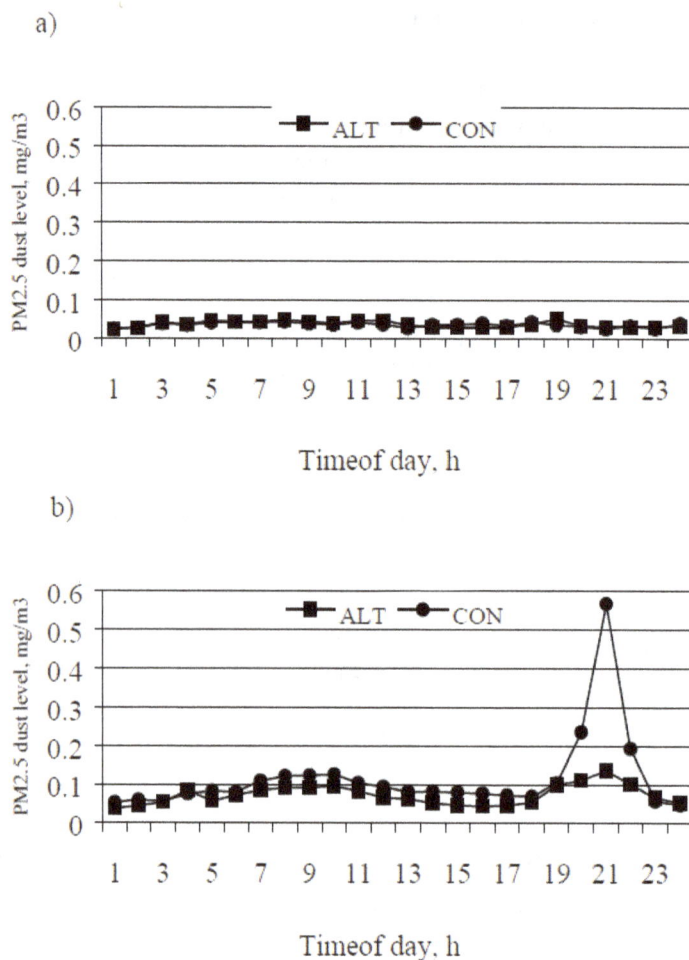

Figure 2. Average PM$_{2.5}$ (particulate matter, <2.5 μm) concentrations over 24 h in mg/m^3 in a West-Texas feedlot under 2 different feeding time regimens (ALT = fed at 0700, 1000 and 1200 h vs. CON = fed at 0700, 1000 h and 1830 h). PM$_{2.5}$ was measured over a period of 7 days in April 2000. Panel (**a**) shows upwind PM$_{2.5}$ concentration, which was 0.035 mg/m^3 in ALT versus 0.036 mg/m^3 in CON (Pooled SE; SEM = 0.006, Treatment p = 0.87, Treatment by time p = 0.08). Panel (**b**) shows average downwind PM$_{2.5}$ concentrations, which was 0.072 mg/m^3 in ALT vs. 0.115 mg/m^3 in CON (SEM = 0.007, Treatment p < 0.01, Treatment by time p < 0.01).

Table 5. Performance of cattle under two different feeding time regimens (ALT = fed at 0700, 1000, 1830 h vs. CON = 0700, 1000 and 1200 h) over a period of 152 days on feed.

Measure	Mean			
	CON	ALT	SEM [a]	p-Value
Number of pens	7	7	-	-
Number of cattle	1228	1585	-	-
Initial BW, kg	354.9	354.8	1.18	0.93
Final BW, kg	570.9	563.8	3.05	0.14
ADG, kg/day	1.42	1.36	0.02	0.095
ADG, kg/day, with DMI as a covariate [b]	1.39	1.39	0.02	0.88
Feed:gain ratio	6.13	6.21	0.10	0.61
DMI, kg/day	8.71	8.40	0.06	0.004

[a] SEM = Standard error means. [b] These means statistically adjust the raw means as if DMI was identical among CON and ALT cattle.

4. Discussion

It is generally accepted that hot and dry weather is conducive to detachment of particles from the feedlot pen surface [14]. The problem of high particulate matter concentrations are most severe during the late afternoon and early evening hours, when the ambient temperatures are highest and the relative humidity lowest. The moisture level of the manure pad in the feedlot pen, vapor pressure in the air, and precipitation undoubtedly affect particulate matter concentrations [14,15]. The cohesion between particles is lowest during dry periods and during those times, detachment of particles from the ground is easiest [16]. However, additional work is needed to clarify these potential relationships.

Other PM work indicated that the high downwind PM concentrations which occur in feedlots in the evening are affected by a strong increase in cattle activity [16,17]. We hypothesized in the present study that the common feeding practice of only feeding cattle in the morning impacts this problem. A change from conventional to more crepuscular feeding times (dusk, noon, and dawn) was proposed to change PM-generating behavior into those that are less active, and therefore generate less particulate matter. Particulate matter-generating behaviors (like agonistic and bulling behaviors) were much lower in the alternative feeding time regime than in the conventional control. Cattle have a strong feeding motivation around dawn and dusk [17], and if feed is unavailable, we hypothesized that cattle will replace feeding with locomotion, agonistic, or bulling behavior.

Correlations between behavior and $PM_{2.5}$ generation do not indicate cause and effect. However, one can see from our data that two behaviors (agonistic behaviors and standing) had a significant (though not perfect) correlation with $PM_{2.5}$ generation (Table 3). These correlations between behavior and fine particle generation support the hypothesis that active behaviors stir up $PM_{2.5}$ while less-active behaviors (e.g., feeding) do not. Lying down is negatively correlated with dust levels because when animals lay down, less $PM_{2.5}$ is generated and when they are not lying down, they may be active fighting or standing which do generate $PM_{2.5}$. A key finding of this work is the concept that cattle behavior contributes to $PM_{2.5}$ generation in a meaningful way. Furthermore, when cattle management/feeding practices are changed to reduce active behaviors, $PM_{2.5}$ generation was being reduced.

The findings of this study were consistent with the hypothesis that active behaviors are associated with $PM_{2.5}$ generation. At dusk, when the majority of agonistic and locomotive behaviors occur, $PM_{2.5}$ concentrations peaked. By altering feeding times, the agonistic behaviors were reduced and consequently $PM_{2.5}$ concentrations were also reduced. Altered feeding schedule clearly caused reduced $PM_{2.5}$ concentrations. Behavioral data supports the hypothesis that increasing feeding behaviors and reducing agonistic behaviors in the evening will reduce $PM_{2.5}$ generation. Further work is needed to quantify the PM distribution generated by cattle feedlots. It would be interesting to know PM_5 and PM_{10} concentrations in this production system and to see if our new management practice might change the distribution of particles of various sizes.

Conducting in-field management studies on $PM_{2.5}$ movement necessitates accounting for wind direction and has the limitations of the physical location of pens within the feedlot. Adjoining pens/experimental units can influence each other and thus, the experimental units cannot be totally independent. However, because behaviors were different between treatments, it was clear that our management change (altered feeding times) caused changes in cattle behavior and dust generation that were larger than any effects that adjoining pens may have caused.

Future studies should determine the relationships between feeding levels and $PM_{2.5}$ generation. Feeding a high proportion of the daily ration in the early evening might alter the feeding behavior of cattle the next morning, which might affect management decisions on allotment of feed to each pen.

In the USA, $PM_{2.5}$ is regulated by the federal and state agencies and cattle feedlots can run the risk of exceeding the thresholds. Approaches are needed to reduce $PM_{2.5}$ emissions from confined cattle feeding operations. The present research may suggest a management practice that may reduce $PM_{2.5}$ emissions from confined animal feeding operations. While this work was conducted in a commercial environment, more research is needed to refine this approach, independently confirm its efficacy, and understand how this approach may impact labor efficiency and profitability.

5. Conclusions

In summary, when the feeding of cattle in a feedlot is managed to reflect biological and behavioral motivations for feed consumption, behaviors that affect the generation of $PM_{2.5}$ were decreased. The study showed that cattle behaviors are an important factor and perhaps the main reason for high $PM_{2.5}$ levels in the evenings. Use of an altered schedule like the one described herein may decrease the generation of $PM_{2.5}$ by altering cattle behavior. Use of a behavioral management schedule that is more consistent with the natural cattle feeding cycle might improve human and animal health and well-being.

Implications

Crepuscular cattle feeding patterns have led to significantly lower $PM_{2.5}$ concentrations compared to common feeding practices (0700, 1000, 1200 h). By changing cattle feeding patterns, a producer may be able to redirect $PM_{2.5}$ generating behaviors to more environmentally benign behaviors, thereby lowering $PM_{2.5}$ concentrations in feedlots.

Acknowledgments: The authors thank Adam Lewis with USDA-ARS and personnel at a commercial feedlot who wish to remain anonymous. This work was supported by a specific cooperative agreement between Texas Tech University and USDA-ARS, and by the German Bundesministerium für Forschung und Technik (Deutscher Akademischer Austausch Dienst—DAAD Program).

Author Contributions: Frank M. Mitloehner conducted the field study and wrote the first draft manuscript. Jeff W. Dailey and Julie L. Morrow provided assistance in analysis of the behavioral data and both revised draft versions. John J. McGlone served as principal investigator of this study. He provided substantive input during the conduct of the study as well as in the revision of draft versions.

Conflicts of Interest: The authors declare no conflict of interest.

References

1. Plummer, L.E.; Pinkerton, K.E.; Reynolds, S.; Meschke, S.; Mitloehner, F.M.; Bennett, D.; Smiley-Jewell, S.; Schenker, M.B. Aerosols in the agricultural setting. *J. Agromed.* **2009**, *14*, 413–416. [CrossRef] [PubMed]
2. Garcia, J.; Bennett, D.; Schenker, M.; Mitloehner, F.M. Occupational exposure to particulate matter and endotoxin for California dairy workers. *Int. J. Hyg. Environ. Health* **2012**, *216*, 56–62. [CrossRef] [PubMed]
3. Garcia, J.; Bennett, D.H.; Tancredi, D.; Schenker, M.B.; Mitchell, D.; Mitloehner, F.M. A survey of particulate matter on California dairy. *J. Environ. Qual.* **2013**, *42*, 40–47. [CrossRef] [PubMed]
4. Wilson, S.C.; Morrow-Tesch, J.; Straus, D.C.; Cooley, J.D.; Wong, W.C.; Mitloehner, F.M.; McGlone, J.J. Airborne microbial flora in a cattle feedlot. *Appl. Environ. Microbiol.* **2002**, *68*, 3238–3242. [CrossRef] [PubMed]
5. Pope, C.A.; Burnett, R.T.; Thurston, G.D.; Thun, M.J.; Calle, E.E.; Krewski, D.; Godleski, J.J. Cardiovascular mortality and long-term exposure to particulate air pollution—Epidemiological evidence of general pathophysiological pathways of disease. *Circulation* **2004**, *109*, 71–77. [CrossRef] [PubMed]
6. Schinasi, L.; Horton, R.A.; Guidry, V.T.; Wing, S.; Marshall, S.W.; Morland, K.B. Air pollution, lung function, and physical symptoms in communities near concentrated swine feeding operations. *Epidemiology* **2011**, *22*, 208–215. [CrossRef] [PubMed]
7. Yamazaki, S.; Shima, M.; Ando, M.; Nitta, H.; Watanabe, H.; Nishimuta, T. Effect of hourly concentration of particulate matter on peak expiratory flow in hospitalized children: A panel study. *Environ. Health* **2011**, *10*, 15. [CrossRef] [PubMed]
8. Madl, A.K.C.C.; Pinkerton, K.E. Particle toxicities. In *Com-Prehensive Toxicology*, 2nd ed.; Mcqueen, C.A., Ed.; Elsevier Ltd.: Oxford, UK, 2010.
9. Liebers, V.; Bruning, T.; Raulf-Heimsoth, M. Occupational endotoxin-exposure and possible health effects on humans. *Am. J. Ind. Med.* **2006**, *49*, 474–491. [CrossRef] [PubMed]

10. Lott, S.C. Australian feedlot hydrology. Part I. In Proceedings of the Feedlot Waste Management Conference, Gold Coast, QLD, Australia, 12–14 June 1995.

11. Arnold, G.W.; Dudzinski, M.L. *Ethology of Free-Ranging Domestic Animals*; Elsevier: Amsterdam, The Netherlands, 1978.

12. Mitloehner, F.M.; Laube, R.B. Chronobiological indicators of heat stress in Bos indicus cattle in the tropics. *J. Anim. Vet. Adv.* **2003**, 2, 654–659.

13. Mitloehner, F.M.; Morrow-Tesch, J.L.; Wilson, S.C.; Dailey, J.W.; McGlone, J.J. Behavioral sampling techniques for feedlot cattle. *J. Anim. Sci.* **2001**, 79, 1189–1193. [CrossRef]

14. Miller, D.N.; Berry, E.D. Cattle feedlot soil moisture and manure content. *J. Environ. Qual.* **2005**, 34, 644–655. [CrossRef] [PubMed]

15. Miller, D.N.; Woodbury, B.L. Simple protocols to determine dust potentials from cattle feedlot soil and surface samples. *J. Environ. Qual.* **2003**, 32, 1634–1640. [CrossRef] [PubMed]

16. Auvermann, B.; Bottcher, R.; Heber, A.; Meyer, D.; Parnell, C.B., Jr.; Shaw, B.; Worley, J. *Particulate Matter Emissions from Animal Feeding Operations*; White Paper for the National Center for Manure and Animal Waste Management; Midwest Plan Service: Ames, IA, USA, 2001.

17. Mitloehner, F.M.; Galyean, M.L.; McGlone, J.J. Shade effects on performance, carcass traits, physiology, and behavior of heat-stressed feedlot heifers. *J. Anim. Sci.* **2002**, 80, 2043–2050. [CrossRef]

12

Relationship between Deck Level, Body Surface Temperature and Carcass Damages in Italian Heavy Pigs after Short Journeys at Different Unloading Environmental Conditions

Agnese Arduini [1,*], Veronica Redaelli [1], Fabio Luzi [2], Stefania Dall'Olio [1], Vincenzo Pace [3] and Leonardo Nanni Costa [1]

[1] Department of Agricultural and Food Sciences, School of Agriculture and Veterinary Medicine, University of Bologna, Via Fanin 50, Bologna 40127, Italy; vereda@tin.it (V.R.); stefania.dallolio@unibo.it (S.D.); leonardo.nannicosta@unibo.it (L.N.C.)

[2] Department of Veterinary Science and Public Health, Faculty of Veterinary Science, University of Milan, Via Celoria 10, Milan 20133, Italy; fabio.luzi@unimi.it

[3] OPAS, Pig Farmer Association, Strada Ghisiolo 57, San Giorgio, Mantua 46030, Italy; vincenzo.opas@coopgsp.it

* Correspondence: agnese.arduini@unibo.it

Academic Editors: John J. McGlone and Anna K. Johnson

Simple Summary: Transport duration and thermal conditions can negatively affect pig welfare and carcass quality. The effects of short journeys (30 min) in different thermal-humidity conditions on the body surface temperature of live heavy pigs and carcass skin damage were examined. Body temperature increased with increasing Temperature Humidity Index (THI) class. The highest and lowest body surface temperatures were found in pigs located on the middle and upper decks, respectively. THI class significantly affected skin damage scores, which increased with increasing THI class. Even at relatively low temperatures and THI, the results of this study suggested the need to increase the control of environmental conditions in the truck during short-distance transport of pigs, in order to improve welfare and reduce loss of carcass value.

Abstract: In order to evaluate the relationships between deck level, body surface temperature and carcass damages after a short journey (30 min), 10 deliveries of Italian heavy pigs, including a total of 1400 animals from one farm, were examined. Within 5 min after the arrival at the abattoir, the vehicles were unloaded. Environmental temperature and relative humidity were recorded and a Temperature Humidity Index (THI) was calculated. After unloading, maximum temperatures of dorsal and ocular regions were measured by a thermal camera on groups of pigs from each of the unloaded decks. After dehairing, quarters and whole carcasses were evaluated subjectively by a trained operator for skin damage using a four-point scale. On the basis of THI at unloading, deliveries were grouped into three classes. Data of body surface temperature and skin damage score were analysed in a model including THI class, deck level and their interaction. Regardless of pig location in the truck, the maximum temperature of the dorsal and ocular regions increased with increasing THI class. Within each THI class, the highest and lowest body surface temperatures were found in pigs located on the middle and upper decks, respectively. Only THI class was found to affect the skin damage score ($p < 0.05$), which increased on quarters and whole carcasses with increasing THI class. The results of this study on short-distance transport of Italian heavy pigs highlighted the need to control and ameliorate the environmental conditions in the trucks, even at relatively low temperature and THI, in order to improve welfare and reduce loss of carcass value.

Keywords: pigs; transport; distance; body surface temperature; carcass; damage

1. Introduction

The transport to the slaughterhouse is considered an important stressor for slaughter pigs, which may have deleterious effects on health and welfare, as well as carcass and pork quality [1]. Several studies have been conducted to assess the influence of factors connected to the transport, including loading density, distance and duration of journey, handling treatment, trailer design, loading method, environmental conditions and internal microclimate [2]. In particular, the thermal environment affects physiological and behavioural responses of transported pigs [3]. Warm environmental conditions are associated with a higher risk of fatigue, open-mouth breathing and death in-transit or at arrival [4]. Moreover, both cold and heat stress affect muscle glycogen stores leading to an increased incidence of pale soft exudative (PSE) or dark firm and dry meat defects [5]. Environmental conditions during transport, that also affect skin blemishes and meat quality, include the position of the animal inside the vehicle [6,7]. Pigs located in the front and rear compartments or in the upper and lower decks showed an increased number of carcass skin bruises and a reduced pork quality [8]. Despite several studies on the influence of the environmental conditions during long-distance transports on pig welfare and carcass quality, few studies have investigated these effects during short-distance transports. Short-distance transports are very common in many European regions with high concentrations of piggeries and slaughter plants [9]. Gajana et al. [10], Guardià et al. [11] and Perez et al. [12] observed a higher incidence of PSE meat in pigs that had been transported a short duration compared to pigs transported longer distances. Barton Gade and Christensen [13] reported an increased risk of skin damage during short-distance transports (2–3 h). Gispert et al. [14] also found higher skin damage scores in short-distance transports (<2 h) compared to long-distance transports (>2 h). Conversely, Mota-Rojas et al. [15] found that the frequency of bruised carcasses increased with journey duration. Hence, there is a need to increase the knowledge on the relationships between short-distance transport and skin damages. An important topic in animal welfare study concerns the measure of stress avoiding invasive methods. Infrared thermography may be considered a reliable and non-invasive tool to evaluate the stress impact of different management practices at the farm and at slaughter [16]. The aim of this study was to evaluate the relationship between the deck level, dorsal and ocular region surface temperature and carcass damage after a short duration transport of Italian heavy pigs destined for the dry-cured industry.

2. Experimental Section

2.1. Data Collection

This study was carried out on data collected from 1400 crossbred (Duroc × (Landrace × Large White)) Italian heavy pigs (live weights average ± s.d.: 171.1 ± 6.1 kg) provided in 10 batches supplied by the same farm on 10 different days, randomly chosen between January and June 2014. Each batch consisted of 140 pigs 9 months old, according to the denomination of protected origin dry-cured ham Parma Consortium [17]. The plant was located in Northern Italy with a chain speed of 280 pigs/h.

2.2. Pre-Slaughter Conditions and Slaughterhouse

The trucks were stocked according to European livestock transport rule EC Regulation No. 1/2005 [18] with an available surface of about 0.73 m^2/pig. The pigs were transported on rural and secondary roads with a journey time of 31 ± 5 min at an average speed of 30 km/h. The transport was always carried out using a truck from Carrozzeria Pezzaioli (Montichiari, Italy), composed of a main lorry and a trailer, each one equipped with three hydraulic decks (Figure 1) containing 23–24 pigs/deck. Lorries and trailers had both natural and mechanical ventilation systems, with automatic fans placed on the left side of both compartments. The fans, nine in each truck, were 225 mm in diameter with a 11,700 m²/h flow. Pigs were off feed for 12 h before transport. Loading was carried out at around 06:00 a.m. by three farm operators, avoiding mixing between unfamiliar pens. The farm operators went out to one pen at a time to drive pigs toward the loading platform, using a plastic stick. The loading procedures lasted approximately 45 min. A mobile ramp (length 6.0 m, width 0.7 m, with 1.0 m solid side walls and adjustable height) was used to load pigs into the truck. Within 5 min after the arrival at the abattoir, the pigs were unloaded using a fixed platform (length 9.3 m, width 2.7 m, 1.0 m solid side walls) that was height-adjusted to the level of the lower deck by the lairage manager and the driver. Each deck was unloaded within 2 min and the complete unloading procedures lasted approximately 12 min. The lorry was always unloaded before the trailer and the decks were unloaded sequentially, starting with the lower deck, as shown in Figure 1.

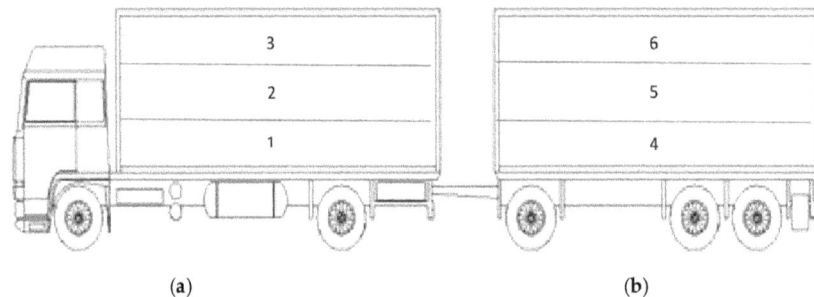

(a)   (b)

Figure 1. Schematic drawing of the truck with hydraulic decks used for pig transportation. The lorry was always unloaded before the trailer and decks were unloaded sequentially, starting with the lower deck. (**a**) LORRY; (**b**) TRAILER.

During the unloading of each deck, environmental temperature (°C) and relative humidity (%) were recorded using a Gemini Tinytag Ultra 4500 Thermal Sensor (Gemini Data Logger Ltd., Chichester, West Sussex, UK) located on a windowsill close to the platform, at the entrance of the resting pens. A Temperature Humidity Index (THI) was then calculated according to NRC [19] using the formula: THI = {(1.8 × T + 32) − (0.55 − (0.0055 × RH))} × {(1.8 × (1.8 × T + 32)) − 26}, in which T is the temperature and RH is the relative humidity. Order and date of deliveries and temperature (T), relative humidity (RH) and THI measured at each delivery during unloading are presented in Table 1.

Table 1. Identification (ID) and date of deliveries and outdoor temperature (T), relative humidity (RH) and Temperature Humidity Index (THI) recorded at unloading. The sensor was located close to the platform crossed by the pigs to reach the resting area.

Delivery ID	Date (yy/mm/dd) *	T (°C)	RH (%)	THI
1	14/01/28	5.6	91.2	42.9
2	14/02/11	5.8	94.1	42.9
3	14/03/11	9.5	70.4	50.6
4	14/03/18	7.0	79.0	46.1
5	14/03/25	4.0	72.0	42.1
6	14/04/01	14.7	66.9	58.4
7	14/04/15	14.2	77.8	57.6
8	14/05/20	19.6	69.0	65.7
9	14/05/27	17.6	80.9	63.1
10	14/06/10	22.0	51.0	67.9

* yy/mm/dd: year/month/day.

At the plant, pigs were driven with plastic sticks or rubber boards to resting pens and they were allowed to rest for 20 to 30 min. During this period, pigs were not mixed with unfamiliar animals. After the rest, the pigs were showered and driven through a single passageway to the stunning cage. Stunning was manually done by electrical tongs (head only; 170 V, 1.3 A). Carcasses were horizontally exsanguinated for 3 min, then hanged for 10 min before being immersed in a scalding tank for dehairing at 62 °C for 10 min. After dehairing, skin damages were subjectively assessed by the same trained technician, using a four-point scale (1 = none to 4 = severe) based on the scale developed by the Danish Meat Research Institute (DMRI) [20]. The DMRI scale was used to score all skin lesions on the front (head included), middle and hind quarters of each carcass. Moreover, a skin damage score for the whole carcass was calculated using the highest score assigned to each quarter [20]. The carcasses were then eviscerated, split, hot-boned and sectioned in primal cuts.

2.3. Thermal Imaging

During the unloading of each deck, as the pigs were driven along the platform, the maximum surface temperatures were recorded on the dorsal and ocular regions using an Avio thermoGear Nec G120 EX thermal camera (Nippon Avionics Co., Ltd., Tokyo, Japan). Several studies have found that these regions show changes in maximum surface temperatures in response to acute stress and variation in environmental conditions [21,22]. The camera was calibrated manually before to carry out measurements on pigs from each delivery. The camera was located at the entrance of the lairage pens at about 3 m from the unloading point and at a height of 1.80 m. The skin emissivity was manually set in the camera at 0.96 before each unloading. Thermal images were downloaded to a computer and examined using NEC InfRec Analyzer and Grayess IRT Analyzer software (Nippon Avionics Co., Ltd., Tokyo, Japan). A total of 7000 readable thermal images including 1222 pigs were analysed to determine the maximum surface temperatures within the dorsal and ocular regions. An example of the examined thermal images is shown in Figure 2.

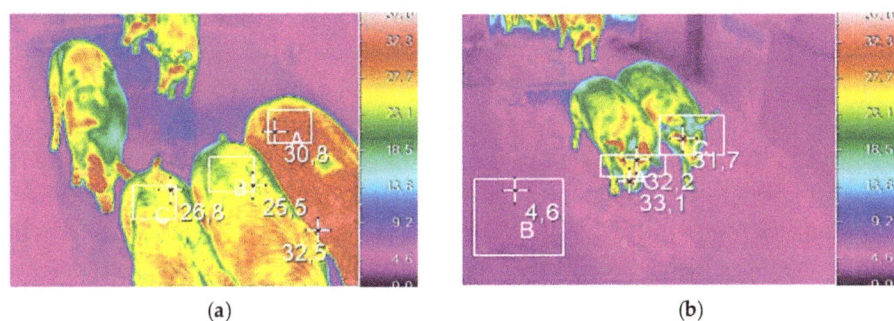

Figure 2. Examples of thermal images of the dorsal (**a**) and ocular (**b**) regions recorded during the unloading of Italian heavy pigs at the slaughterhouse after transport of approximately 30 min under commercial conditions. The white rectangles indicate the areas in which the maximum temperatures were recorded.

2.4. Statistical Analysis

For the statistical analyses, a classification of deliveries on the basis of THI was done using the CLUSTER procedure of SAS (SAS Institute, Cary, NC, USA) [23]. Using a dendogram analysis, three clusters were identified. The FASTCLUS procedure of SAS [23] was used in order to classify the deliveries into one of the three clusters previously defined. In this procedure, observations that are very close to each other are assigned to the same cluster by an algorithm for minimizing the sum of squared distances from the cluster means [23]. Deliveries classification and means and standard deviations of environmental temperature, relative humidity and THI for each THI class are reported in Table 2. All data were tested for normality by using PROC UNIVARIATE of SAS [23]. A preliminary analysis was conducted to assess differences between the lorry and trailer. No significant differences ($p > 0.05$) were found, therefore this source of variation was not included in subsequent statistical analyses. Data of maximum surface temperatures were analysed using the GLIMMIX procedure of SAS using a model including THI class, deck level and their interaction. GLIMMIX was also used to analyse the effects of the same sources of variation on skin damage scores recorded on each quarter separately as well as on the whole carcass. Because these data approximated a Poisson distribution, the GLIMMIX procedure's POISSON option was used. The ILINK option was used to back-transform least squares means of the skin damage score. The differences in least squares means were evaluated using Tukey-Kramer's test. The level for statistical significance used was $p < 0.05$ in all analyses.

Table 2. Distribution based on the Temperature Humidity Index (THI) of the ten deliveries of Italian heavy pigs transported approximately for 30 min under commercial conditions. For each class of THI, identification (ID) of the deliveries, number of pigs, mean and standard deviation (s.d.) of outdoor temperature (T), relative humidity (RH) and THI at unloading are shown.

THI Class *	Deliveries ID	Pigs	T (°C)		RH (%)		THI	
		No	Mean	s.d.	Mean	s.d.	Mean	s.d.
1	1, 2, 4, 5	560	5.6	1.1	76.6	2.8	43.5	1.5
2	3, 6, 7	420	12.8	2.4	71.7	4.6	55.5	3.5
3	8, 9, 10	420	19.7	1.8	67.0	12.3	65.6	2.0

* THI classes were obtained by the CLUSTER procedure on the basis of THI values and the deliveries were allocated into the classes by the FASTCLUS procedure of SAS [23].

3. Results and Discussion

THI class, deck level and their interaction significantly influenced the maximum surface temperatures of the dorsal region ($p < 0.05$). The interaction effect on these temperatures is shown in Table 3. Within each deck, the surface temperatures increased significantly ($p < 0.05$) with increasing THI class. This result agrees with findings of several studies reviewed by Soerensen and Pedersen [24] who pointed out that body superficial temperature increased at high ambient temperature and decreased at low ambient temperatures. A significant effect of deck level was observed in the first THI class only ($p < 0.05$) where the mean value recorded on pigs located on the upper deck of the trailer (deck 6) was significantly lower compared to the middle and lower decks of the whole truck. In the second THI class, there was a tendency in pigs located on the upper deck of the trailer (deck 6) to show the lowest surface temperature while in the third class, the lowest mean values were recorded on pigs located in the lower deck of the trailer (decks 4). Probably, due to a short-distance transport time, the variation of ambient temperature and internal air flow between decks within THI classes had a weak impact on the thermoregulation of pigs.

Table 3. Effect of the interaction between the class of the Temperature Humidity Index (THI) and deck level on the maximum surface temperature (°C) recorded at unloading by a thermal camera on the dorsal region of Italian heavy pigs transported approximately for 30 min under commercial conditions (least squares means).

THI Class *	Deck Level						SE
	1	2	3	4	5	6	
1	28.6 [x ab]	29.1 [x ab]	27.8 [x ab]	28.7 [x ab]	29.5 [x a]	27.3 [x b]	0.26
2	31.1 [y]	31.6 [y]	31.2 [y]	30.9 [y]	31.1 [y]	30.5 [y]	0.30
3	34.4 [z]	35.0 [z]	34.2 [z]	33.7 [z]	34.3 [z]	34.1 [z]	0.34

[a, b]: different superscript letters in the same row are different at $p < 0.05$; [x, y, z]: different superscript letters in the same column are different at $p < 0.05$. SE: standard error. * THI classes included the following deliveries (ID): 1, 2, 4 and 5 in class 1; 3, 6 and 7 in class 2; 8, 9 and 10 in class 3.

In terms of the maximum surface temperature of the ocular region, an interaction between THI class and deck level was again observed (Table 4). As in the dorsal region, the maximum surface temperatures of the ocular area increased with increasing THI class. A significant effect of deck ($p < 0.05$) was observed in the first and second THI classes only. In the first THI class, the highest mean values of ocular surface temperature were recorded on pigs located on the middle deck of the lorry (deck 2) and in the lower deck of the trailer (deck 4), whereas the lowest values were found on subjects located on the upper deck (decks 3). In the second THI class, the lowest mean values were found in pigs located on the upper deck (deck 6), whereas the highest values were observed in pigs transported in the middle decks of trailers (deck 5). A tendency towards a higher temperature on lorry decks 2 and 3 was observed in the third THI class.

Table 4. Effect of the interaction between the class of the Temperature Humidity Index (THI) and deck level on the maximum surface temperature (°C) recorded at unloading by a thermal camera on the ocular region of Italian heavy pigs transported approximately for 30 min under commercial conditions (least square means).

THI Class *	Deck Level						SE
	1	2	3	4	5	6	
1	32.8 $^{x\,ab}$	33.2 $^{x\,a}$	32.0 $^{x\,b}$	33.2 $^{x\,a}$	33.0 $^{x\,ab}$	32.4 $^{x\,ab}$	0.60
2	33.7 $^{y\,ab}$	34.2 $^{y\,ab}$	33.7 $^{y\,ab}$	33.8 $^{y\,ab}$	34.5 $^{y\,a}$	33.5 $^{y\,b}$	0.74
3	35.1 ^{z}	35.4 ^{z}	35.3 ^{z}	35.1 ^{z}	35.1 ^{z}	35.1 ^{z}	0.87

[a, b]: different superscript letters in the same row are different at $p < 0.05$; [x, y, z]: different superscript letters in the same column are different at $p < 0.05$. SE: standard error. * In THI classes, the following deliveries (ID) were included: 1, 2, 4 and 5 in class 1; 3, 6 and 7 in class 2; 8, 9 and 10 in class 3.

In general, in the present study, the maximum surface temperatures recorded in the ocular region were slightly lower compared to those recorded in the same region on pigs restrained in cages [21,24]. This is probably due to differences in the distance [25] between the thermal camera and the pigs at unloading compared to pigs restrained into cages.

For the skin damages, only the THI class had a significant effect ($p < 0.05$) on scores recorded both in individual quarters and the whole carcass (Table 5). Even at relatively low temperatures and THI, the general pattern observed was an increase in the skin damage score in all quarters with increasing THI class. In the hind and front quarters, as well as in the whole carcass, the mean score of the third THI class was significantly higher than those of the first and second classes ($p < 0.05$), which were not significantly different. In the middle quarter, the mean scores of the third THI class were also higher than the other two classes, and the middle THI class was significantly higher than the lowest THI class ($p < 0.05$). Probably, warmer environments resulted in pigs being more active and prone to hits against loading and unloading facilities. These results agree with Dalla Costa et al. [5] and Eldridge and Winfield [26] who found that environmental factors, such as temperature and humidity, affect the incidence of skin bruises. In a recent study on the effects of season and location inside the truck on pig behaviour, Torrey et al. [27] observed more slips, falls, overlaps and backward at unloading in summer than in winter. Also in cattle, skin damage scores were found to be higher in warmer environments [28]. In particular, Mpakama [29] showed that higher temperatures, especially in summer, increased the risk of skin bruises on arrival at the plant.

Table 5. Effect of the Temperature Humidity Index (THI) class on the skin damage score [1] of single quarters and whole carcass of Italian heavy pigs (least squares means).

Skin Damage Score	THI Class			SE
	1	2	3	
Single quarters:				
-hind	2.07 ^{b}	2.26 ^{b}	2.59 ^{a}	0.07
-middle	2.56 ^{c}	2.83 ^{b}	3.50 ^{a}	0.08
-front	2.10 ^{b}	2.14 ^{b}	2.58 ^{a}	0.07
Whole carcass	2.75 ^{b}	2.98 ^{b}	3.58 ^{a}	0.08

[1] four-point scale: 1 = none to 4 = severe; [a, b, c]: different superscript letters in the same row are different at $p < 0.05$. SE: standard error.

It could be argued that maintaining pigs at low space and high THI in a stationary vehicle at the slaughterhouse can lead to aggression even among well-acquainted animals. It is unlikely that this occurrence can explain the effect of THI class on the increase of skin damage because of the short time spent to complete unloading procedures and the behaviour of familiar heavy pigs. Martelli et al. [30] found very low incidence of aggressive interactions in well-acquainted Italian heavy pigs kept at different light intensity. Moreover, during all deliveries, there was no evidence of aggressions among pigs in the stationary vehicles.

Deck level did not significantly affect skin damage scores (data not shown). A tendency towards higher skin damage scores was found in pigs transported on the trailer compared to those located on the lorry. This tendency could be explained by the fact that the trailer is subjected to more vibrations and movements compared to the lorry.

4. Conclusions

The results of this study on short-distance transport of Italian heavy pigs confirm that different environmental conditions, even when experienced during a limited time, affect surface body temperatures and carcass skin damages. The location of the pigs in the vehicle interacts with environmental conditions in their effects on surface body temperatures, but not on carcass damage scores. Thermal and humidity conditions played an important role on the skin damage score which appeared to increase with increasing THI. If the effect of THI increase on the risk of skin damages is confirmed by further studies, then the control of environmental conditions during short-distance transport of pigs will be one of the main concerns from a welfare perspective. However, more research is needed to determine the effect of short-time transport on the stress and carcass damages in heavy pigs during different environmental conditions, such as extreme THI values.

Acknowledgments: The authors wish to acknowledge the technical assistance of quality assurance staff of the abattoir for data collected at the slaughterhouse. This research was supported by Regione Lombardia, Programma di Sviluppo Rurale 2007–2013, Misura 124.

Author Contributions: Agnese Arduini, Leonardo Nanni Costa, Veronica Redaelli and Fabio Luzi conceived, designed and performed the experiment, collecting data on field. Vincenzo Pace performed technician evaluation during slaughters. Agnese Arduini, Leonardo Nanni Costa and Veronica Redaelli analyzed the data and contributed to materials and analysis tools together Fabio Luzi and Stefania Dall'Olio.

Conflicts of Interest: The authors declare no conflict of interest.

References

1.   Bench, C.; Schaefer, A.L.; Faucitano, L. The welfare of pigs during transport. In *The Welfare of Pigs—From Birth to Slaughter*; Faucitano, L., Schaefer, A.L., Eds.; Wageningen Academic Publishers: Wageningen, The Netherlands, 2008; pp. 161–195.

2.   Brown, J.A.; Samarakone, T.S.; Crowe, T.; Bergeron, R.; Widowski, T.; Correa, J.A.; Faucitano, L.; Torrey, S.; Gonyou, H.W. Temperature and humidity conditions in trucks transporting pigs in two seasons in Eastern and Western Canada. *Trans. ASABE* **2011**, *54*, 2311–2318. [CrossRef]

3.   Warris, P.D. The welfare of slaughter pigs during transport. *Anim. Welf.* **1998**, *7*, 365–381.

4.   McGlone, J.; Johnson, A.; Sapkota, A.; Kephart, R. Market pig transport. In *Allen D. Leman Swine Conference*; Veterinary Continuing Education: Minneapolis, MN, USA, 2012; Volume 39, pp. 169–176.

5.   Dalla Costa, O.A.; Faucitano, L.; Coldebella, A.; Ludke, J.V.; Peloso, J.V.; Dalla Roza, D.; Paranhos da Costa, M.J.R. Effects of the season of the year, truck type and location on truck on skin bruises and meat quality in pigs. *Livest. Sci.* **2007**, *107*, 29–36. [CrossRef]

6.   Guise, H.J.; Penny, R.H.C. Factors influencing the welfare and carcass and meat quality of pigs: 1. The effects of stocking density in transport and the use of electric goads. *Anim. Prod.* **1989**, *49*, 511–515. [CrossRef]

7.   Barton-Gade, P.A.; Christensen, L.; Brown, S.N.; Warriss, P.D. Effect of tier ventilation during transport on blood parameters and meat quality in slaughter pigs. In *EU-Seminar: New Information on Welfare and Meat Quality of Pigs as Related to Handling, Transport and Lairage Conditions*; Landbauforschung Völkenrode: Mariensee, Kulmbach, Germany, 1996; pp. 101–116.

8.   Scheeren, M.B.; Gonyou, H.W.; Brown, J.; Weschenfelder, A.V.; Faucitano, L. Effect of transport time and location within truck on skin bruises and meat quality of market pigs in two seasons. *Can. J. Anim. Sci.* **2014**, *94*, 71–78. [CrossRef]

9.   Marquer, P.; Rabade, T.; Forti, R. Pig Farming in the European Union: Considerable Variations from One Member State to Another. Eurostat, Statistic in Focus 15/2014. Available online: http://ec.europa. eu/eurostat/statistics-explained/index.php/Pig_farming_sector_-_statistical_portrait_2014 (accessed on 1 September 2016).

10.   Gajana, C.S.; Nkukwana, T.T.; Marume, U.; Muchenje, V. Effects of transportation time, distance, stocking density, temperature and lairage time on incidences of pale soft exudative (PSE) and the physico-chemical characteristics of pork. *Meat Sci.* **2013**, *95*, 520–525. [CrossRef] [PubMed]

11.   Guàrdia, M.D.; Estany, J.; Balash, S.; Oliver, M.A.; Gispert, M.; Diestre, A. Risk assessment of DFD meat due to pre-slaughter conditions and RYR1 gene in pigs. *Meat Sci.* **2005**, *70*, 709–716. [CrossRef] [PubMed]

12.   Peréz, M.P.; Palaciö, J.; Santolaria, M.P.; Acena, M.C.; Chacón, G.; Gascón, M.; Calvo, P.; Zaragoza, S.; Beltran, J.A.; Garcia-Belenguer, S. Effect of transport time on welfare and meat quality in pigs. *Meat Sci.* **2002**, *61*, 425–433. [CrossRef]

13.   Barton-Gade, P.; Christensen, L. Effect of different loading densities during transport on welfare and meat quality in Danish slaughter pigs. *Meat Sci.* **1998**, *48*, 237–247. [CrossRef]

14.   Gispert, M.; Faucitano, L.; Oliver, M.A.; Guàrdia, M.D.; Coll, C.; Siggens, K.; Harvey, K.; Diestre, A. A survey on pre-slaughter conditions, halothane gene frequency, and carcass and meat quality in five Spanish pig commercial abattoirs. *Meat Sci.* **2000**, *55*, 97–106. [CrossRef]

15.   Mota-Rojas, D.; Becerril, M.; Lemus, C.; Sánchez, P.; González, M.; Olmos, S.A.; Ramirez, R.; Alonso-Spilsbury, M. Effects of mid-summer transport duration on pre and post-slaughter performance and pork quality in Mexico. *Meat Sci.* **2006**, *73*, 404–412. [CrossRef] [PubMed]

16.   Stewart, M.; Schaefer, A.L.; Haley, D.B.; Colyn, J.; Cook, N.J.; Stafford, K.J.; Webster, J.R. Infrared thermography as a non-invasive method for detecting fear-related responses of cattle to handling procedures. *Anim. Welf.* **2008**, *17*, 387–393.

17.   Disciplinare del Prosciutto di Parma. Available online: http://www.prosciuttodiparma.com/en_UK/home (accessed on 10 September 2016).

18.   The Council of the European Union. *Council Regulation (EC) No. 1/2005. No. 1/2005 of 22 December 2004 on the Protection of Animals during Transport and Related Operations and Amending Directives 64/432/EEC and 93/119/EC and Regulation (EC) No. 1255/97*; The Council of the European Union: Brussels, Belgium, 2005. Available online: https://www.agriculture.gov.ie/media/migration/animalhealthwelfare/ transportofliveanimals/Council%20Regulation%201%20of%202005.pdf (accessed on 25 November 2016).

19.   National Research Council. *A Guide to Environmental Research on Animals*; National Academy of Sciences: Washington, DC, USA, 1971.

20.   Barton Gade, P.A.; Warriss, P.D.; Brown, S.N.; Lambooij, E. Methods of improving pig welfare and meat quality by reducing stress and discomfort before slaughter—Methods of measuring meat quality. In *EU-Seminar: New Information on Welfare and Meat Quality of Pigs as Related to Handling, Transport and Lairage Conditions*; Landbauforschung Völkenrode: Mariensee, Kulmbach, Germany, 1996; Volume 166, pp. 23–34.

21.   Nanni Costa, L.; Redaelli, V.; Magnani, D.; Cafazzo, S.; Amadori, M.; Razzuoli, E.; Verga, M.; Luzi, F. Preliminary study on the relationship between skin temperature of piglet measured by infrared thermography and environmental temperature in a vehicle in transit. In *Veterinary Science. Current Aspects in Biology, Animal Pathology, Clinic and Food Hygiene*; Pugliese, A., Gaiti, A., Boiti, C., Eds.; Springer: Berlin/Heidelberg, Germany, 2012; pp. 193–198.

22.   Weschenfelder, A.V.; Torrey, S.; Devillers, N.; Crowe, T.; Bassols, A.; Saco, Y.; Pineirõ, M.; Saucier, L.; Faucitano, L. Effect of trailer design on animals welfare parameters and carcass and meat quality of three Pietrain crosses being transported over short distance. *Livest. Sci.* **2013**, *157*, 234–244. [CrossRef]

23.   SAS Institute, Inc. *Statistical Analysis System. Version 9.4*; SAS Institute, Inc.: Cary, NC, USA, 2013.

24.   Soerensen, D.D.; Pedersen, L.J. Infrared skin temperature measurements for monitoring health in pigs: A review. *Acta Vet. Scand.* **2015**, *57*, 5. [CrossRef] [PubMed]

25. Westermann, S.; Buchner, H.H.F.; Schramel, J.P.; Tichy, A.; Stanek, C. Effects of infrared camera angle and distance on measurement and reproducibility of thermographically determined temperatures of the distolateral aspects of the forelimbs in horses. *J. Am. Vet. Med. Assoc.* **2013**, *242*, 388–395. [CrossRef] [PubMed]

26. Eldridge, G.A.; Winfield, C.G. The behaviour and bruising of cattle during transport at different space allowances. *Aust. J. Exp. Agric.* **1988**, *28*, 695–698. [CrossRef]

27. Torrey, S.; Bergeron, R.; Faucitano, L.; Widowski, T.; Lewis, N.; Crowe, T.; Correa, J.A.; Brown, J.; Gonyou, H.W. Transportation of market-weight pigs. 2. Effect of season and animal location in the truck on behaviour with a 8 hour transport. *J. Anim. Sci.* **2013**, *91*, 2872–2878. [CrossRef] [PubMed]

28. Strappini, A.C.; Frankena, K.; Gallo, C.; Metz, J.; Kemp, B. Prevalence and risk factors for bruises in Chilean bovine carcasses. *Meat Sci.* **2010**, *86*, 859–864. [CrossRef] [PubMed]

29. Mpakama, T. Bruising in Slaughter Cattle: Its Relationship with Creatine Kinase (CK) Levels and Meat Quality. Master's Thesis, University of Fort Hare, Alice, South Africa, 3 December 2012.

30. Martelli, G.; Boccuzzi, R.; Grandi, M.; Mazzone, G.; Zaghini, G.; Sardi, L. The effect of two different light intensities on the production and behavioural traits of Italian heavy pigs. *Berl. Munch. Tierarztl. Wochenschr.* **2010**, *123*, 457–462. [PubMed]

13

The Impact of Stakeholders' Roles within the Livestock Industry on Their Attitudes to Livestock Welfare in Southeast and East Asia

Michelle Sinclair, Sarah Zito [†] and Clive J. C. Phillips *

Centre for Animal Welfare and Ethics, School of Veterinary Sciences, The University of Queensland, Gatton, Queensland 4343, Australia; m.sinclair6@uq.edu.au (M.S.); s.zito@uq.edu.au (S.Z.)
* Correspondence: c.phillips@uq.edu.au
† Current address: Royal New Zealand Society for the Prevention of Cruelty to Animals, New Lynn, Auckland 0640, New Zealand.

Academic Editor: Paul Koene

Simple Summary: Improving stakeholder attitudes to livestock welfare may help to facilitate the better welfare that is increasingly demanded by the public for livestock. Knowledge of the existing attitudes towards the welfare of livestock during transport and slaughter provides a starting point that may help to target efforts. We compared the attitudes of different stakeholders within the livestock industries in east (E) and southeast (SE) Asia. Farmers were more motivated to improve animal welfare during transport and slaughter by peer pressure, business owners by monetary gain, and business managers by what is prescribed by their company. Veterinarians showed the most support for improving animal welfare. The results suggest that the role that stakeholders play in their sector of the livestock industry must be considered when attempting to change attitudes towards animal welfare during transport and slaughter.

Abstract: Stakeholders in the livestock industry are in a position to make critical choices that directly impact on animal welfare during slaughter and transport. Understanding the attitudes of stakeholders in livestock-importing countries, including factors that motivate the stakeholders to improve animal welfare, can lead to improved trade relations with exporting developed countries and improved animal welfare initiatives in the importing countries. Improving stakeholder attitudes to livestock welfare may help to facilitate the better welfare that is increasingly demanded by the public for livestock. Knowledge of the existing attitudes towards the welfare of livestock during transport and slaughter provides a starting point that may help to target efforts. This study aimed to investigate the animal welfare attitudes of livestock stakeholders (farmers, team leaders, veterinarians, business owners, business managers, and those working directly with animals) in selected countries in E and SE Asia (China, Thailand, Viet Nam, and Malaysia). The factors that motivated them to improve animal welfare (in particular their religion, knowledge levels, monetary gain, the availability of tools and resources, more pressing community issues, and the approval of their supervisor and peers) were assessed for their relationships to stakeholder role and ranked according to their importance. Stakeholder roles influenced attitudes to animal welfare during livestock transport and slaughter. Farmers were more motivated by their peers compared to other stakeholders. Business owners reported higher levels of motivation from monetary gain, while business managers were mainly motivated by what was prescribed by the company for which they worked. Veterinarians reported the highest levels of perceived approval for improving animal welfare, and all stakeholder groups were least likely to be encouraged to change by a 'western' international organization. This study demonstrates the differences in attitudes of the major livestock stakeholders towards their animals' welfare during transport and slaughter, which advocacy organisations can use to tailor strategies more effectively to improve animal welfare. The results suggest that animal welfare initiatives are more likely to engage their target audience when tailored to specific stakeholder groups.

Keywords: animal welfare; attitudes; slaughter; transportation; livestock stakeholders; Asia

---

1. Introduction

Agribusiness is a large and important global industry that impacts on the lives of over 25 billion animals annually (excluding fish and invertebrates) [1], far larger than that of any other industry. Slaughter and transport are key events for the welfare of the animals involved. As well as impacting the animals, adverse welfare events occurring during slaughter and transport activate adrenergic mechanisms within the body, resulting in increased muscle glycogenolysis and reduced carcass quality [2]. Slaughtermen, livestock transporters, business owners, business managers, farmers, and vets are required to make decisions within their roles that have the ability to improve or jeopardize the welfare of the animals in their care. According to the Theory of Planned Behavior, understanding attitudes is the precursor to understanding human behavior [3]. Understanding the factors that motivate human behavior is of critical importance when trying to encourage behavioral changes that will improve animal welfare. The benefit of understanding the target audience is well understood in terms of improved engagement with a product in marketing spheres [4], but the same understanding seems to rarely have been prioritized when encouraging engagement with an idea, message, or practice in social progress initiatives.

An understanding of the attitudes of and factors motivating specific groups of stakeholders within an industry could potentially provide advice on how to tailor initiatives for the individuals in each stakeholder group to best encourage improvement in animal welfare.

The effects of nation and culture on attitudes towards animal welfare and the discovery of national differences in motivating factors have been previously reported [5]. That study suggested that progress initiatives in not-for-profit advocacy groups would benefit from being designed for individual nations, using a knowledge of specific attitudes and motivating factors in different regions and cultures. Other research has also yielded evidence of geo-political influences on attitudes to animal welfare related topics. For example, significant consistencies were found in attitudes to animals in university students across 12 Eurasian countries, based on the geo-political region of the students, rather than on other demographic factors such as religion, ethnicity, or age [6]. Similarly, the attitudes of the public in Germany, the USA, and Japan towards animals differ significantly [7].

The nature of a person's involvement with the livestock industry has been associated with differing attitudes to animal welfare. For example, discord in attitudes to animal welfare exists in Belgium between farmers, who reported satisfactory levels of farm animal welfare, and the public, who described the current state of farm animal welfare as 'problematic' [8]. This highlights the importance of understanding and improving the attitudes to animal welfare of each key stakeholder group within the industry. Understanding the attitudes and resulting behaviors of the stakeholders directly involved in handling animals is of particular importance given the direct impact that their attitude has on animal welfare [9–11]. The consumers' growing demand for high welfare products in developed countries [8] has implications if products come from international trade with countries that have lower welfare practices [12].

There are no reports of attitudes of stakeholders in different livestock industry roles within Asia. When livestock are sent there from developed countries, such as Australia, there is considerable concern by those internal and external to the industry that advocate, on behalf of the animals, that the animal welfare standards are poor [13]. Asia is responsible for 39% of global livestock production [1], and the industry is growing rapidly on that continent. In addition to supplying the domestic market, Asian producers are now also exporting animal products, such as Thai chicken exports to the European Union. Thus the export markets include nations with legislated welfare requirements and consumers who demand products with high standards of animal welfare. This is a critical time for the development of the livestock industry in many Asian countries, yet little is known about the attitudes towards animal welfare of the people who work within the industry.

While the attitudes of the people concerned with livestock (e.g., veterinary and animal science students [14]) towards animal welfare have been compared between Asian countries, there have been no comprehensive studies of the attitudes of different industry stakeholders towards livestock welfare during transport and slaughter. The aim of this study was to assess both their attitudes to animal welfare and the factors that motivate or act as barriers to improving animal welfare. This information could potentially facilitate the tailoring of animal welfare initiatives to specific stakeholder groups in order to improve stakeholder engagement and address the key welfare issues.

2. Methods

Trainers ($n = 44$) with relevant livestock industry knowledge in four key E and SE Asian countries attended one of four two-day workshops (one in each country) presented by four international experts in livestock transport and slaughter. Each workshop included a presentation and explanation of the translated educational resources that were prepared for this project (www.animalwelfarestandards.org). The trainers then delivered forty-four one-day regional workshops to stakeholders (about 25 participants in each) in the livestock transport and slaughter industry in geographically-relevant locations of People's Republic of China (hereafter China, trainer $n = 16$), Malaysia ($n = 6$), Thailand ($n = 11$), and the Socialist Republic of Viet Nam (hereafter Viet Nam, $n = 11$). These countries were selected because of their important role in global livestock import and export industries and in order to investigate attitudes across countries with diverse religious and cultural attributes. Stakeholders were invited to the workshops and also to participate in the research by the workshop trainers, with the only selection criteria being that they must be employed and involved in the local livestock slaughter and transport industry. The selection criteria to attend the training and participate in the research were given to the trainers, who then invited local stakeholders, most commonly by approaching local businesses and local contacts.

The invited participants, comprised of individuals involved in animal production industries in their country of residence included slaughtermen, transporters, livestock slaughter and transport business owners and managers, senior livestock veterinarians, and government veterinary representatives.

They were surveyed using a paper-based questionnaire at the start of the slaughter and transport workshops, which had been developed in English through consultation with academic and industry experts in the animal welfare field and through extensive literature review. It was translated into Bahasa, Mandarin, Thai, and Vietnamese and then back translated to ensure consistency of meaning. This questionnaire was also administered to the trainers at the start of their workshops, so that they were familiar with it and because they were also deemed to effectively be stakeholders in the industry. These were incorporated with the stakeholders' responses, increasing the total number of respondents to 1066.

In the questionnaire, respondent demographics were first obtained, including sex, age, residential area, religion, their self-identified role within the industry, and how their industry knowledge was gained (formal qualifications or otherwise). The options for identified role (and the number of representatives) were: working directly with animals ($n = 345$); team leaders, supervising people who work directly with animals ($n = 147$); business owners ($n = 55$); business managers ($n = 91$); farmers ($n = 179$); veterinarians, who were directly involved in treating animals ($n = 107$); and veterinarians working for the government as an advisor ($n = 138$).

The rest of the questionnaire consisted of four key question sets with responses to each question being measured on a Likert scale from 'strongly disagree' to 'strongly agree'.

The first non-demographic set of questions focused on general attitudes to animal welfare, including:

- the importance placed on animal welfare during slaughter and transport
- how satisfactory animal welfare in the respondents' workplace was believed to be

- whether the respondent intended or felt confident to make animal welfare improvements in their workplace
- whether the respondent had tried to make animal welfare improvements in the past

The second question set investigated the key factors influencing the stakeholders' evaluation of animal welfare during slaughter and transport. These included religion, personal beliefs, the extent to which there are more pressing issues in the community, personal and community monetary gain, importance within the workplace and amongst peers, knowledge, and the relevant laws.

The third question set focused on the respondents' evaluation of their ability to improve animal welfare during slaughter and transport and the factors that may enable or hinder their ability to effect improvement. These included the same factors as the second question set, but with the addition of company approval of improving animal welfare, physical workspace, available tools and resources, and vehicle design (for transport only).

The final question set focused on sources of encouragement to improve animal welfare and which sources respondents were more likely to respond to favorably. Those investigated were:

- prescription by local government, local organizations, local law enforcement, and 'western' international organizations
- prescription by law, workplace, supervisor, and community elders
- the respondent seeing moral or monetary gain in change or seeing others making the change

The survey was reviewed by a panel of sociological researchers, piloted with nationals from each participating country and amended to ensure comprehension and relevance.

Once at the workshop, stakeholders were asked by their trainer if they would participate in the research; the only selection criteria were that they must be employed and involved in the local livestock slaughter and transport industry.

3. Statistical Analysis

Multivariable logistic regression analyses were performed using the statistical package Minitab to assess the significance of the relationships between the respondent demographics (with nation, stakeholder role, age, sex, religion, residential zone, and knowledge acquisition method as the independent variables) and the distribution of the Likert scale responses for each question (the dependent variable). Religiosity and length of time in the industry were excluded from the model as their inclusion prevented it from converging after 20 iterations. Models of attitudinal statements utilized all seven stakeholder groups identified, but, when evaluating influences on attitudes, the stakeholder groups were reduced to four logical groups to improve the effectiveness of the logistic regression modelling process; business owners/managers (n = 127), private practice/government veterinarians (n = 207), the team leader and the staff working directly with animals (n = 423), and farmers (n = 153). The reference category in both cases was chosen as the most numerous response category (i.e., those working directly with animals in the case of seven groups and the team leader and those working directly with animals in the case of the four groups).

The least squared means of rated importance for each question were determined for each stakeholder group. The importance rankings of factors influencing attitudes to animal welfare were determined using the Fisher Least Significant Difference (LSD) Method, and 95% confidence intervals were determined using the original seven categories of stakeholders. The residuals were checked to ensure they approximated normality. The probability values were considered significant at $p < 0.05$.

This paper focuses on the influence of the stakeholders' role within the livestock industry on attitudes to animal welfare and the factors that motivate or act as barriers to improving animal welfare. It compares the responses of stakeholders working directly with the animals, supervising other staff members within the industry, business owners or managers within the industry, and livestock veterinarians and farmers. These stakeholders were from China, Malaysia, Thailand, and Vietnam, with the differences between the four nations presented separately [5].

4. Results

All of the stakeholders participating in the workshops completed the questionnaire at the start of the 44 workshops, yielding 1022 respondents (100% response rate). Three surveys with incomplete data were excluded from analysis, therefore 1019 responses were analysed from the workshop attendees, plus those of the 44 trainers (total n = 1063).

The majority of respondents (n = 684; 69%) were male and aged between 26 and 35 (n = 361; 36%) or 36–45 (n = 248; 25%), with 16% (n = 166) being under 25, 15% (n = 150) between 46–55, and 6% (n = 63) over 56. The majority of the respondents (n = 563; 60%) reported that they gained their knowledge through formal qualifications in agriculture and 37% (n = 354) through farm employment. Most respondents resided in rural (n = 421; 42.5%) or urban (n = 398; 40%) areas, with just 17% (n = 168) residing in a metropolitan area. Of the 991 respondents who identified their theological affiliation, 43% (n = 431) identified as Buddhist, 37% (n = 370) as atheist, 7% (n = 76) as Muslim, and 4% (n = 43) as Christian.

4.1. Attitudes to Animal Welfare during Slaughter and Transport

Respondents who were team leaders and business owners agreed more that the welfare of the animals during slaughter was important to them compared to the respondents working directly with the animals (Table 1). Compared to the respondents working directly with the animals during slaughter and transport, the farmers disagreed more that the welfare of the animals during slaughter and transport was important to them.

Table 1. Least square means of the Likert scale responses for statements about animal welfare during transport and slaughter in industry respondents from China (n = 381), Thailand (n = 307), Malaysia (n = 124), and Vietnam (n = 210). Results indicate the odds ratio, confidence interval, and probability of stakeholders working directly with animals compared with each of the six other groups, in turn, agreeing with the 6 statements in bold.

	Mean Likert Scale Response Value [1]	Odds Ratio [2]	95% Confidence Interval [2]	p Value [2]
The welfare of the animals during slaughter is important to me.				
Working directly with the animals	3.93			
Team Leader: supervising people who work directly with the animals	4.27	0.65	0.43–0.98	0.04
Business owner	4.22	0.53	0.29–0.99	0.04
Business Manager	4.05	0.83	0.51–1.35	0.45
Farmer	3.75	2.07	1.33–3.21	<0.001
Veterinarian who treats animals hands on	4.23	0.65	0.41–1.05	0.07
Veterinarian working for the government as an advisor	4.32	0.87	0.52–1.47	0.59
The welfare of the animals during transport is important to me.				
Working directly with the animals	3.95			
Team Leader: supervising people who work directly with the animals	4.27	0.7	0.46–1.07	0.09
Business owner	4.31	0.65	0.35–1.19	0.16
Business Manager	4.15	0.73	0.45–1.20	0.22
Farmer	3.86	2.15	1.38–3.33	0.00
Veterinarian who treats animals hands on	4.24	0.59	0.37–0.95	0.02
Veterinarian working for the government as an advisor	4.23	0.8	0.48–0.06	0.41
The welfare of the animals while being slaughtered is satisfactory in my workplace.				
Working directly with the animals	3.23			
Team Leader: supervising people who work directly with the animals	3.60	0.68	0.45–1.01	0.05
Business owner	3.68	0.45	0.25–0.82	<0.001
Business Manager	3.59	0.45	0.28–0.73	<0.001
Farmer	3.26	1.18	0.77–1.80	0.45
Veterinarian who treats animals hands on	3.41	0.83	0.53–1.30	0.42
Veterinarian working for the government as an advisor	3.68	0.75	0.45–1.24	0.26

Table 1. *Cont.*

	Mean Likert Scale Response Value [1]	Odds Ratio [2]	95% Confidence Interval [2]	*p* Value [2]
The welfare of the animals while being transported is satisfactory in my workplace.				
Working directly with the animals	3.28			
Team Leader: supervising people who work directly with the animals	3.52	0.85	0.57–1.28	0.44
Business owner	3.62	0.51	0.28–0.92	0.02
Business Manager	3.53	0.56	0.35–0.91	0.01
Farmer	3.47	1.21	0.79–1.85	0.39
Veterinarian who treats animals hands on	3.43	0.84	0.53–1.32	0.44
Veterinarian working for the government as an advisor	3.66	0.85	0.51–1.41	0.52
Most people who are important to me would approve of me making improvements to the welfare of the animals in my care.				
Working directly with the animals	3.68			
Team Leader: supervising people who work directly with the animals	3.84	0.98	0.65–1.48	0.91
Business owner	3.83	0.94	0.51–1.71	0.83
Business Manager	3.65	1.04	0.64–1.69	0.86
Farmer	3.73	1.44	0.93–2.22	0.10
Veterinarian who treats animals hands on	3.96	0.59	0.37–0.94	0.02
Veterinarian working for the government as an advisor	3.86	0.98	0.58–1.65	0.94
In the past I have tried to make improvements to the welfare of the animals in my care.				
Working directly with the animals	3.70			
Team Leader: supervising people who work directly with the animals	3.91	0.85	0.55–1.31	0.47
Business owner	4.14	0.42	0.22–0.79	<0.001
Business Manager	3.92	0.61	0.36–1.02	0.06
Farmer	3.81	1.15	0.73–1.82	0.54
Veterinarian who treats animals hands on	3.73	0.76	0.47–1.25	0.27
Veterinarian working for the government as an advisor	3.52	0.96	0.56–1.62	0.86

[1] The Likert scale was measured from 1 (strongly disagree) to 5 (strongly agree); [2] Probability that response for that stakeholder differs from that of those working directly with animals; derived from multivariable ordinal logistic regression models including all demographic factors.

Compared to respondents working directly with the animals during slaughter, veterinarians who practised in the livestock industry agreed more that the welfare of the animals during transport was important to them and that most people who were important to them would approve of them making improvements to the welfare of the animals in their care.

Respondents who were business owners and business managers agreed more that the welfare of animals during slaughter and transport was satisfactory in their workplace, compared to respondents working directly with the animals during slaughter and transport. Business owners agreed more that they had tried to make improvements to the welfare of the animals in their care, compared to respondents working with the animals during slaughter and transport.

4.2. Influencing Factors

Compared to respondents working directly with the animals, farmers agreed less that 'the importance of the welfare of animals to the company they work for' was a key factor influencing their personal evaluation of animal welfare or a factor influencing their perceived ability to improve animal welfare during slaughter and transport (Table 2). Conversely, farmers agreed more than those working directly with the animals during slaughter and transport that the importance of animal welfare to those who worked with them influences their personal evaluation of the welfare of animals during slaughter. Farmers also agreed more that the importance of animal welfare to those they work with was one of the main factors influencing their ability to make improvements to animal welfare during transport, as compared to respondents working directly with the animals or team leaders. Farmers agreed less that personal monetary gain, their knowledge of animal welfare, their workspace, and the availability of tools and resources were influencing factors when considering their ability to improve animal welfare during slaughter, as compared with respondents working directly with the animals.

Table 2. Least square means of Likert scale responses for the statements about influencing factors in the personal evaluation of, and the ability to, improve animal welfare during transport and slaughter, by industry respondents from China ($n = 381$), Thailand ($n = 307$), Malaysia ($n = 124$), and Vietnam ($n = 210$). Results indicate the odds ratio, confidence interval, and probability of stakeholders working directly with the animals differing from each of three other composite groups, in the importance of different influences on animal welfare issues in their workplace.

	Mean Likert Scale Response Value [1]	Odds Ratio [2]	95% Confidence Interval [2]	p Value [2]
The following factors influence my personal evaluation of animal welfare during slaughter and transport				
Importance to peers				
Working directly with the animals (including team leaders)	3.68			
Business owner + business managers	3.76	0.80	0.54–1.19	0.26
Farmer	3.69	1.66	1.08–2.55	0.02
Veterinarian (private and government)	3.66	1.05	0.72–1.53	0.8
Importance of animal welfare to the company I work for				
Working directly with the animals (including team leaders)	3.74			
Business owner + business managers	3.75	1.01	0.68–1.49	0.96
Farmer	3.50	1.79	1.18–2.72	0.00
Veterinarian (private and government)	3.74	0.87	0.60–1.27	0.47
The following factors impact my ability to make improvements to welfare during slaughter				
Monetary gain				
Working directly with the animals (including team leaders)	3.42			
Business owner + business managers	3.40	1.10	0.75–1.60	0.62
Farmer	3.66	1.65	0.43–0.98	0.04
Veterinarian (private and government)	3.20	1.40	0.98–2.01	0.06
Company approval				
Working directly with the animals (including team leaders)	3.75			
Business owner + business managers	3.77	0.93	0.63–1.38	0.73
Farmer	3.55	2.17	1.42–3.31	0.00
Veterinarian (private and government)	3.60	1.23	0.85–1.80	0.27
My personal knowledge				
Working directly with the animals (including team leaders)	3.79			
Business owner + business managers	3.69	1.30	0.88–1.94	0.19
Farmer	3.58	1.63	1.06–2.52	0.02
Veterinarian (private and government)	3.83	1.10	0.74–1.62	0.64
Workspace				
Working directly with the animals (including team leaders)	3.69			
Business owner + business managers	3.66	1.16	0.78–1.73	0.45
Farmer	3.65	1.92	1.25–2.97	0.00
Veterinarian (private and government)	3.64	1.13	0.77–1.66	0.53
Available tools and resources				
Working directly with the animals (including team leaders)	3.83			
Business owner + business managers	3.87	0.91	0.61–1.36	0.65
Farmer	3.62	1.98	1.29–3.04	0.00
Veterinarian (private and government)	3.76	0.97	0.66–1.42	0.85
The following factors impact my ability to make improvements to welfare during transport				
Company approval				
Working directly with the animals (including team leaders)	3.86			
Business owner + business managers	3.75	1.28	0.86–1.91	0.22
Farmer	3.74	1.85	1.20–2.84	0.00
Veterinarian (private and government)	3.78	1.14	0.77–1.67	0.51

Table 2. *Cont.*

	Mean Likert Scale Response Value [1]	Odds Ratio [2]	95% Confidence Interval [2]	p Value [2]
Importance to peers				
Working directly with the animals (including team leaders)	3.70			
Business owner + business managers	3.59	1.00	0.67–1.48	0.98
Farmer	3.75	1.72	1.12–2.65	0.01
Veterinarian (private and government)	3.76	1.09	0.75–1.60	0.64
Workspace				
Working directly with the animals (including team leaders)	3.64			
Business owner + business managers	3.41	1.65	1.11–2.43	0.01
Farmer	3.82	0.92	0.59–1.43	0.70
Veterinarian (private and government)	3.63	0.98	0.67–1.43	0.90

[1] The Likert scale was measured from 1 (strongly disagree) to 5 (strongly agree); [2] Probability that response for that stakeholder differs from that of those working directly with animals; derived from multivariable ordinal logistic regression models including all demographic factors.

Compared to respondents working directly with the animals or team leaders, business owners and managers agreed less that their work space was one of the main factors influencing their ability to make improvements to animal welfare during transport.

4.3. Sources of Influence to Improve Animal Welfare

Respondents in all roles strongly agreed that they were more likely to change their practices if they were prescribed by law and if they saw moral value in changing them and least likely if prescribed by an international organization (Table 3). Business owners and farmers were as likely to change if they saw the potential for monetary gain as they were for reasons of moral value and the law, whereas monetary gain was of little influence for the other groups. Business managers, farmers, and government veterinarians ranked the importance of company prescriptions as high as moral value and the law, whereas this was a secondary influence for those working directly with animals, team leaders, business owners, and private practice veterinarians.

Table 3. Differences between stakeholder groups in the importance rankings of factors influencing attitudes to animal welfare in Chinese (*n* = 381), Thai (*n* = 307), Malaysian (*n* = 124), and Vietnamese (*n* = 210) industry respondents.

Stakeholder	I Am More Encouraged to Change My Practices by …
Working directly with the animals	Law [a], Moral value [a,b], Local gov [b,c], Police [c], Workplace [c,d], Local org [c,d,e], Supervisor [d,e,f], Money gain [e,f], Peers [f], Comm leader [f], Intl org [g]
Team Leader	Moral value [a], Law [a], Workplace [b], Local gov [b], Police [b], Local org [b,c], Supervisor [b,c,d], Money gain [b,c,d], Peers [b,c,d], Comm leader [c,d], Intl org [d]
Business owner	Law [a], Moral value [a,b], Money gain [a,b,c], Local gov [a,b,c], Workplace [b,c,d], Police [b,c,d], Local org [b,c,d], Peers [c,d,e], Supervisor [d,e], Intl org [d,e], Comm leader [e]
Business Manager	Moral value [a], Law [a,b], Workplace [a,b,c], Local gov [a,b,c], Local org [a,b,c,d], Supervisor [a,b,c,d], Police [b,c,d], Peers [b,c,d], Comm leader [c,d], Money gain [c,d], Intl org [d]
Farmer	Moral value [a], Law [a,b], Local org [a,b], Money gain [a,b], Local gov [a,b], Workplace [a,b,c], Peers [a,b,c], Police [b,c], Comm leader [c], Intl org [c], Supervisor [c]
Private practice veterinarian	Law [a], Moral value [a], Local gov [a,b], Workplace [b,c], Local org [b,c], Police [b,c], Supervisor [c,d], Comm leader [d], Peers [d], Money gain [d], Intl org [d]
Government veterinarian	Law [a], Moral value [a], Workplace [a,b], Police [a,b], Local gov [b,c], Local org [b,c,d], Supervisor [c,d,e], Intl org [d,e,f], Peers [e,f], Comm leader [f], Money gain [f]

Factors within stakeholder groups with different superscripts are significantly different (*p* < 0.05); Legend: 'if changes are prescribed by … '; local government ('local gov'), a local organization ('local org'), local law enforcement ('police'), a 'western' international organization ('intl org'), the law ('law'), my company ('workplace'), my supervisor ('supervisor'), or my community elder or community leader ('comm leader'); 'I see … '; moral value in changing practices ('moral value'), personal monetary gain from changing practices ('money gain'), or others making the change ('peers').

5. Discussion

This study has demonstrated significant relationships between attitudes to animal welfare and the roles of stakeholders within the livestock industry. The results have implications for the development of initiatives focused on improving animal welfare in these regions; initiatives may be more engaging and successful if they are targeted to specific stakeholder groups, as well as tailored by country [5]. We have also demonstrated that legislation and 'seeing moral value' in implementing animal welfare change is shared by several roles; however some important differences exist. Many of these key role differences are in contrast to those working directly with the animals during slaughter and transport.

5.1. Business Owners, Team Leaders and Managers

Team leaders and business owners attributed higher levels of importance to the welfare of animals in transport and slaughter as compared to stakeholders in other roles. This high level of importance placed on animal welfare may represent a greater level of understanding and awareness of the concept of animal welfare, its importance to buyers and consumers, and its implications for income. This occurs as the more senior stakeholders, leaders, and owners are tasked with making decisions for the business, the animals, and other stakeholders working with the animals. The apparent importance placed on animal welfare by this group represents a promising opportunity to influence animal welfare improvements in business from the top down.

Business owners and managers also had a more positive opinion of animal welfare in their workplace, compared to respondents working directly with animals, as they more commonly reported that animal welfare was satisfactory during both slaughter and transport in their workplace. It is possible that business owners and managers feel compelled to report high levels of regard for animal welfare, given their senior roles within industry and the need to create and maintain a positive image for their business. Business owners have greater stakes in the viability and success of their business (and therefore business image) than those working in less senior roles, which may explain the high importance placed on monetary gain as a factor influencing business owners to improve animal welfare. It is of note that business managers were more likely to change their practices to improve animal welfare under the influence of company prescriptions, as compared with owners. This may be explained by the common structure of business operations that often sees business owners as responsible for setting company prescriptions and holds business managers primarily accountable for ensuring that what is prescribed is implemented within the operation.

Business owners and managers were also more likely to report that they had tried to improve animal welfare in the past than those working hands on with the animals. These stakeholders may feel significantly more empowered to engender change, but it is possible that this response was biased by a desire to embody the most desirable business image. Business managers did not see their workspace as an issue when considering their ability to improve animal welfare, whereas people working directly with animals did. This indicates that business managers believe they have or have provided all the necessary tools to improve animal welfare in their business, and this belief is consistent with their positive opinion of animal welfare in their workplace.

These findings suggest that building awareness amongst business managers, owners, and supervisors about the benefits of improving animal welfare may increase the likelihood of engaging business owners and managers in encouraging employees in efforts to improve animal welfare. Business owners could be encouraged to incorporate higher welfare standards into key performance indicators and initiate company-based training workshops to facilitate and empower improvements to animal welfare during slaughter and transport in their business. Since company prescription was an important motivator for business managers to improve animal welfare, once business owners set higher welfare standards for the company, business managers are likely to engage with implementing these changes.

5.2. Farmers

Farmers placed a lower importance on animal welfare during transport and slaughter compared with other stakeholders; this may be because they are less likely to be involved in these processes. This may also explain why farmers reported that monetary gain, company approval, their knowledge levels, and the availability of tools and resources were less likely to influence their ability to make improvements to animal welfare during slaughter. Farmers also reported that company prescriptions did not influence their ability to improve animal welfare but reported a significantly greater influence of peer acceptance on their evaluation of animal welfare and their ability to make improvements to animal welfare, compared to those working directly with the animals during slaughter and transport. This finding is consistent with a study of Danish dairy farmers that showed social and peer influences to be the most important motivator to comply with environmental policy, outranked only by civil duty [15]. Similarly, a study of Welsh and English cattle farmers found non-supportive peer practices and norms to be a major barrier to the implementation of zoonotic control programs [16]. This could be explained by farmers' operational and geographic isolation, in which their neighboring farmers and peers may provide their nearest or only point of reference and also the most personally meaningful. This suggests that farmers may be more readily engaged in initiatives that share welfare practices and knowledge from farmer to farmer. This is supported by the results of another study that found that farmers' involvement in active peer dialogue networks to be improved their capacity to innovate [17].

5.3. Veterinarians

Veterinarians working with animals in the field reported that the welfare of the animals was more important than did those working hands-on in slaughter and transport and had more respect for peer approval when looking to improve animal welfare. This supports the notion that animal welfare is seen as an inherent role and responsibility of a veterinarian and the stance of the World Animal Health Organisation (OIE) that the world community of veterinarians is dedicated to improving animal welfare [18]. In addition, veterinarians are focused on animal centric measurements and diagnostics, and may therefore be more acutely aware of and knowledgeable about suffering.

Given the high importance of perceived peer acceptance for actively attempting to improve animal welfare reported by veterinarians, these stakeholders have great potential to be advocates for the animals and drivers of change within the livestock industry. The ability to effectively undertake this role as a driver of animal welfare improvements may be hampered by a conflict of interest for veterinarians working in a private livestock enterprise, where future income may rely on acquiescence with current practice and not entering into conflict with business owners [19]. Thus monetary gain was attributed greater importance by veterinarians who work directly with livestock within a private enterprise, compared to government veterinarians who attributed more importance to company prescriptions, such as policies and standards. This suggests that veterinarians may be best placed to advocate for improved animal welfare when their income is independent of the livestock business that they are advising or monitoring.

The involvement of a 'western' international organization was amongst the least likely of the factors to encourage change for each stakeholder role and was overall the least influential source of encouragement. This is particularly the case for those working directly with livestock during slaughter and transport, but this may be, in large part, due to the decreased likelihood of these stakeholders interacting with an international organization. This potentially results in the perception among these stakeholders that an international organization is unlikely to understand their work and so would not be in a position to influence or interfere with their practices. This suggests that improvements to animal welfare may be best initiated locally and within companies.

The potential limitations of this study include response biases towards perceived preferred answers by the respondent on a sensitive issue. Attempts to mitigate this issue were made through the confidential nature of the survey, a request to be honest, and conducting of the survey before any training content was shared. This was also intended to mitigate any trainer bias in the results.

We also acknowledge that there are other factors influencing the attitudes expressed in this survey, in particular each respondent's country (evaluated in [5]), but expect that the close geographical proximity of the four countries leads to greater similarity than between unconnected 'Western' and developing countries.

6. Conclusions

This study demonstrated that the attitudes of industry stakeholders in the Asia Pacific region to animal welfare during slaughter and transport are influenced by each stakeholder's role within the industry. This is particularly the case in regard to the influence of peers, monetary gain, and the company. Legislation and seeing moral value in changes to animal welfare were key motivators to change practices across all stakeholder roles. Key differences between stakeholder groups need to be understood and incorporated in animal welfare initiatives aimed at each target audience to maximize engagement and success. Livestock stakeholders are in a position to make daily decisions that directly affect the welfare of animals during slaughter and transport. Improved understanding of the stakeholder audience and what motivates them should enable the development of more collaborative and engaging initiatives that are likely to succeed in improving the welfare of animals during the critical moments of slaughter and transport.

Acknowledgments: This study was part of a project led by a collaboration between the University of Queensland in Australia and University Putra Malaysia under the framework of the World Organisation for Animal Health (OIE)'s David Bayvel Collaborating Centre for Animal Welfare and Bioethical Analysis. It was funded by the New Zealand Government Ministry of Primary Industries, the European Commission via OIE, World Animal Protection, Universiti Putra Malaysia (UPM), the Malaysian Government Department of Veterinary Services via UPM, and the Australian Government Department of Agriculture, Fisheries, and Food. The authors also wish to acknowledge Zulkifli Idrus, Duong van Nhiem, Pongchan Na_Lampang, and Wang Yan for coordinating data collection in their respective countries. Ethical approval for this study was granted by the University of Queensland Human Ethics Committee (Project Identification Code: 2015000059).

Author Contributions: Michelle Sinclair developed the study and designed the questions, in consultation with Clive J. C. Phillips, who directed the project. All authors analysed and interpreted the data; the paper was written by Michelle Sinclair in conjunction with Clive J. C. Phillips and Sarah Zito. The funders had no role in the design, analysis, or interpretation of the study.

Conflicts of Interest: The authors declare no conflict of interest.

References

1. Food and Agriculture Organisation. FAOSTAT. 2016. Available online: http://faostat.fao.org (accessed on 20 February 2016).
2. Ferguson, D.M.; Warner, R.D. Have we underestimated the impact of pre-slaughter stress on meat quality in ruminants? *Meat Sci.* **2008**, *80*, 12–19. [CrossRef] [PubMed]
3. Ajzen, I. The theory of planned behavior. *Org. Behav. Hum. Decis.* **1991**, *50*, 179–211.
4. Keshava, S.; Kiran, P.; Nithin, S.J. Audience Discovery and targeted marketing using SAP HANA. In Proceedings of the 2015 IEEE International Advance Computing Conference (IACC), Banglore, India, 12–13 June 2015; pp. 749–753.
5. Sinclair, M.; Zito, S.; Idrus, Z.; Nhiem, D.V.; Wang, Y.; Na_Lampang, P.; Phillips, C.J.C. Stakeholder attitudes to animal welfare during slaughter and transport in SE and E Asia. *Anim. Welf.* **2016**, submitted.
6. Phillips, C.J.C.; Izmirli, S.; Aldavood, S.J.; Alonso, M.; Choe, B.I.; Hanlon, A.; Handziska, A.; Illmann, G.; Keeling, L.; Kennedy, M.; et al. Students' attitudes to animal welfare and rights in Europe and Asia. *Anim. Welf.* **2012**, *21*, 87–100. [CrossRef]
7. Kellert, S.R. Attitudes, knowledge, and behavior toward wildlife among the industrial superpowers: United States, Japan, and Germany. *J. Soc. Issues* **1993**, *49*, 53–69. [CrossRef]
8. Vanhonacker, F.; Verbeke, W.; van Poucke, E.; Tuyttens, F.A. Do citizens and farmers interpret the concept of farm animal welfare differently? *Livest. Sci.* **2008**, *116*, 126–136. [CrossRef]
9. Broom, D.M. The effects of land transport on animal welfare. *Rev. Sci. Tech.* **2005**, *24*, 683–691. [PubMed]

10. Coleman, G.J.; McGregor, M.; Hemsworth, P.H.; Boyce, J.; Dowling, S. The relationship between beliefs, attitudes and observed behaviours of abattoir personnel in the pig industry. *Appl. Anim. Behav. Sci.* **2003**, *82*, 189–200. [CrossRef]

11. Kielland, C.; Skjerve, E.; Østerås, O.; Zanella, A.J. Dairy farmer attitudes and empathy toward animals are associated with animal welfare indicators. *J. Dairy Sci.* **2010**, *93*, 2998–3006. [CrossRef] [PubMed]

12. Blandford, D.; Bureau, J.C.; Fulponi, L.; Henson, S. Potential implications of animal welfare concerns and public policies in industrialized countries for international trade. In *Global Food Trade and Consumer Demand for Quality*; Kluwer: New York, NY, USA, 2002; pp. 77–99.

13. Tiplady, C.; Walsh, D.B.; Phillips, C.J.C. Cruelty to Australian cattle in Indonesian abattoirs—How the public responded to media coverage. *J. Agric. Environ. Ethics* **2012**, *26*, 869–885. [CrossRef]

14. Ling, R.Z.; Zulkifli, I.; Lampang, P.N.; Nhiem, D.V.; Wang, Y.; Phillips, C.J.C. Attitudes of students from southeast and east Asian countries to slaughter and transport of livestock. *Anim. Welf.* **2016**, *25*, 377–387. [CrossRef]

15. May, P.J. Compliance Motivations: Perspectives of Farmers, Homebuilders, and Marine Facilities. *Law Policy* **2005**, *27*, 317–347. [CrossRef]

16. Ellis-Iversen, J.; Cook, A.J.; Watson, E.; Nielen, M.; Larkin, L.; Wooldridge, M.; Hogeveen, H. Perceptions, circumstances and motivators that influence implementation of zoonotic control programs on cattle farms. *Prev. Vet. Med.* **2010**, *93*, 276–285. [CrossRef] [PubMed]

17. Faysse, N.; Sraïri, M.T.; Errahj, M. Local farmers' organisations: A space for peer-to-peer learning? The case of milk collection cooperatives in Morocco. *J. Agric. Educ. Ext.* **2012**, *18*, 285–299. [CrossRef]

18. Edwards, J.D. The role of the veterinarian in animal welfare: A global perspective. In *First Global Conference on Animal Welfare: An OIE Initiative*; OIE: Paris, France; the European Commission: Brussels, Belgium, 2004; pp. 27–32.

19. Arkow, P. Application of ethics to animal welfare. *Appl. Anim. Behav. Sci.* **1998**, *59*, 193–200. [CrossRef]

Permissions

List of Contributors

Filipe Antônio Dalla Costa
Programa de Pós-Graduação em Zootecnia, Faculdade de Ciências Agrárias e Veterinárias, University of São Paulo State UNESP-FCAV, Jaboticabal 14884-900, Brazil
Grupo de Estudos e Pesquisas em Etologia e Ecologia Animal-ETCO, UNESP/FCAV, Jaboticabal 14884-900, Brazil

Letícia S. Lopes
Embrapa Swine and Poultry, BR 153, Km 110, Concórdia 89700-991, Brazil

Osmar Antônio Dalla Costa
Grupo de Estudos e Pesquisas em Etologia e Ecologia Animal-ETCO, UNESP/FCAV, Jaboticabal 14884-900, Brazil
Embrapa Swine and Poultry, BR 153, Km 110, Concórdia 89700-991, Brazil

Jane Williams
Animal Health Research Group, Hartpury University Centre, Gloucester GL19 3BE, UK

Catherine Phillips and Hollie Marie Byrd
Veterinary Nursing Research Group, Hartpury University Centre, Gloucester GL19 3BE, UK

Ilaria Baldelli
Dipartimento di Scienze Chirurgiche e Diagnostiche Integrate (DISC), Università di Genova, 16132 Genova Unità Operativa di Chirurgia Plastica e Ricostruttiva, IRCCS Azienda Ospedaliera Universitaria San Martino -IST Genova, 16132 Genoa, Italy

Alma Massaro
Dipartimento di Antichità, Filosofia, Storia, Geografia (DAFIST), Università di Genova, 16126 Genova, Italy

Susanna Penco and Anna Maria Bassi
Dipartimento di Medicina Sperimentale (DIMES), Università di Genova, 16132 Genova, Italy

Sara Patuzzo
School of Medicine and Surgery, University of Verona, P.le L. A. Scuro 10, 37134 Verona, Italy

Rosagemma Ciliberti
Dipartimento di Scienze della Salute (DISSAL), Università di Genova, 16132 Genova, Italy

Kirsty Le'sniak, Jane Williams, Kerry Kuznik
Centre for Performance in Equestrian Sport, Hartpury College, Gloucester GL19 3BE, UK

Peter Douglas
PE Douglas DWP, Ivybridge, Devon PL21 0NP, UK

Andrew Knight
Centre for AnimalWelfare, Faculty of Humanities and Social Sciences, University ofWinchester, Sparkford Road,Winchester SO22 4NR, UK

Katherine D. Watson
School of History, Philosophy and Culture, Oxford Brookes University, Tonge Building, Gipsy Lane, Oxford OX3 0BP, UK

Herman M. Vermeer, Nienke C. P. M. M. Dirx-Kuijken and Marc B. M. Bracke
Wageningen Livestock Research, Wageningen 6700 AH, The Netherlands

Jessica K. Walker
New Zealand Companion Animal Council, Waiuku, Auckland 2341, New Zealand

Stephanie J. Bruce
Environmental and Animal Sciences Network, Unitec Institute of Technology, Auckland 1025, New Zealand

Arnja R. Dale
Royal New Zealand Society for the Prevention of Cruelty to Animals, 3047 Great North Road, New Lynn, Auckland 0610, New Zealand

Elly Hiby ID and Lex Hiby
Conservation Research Ltd., 110 Hinton Way, Great Shelford, Cambridge CB22 5AL, UK

Patrycia Sato and Marina A.G. von Keyserlingk
AnimalWelfare Program, 2357 Main Mall, Faculty of Land and Food Systems,
University of British Columbia, Vancouver, BC V6T 1Z4, Canada

Maria J. Hötzel
Laboratório de Etologia Aplicada e Bem-Estar Animal, Departamento de Zootecnia e Desenvolvimento Rural, Universidade Federal de Santa Catarina, Florianópolis 88034-001, Brazil

Karen Moore
Faculty of Veterinary and Agricultural Sciences, The University of Melbourne, Parkville, Victoria 3010, Australia
Grains and Livestock Industries, Department of Agriculture and FoodWestern Australia, South Perth, Western Australia 6151, Australia

Frank Dunshea
Faculty of Veterinary and Agricultural Sciences, The University of Melbourne, Parkville, Victoria 3010, Australia

Bruce Mullan and Jae Cheol Kim
Grains and Livestock Industries, Department of Agriculture and Food Western Australia, South Perth, Western Australia 6151, Australia

Frank M. Mitloehner and John J. McGlone
Department of Animal and Food Sciences, Texas Tech University, Lubbock, TX 79409, USA

Jeff W. Dailey and Julie L. Morrow
Livestock Issues Research Unit, USDA-ARS, Lubbock, TX 79409, USA

Agnese Arduini, Veronica Redaelli, Stefania Dall'Olio and Leonardo Nanni Costa
Department of Agricultural and Food Sciences, School of Agriculture and Veterinary Medicine, University of Bologna, Via Fanin 50, Bologna 40127, Italy

Fabio Luzi
Department of Veterinary Science and Public Health, Faculty of Veterinary Science, University of Milan, Via Celoria 10, Milan 20133, Italy

Vincenzo Pace
OPAS, Pig Farmer Association, Strada Ghisiolo 57, San Giorgio, Mantua 46030, Italy

Michelle Sinclair, Sarah Zito and Clive J. C. Phillips
Centre for AnimalWelfare and Ethics, School of Veterinary Sciences, The University of Queensland, Gatton, Queensland 4343, Australia

Index

www.ingramcontent.com/pod-product-compliance
Lightning Source LLC
Chambersburg PA
CBHW080300230326
41458CB00097B/5242